Current Topics in Microbiology and Immunology

Volume 320

Patrick J. Paddison • Peter K. Vogt
Editors

RNA Interference

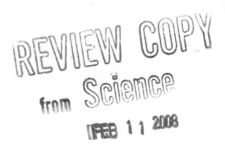

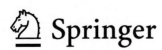 Springer

Patrick J. Paddison
Cold Spring Harbor Fellows Program
Cold Spring Harbor Laboratory
Cold Spring Harbor, NY 11771
e-mail: paddison@cshl.edu

Peter K. Vogt
The Scripps Research Institute
Department of Molecular & Experimental
    Medicine
Division of Oncovirology
10550 N. Torrey Pines Road, BCC-239
La Jolla, CA 92037
USA
e-mail: pkvogt@scripps.edu

Cover Illustration: A model of the small RNA transcriptional silencing complex is shown with the transcription bubble and RNAPII (dark blue), Argonaute 1 (green), and the antisense strand of the small RNA (red) bound to nascent mRNA (also red). An epigenetic regulatory complex composed of Ezh2, DNMT3a, and HDAC-1 is also shown (red, blue and green), remodeling the histone. (Computer graphics courtesy to Paula J. Morris).

ISBN 978-3-540-75156-4   e-ISBN 978-3-540-75157-1

Current Topics in Microbiology and Immunology ISSN 007-0217x

Library of Congress Catalog Number: 72-152360

© 2008 Springer-Verlag Berlin Heidelberg

Cover Design: WMXDesign GmbH, Heidelberg, Germany

Printed on acid-free paper

9 8 7 6 5 4 3 2 1

springer.com

Contents

Contributors

R.C. Allshire
Wellcome Trust Centre for Cell Biology, Institute of Cell Biology,
The University of Edinburgh, Edinburgh EH9 3JR, UK

J.J. Arnold
Department of Biochemistry and Molecular Biology, The Pennsylvania State
University, 201 Althouse Laboratory, University Park, PA 16802, USA

I. Bentwich
Rosetta Genomics Ltd, 10 Plaut Street, Rehovot 76706, Israel,
bentwich@rosettagenomics.com

J.A. Birchler
Division of Biological Sciences, Tucker Hall, University of Missouri, Columbia,
MO 65211, USA, BirchlerJ@Missouri.edu

M.-E.L. Boisvert
Laval University Cancer Research Center, Hôtel-Dieu de Québec (CHUQ),
Québec City, Québec G1R 2J6, Canada

C.E. Cameron
Department of Biochemistry and Molecular Biology, The Pennsylvania State
University, 201 Althouse Laboratory, University Park, PA 16802, USA

X. Chen
Department of Botany and Plant Sciences, University of California, Riverside,
Riverside, CA 92521, USA, xuemei.chen@ucr.edu

S.C.R. Elgin
Department of Biology, Washington University, One Brookings Dr.,
Campus Box 1229, St. Louis, MO 63130, USA, selgin@biology.wustl.edu

H. Fernandez
Division of Biological Sciences, Tucker Hall, University of Missouri, Columbia,
MO 65211, USA

W. Filipowicz
Friedrich Miescher Institute for Biomedical Research, 4002 Basel, Switzerland,
Witold.Filipowicz@fmi.ch

L. Jaskiewicz
Friedrich Miescher Institute for Biomedical Research, 4002 Basel, Switzerland

X. Ji
Macromolecular Crystallography Laboratory, National Cancer Institute, National
Institutes of Health, Frederick, MD 21702-1201, USA, jix@ncifcrf.gov

H.H. Kavi
Division of Biological Sciences, Tucker Hall, University of Missouri, Columbia,
MO 65211, USA

K.V. Morris
Department of Molecular and Experimental Medicine, The Scripps Research
Institute, 10550N, Torrey Pines Road, La Jolla, CA 92037, USA,
kmorris@scripps.edu

K.K.-S. Ng
Department of Biological Sciences, University of Calgary, 2500 University Drive
NW, Calgary, Alberta T2N 1N4, Canada, ngk@ucalgary.ca

Patrick J. Paddison
Cold Spring Harbor Fellows Program, Cold Spring Harbor Laboratory,
Cold Spring Harbor, NY 11771, USA, paddison@cshl.edu

N.C. Riddle
Department of Biology, Washington University, One Brookings Dr.,
Campus Box 1229, St. Louis, MO 63130, USA

M.J. Simard
Laval University Cancer Research Center, Hôtel-Dieu de Québec (CHUQ),
Québec City, Québec G1R 2J6, Canada, Martin.Simard@crhdq.ulaval.ca

P. Svoboda
Institute of Molecular Genetics, Czech Academy of Sciences, Videnska 1083,
14220 Prague, Czech Republic, svobodap@img.cas.cz

W. Xie
Division of Biological Sciences, Tucker Hall, University of Missouri, Columbia,
MO 65211, USA

S.A. White
Wellcome Trust Centre for Cell Biology, Institute of Cell Biology, The University
of Edinburgh, Edinburgh EH9 3JR, UK, Sharon.A.White@ed.ac.uk

RNA Interference in Mammalian Cell Systems

Patrick J. Paddison

Abstract The use of RNA interference (RNAi) to evoke gene silencing in mammalian cells has almost become routine laboratory practice. Through refinement of double-stranded RNA (dsRNA) triggers of RNAi and creation of genome-scale libraries, the first genome-wide loss of function screens have been carried out in mammals. This review discusses some of the key features of RNAi in mammalian systems.

1   Introduction

Since the discovery that DNA was genetic material, a major theme in biological sciences has been to remove or mutate genes to demonstrate their participation in cellular processes and pathways. In model genetic systems, the ability to carry out genetic manipulation has been an enabling feature of countless discoveries, ranging from bacteriophage viral morphogenesis modules (Edgar and Wood 1966) to genes

Patrick J. Paddison
Cold Spring Harbor Fellows Program, Cold Spring Harbor Laboratory,
Cold Spring Harbor, NY 11771, USA
paddison@cshl.edu

P.J. Paddison and P.K. Vogt (eds.), *RNA Interference.*
Current Topics in Microbiology and Immunology 320.
© Springer-Verlag Berlin Heidelberg 2008

required for coordinating the eukaryotic cell cycle (Hartwell et al. 1974; Hartwell and Weinert 1989). Mammalian-based systems, however, have lagged behind, being almost impervious to commonly used gene-targeting techniques and lacking the ability to be "crossed" or "mated" to map genetic elements. As a result, many basic questions regarding the underlying function of molecular pathways have gone unanswered in mammals. This genetic intractability has hit cancer research particularly hard. Until recently, researchers have lacked reliable tools with which to reveal underlying vulnerabilities in cancer cells that, in turn, could be exploited in the clinic. With the advent of RNA interference (RNAi) in mammals, however, this may be about to change.

RNAi emerged out of the pioneering work of Fire, Mello, and colleagues (1998) in the nematode *Caenorhabditis elegans*. Attempting to use antisense RNA to knock down gene expression, they found synergistic effects on gene silencing when antisense and sense RNA strands where delivered together. While at first RNAi seemed a peculiarity of nematodes, double-stranded RNA (dsRNA)-dependent gene silencing has since become one of the biggest surprises in the past decade of research in eukaryotic cells. The core machinery that underlies RNAi is conserved in virtually every experimental eukaryotic system (with the notable exception of *Saccharomyces cerevisiae*) and has been co-opted in most of them to trigger gene silencing (reviewed in Zamore and Haley 2005; Tolia and Joshua-Tor 2007).

With the advent of RNAi in mammals and the refinement of silencing triggers, we have reached a point at which any gene in the human or mouse genome can conceivably be targeted using small dsRNA gene silencing triggers—synthetic small interfering RNAs (siRNAs) or expressed short hairpin RNAs (shRNAs). In the next decade in the biomedical sciences, siRNAs and shRNAs will be employed to: (1) validate disease models in vitro in cell-based systems and in vivo in rodent and primate systems; (2) validate drug activities through the removal of suspected targets; (3) identify new drug candidates in genome-wide, functional genomic screens; and finally (4) combat disease directly, using siRNAs or shRNAs as therapeutic molecules in the clinic. This chapter provides an overview of the RNAi pathway and the extent to which the RNAi pathway has been co-opted in mammals to evoke gene silencing.

2   The RNAi Pathway in Mammals

From the start, RNAi experiments in *C. elegans*, plants, and *Drosophila* suggested a homology-based silencing mechanism that somehow used dsRNA to seek and, in most cases, destroy cognate targets. Uncovering and characterizing many of the components and biochemical determinants of RNAi in invertebrate systems (reviewed in Hannon 2002) has helped translate RNAi into a genetic tool in mammals.

The RNAi pathway likely arose early during eukaryotic evolution as a cell-based defense against viral and genetic parasites. Double-stranded RNA viruses and mobile genetic elements with the potential to form dsRNA structures are ubiquitous in nature and can be subject to RNAi-dependent gene silencing in *C. elegans*, plants, *Drosophila*, yeast, and mammals (reviewed in Zamore and Haley 2005). In addition, elements of the RNAi pathway are also used for regulation of endogenous genes (e.g., during metazoan development), where endogenous, non-coding RNAs are processed and used to seek out targets (e.g., miRNAs). Endogenously expressed small hairpin RNAs regulate gene expression through the RNAi pathway during *C. elegans* development (Reinhart et al. 2000; Grishok et al. 2001; Hutvagner et al. 2001; Ketting et al. 2001; Knight and Bass 2001; reviewed in Hannon 2002). These small hairpin RNAs (~70 nt) are processed into a 21- to 22-nt mature form by Dicer and then used to seek out mRNA targets of similar sequence (generally via imperfect base-pairing interactions). For the two prototypes of this family, *C. elegans* lin-4 and let-7, silencing occurs at the level of protein synthesis (reviewed in Bernstein et al. 2001b). The first small hairpin RNAs were dubbed small temporal RNAs (stRNAs), owing to their role in developmental timing (Lee et al. 1993; Wightman et al. 1993; Ha et al. 1996; Slack et al. 2000). More recently, dozens of orphan hairpins have been identified in *C. elegans*, *Drosophila*, mouse, and humans, which are collectively referred to as microRNAs (miRNAs) (Pasquinelli et al. 2000; Lagos-Quintana et al. 2001; Lau et al. 2001; Lee and Ambros 2001; Mourelatos et al. 2002).

At least three core components of the RNAi pathway appear to be generally required for dsRNA-dependent silencing phenomena in higher eukaryotes: the Drosha, Dicer, and Argonaute (Ago) gene family members. Drosha and Dicer proteins sit atop the RNAi pathway in the first catalytic steps that convert various forms of dsRNA into smaller, guide dsRNAs of 21–25 nt. Both Drosha and Dicer belong to the RNase III family of proteins that cleave dsRNA, leaving a characteristic dsRNA terminal consisting of a 5′ phosphate group and a two-base overhang at the 3′ end (Bernstein et al. 2001a; Lee and Ambros 2001). Drosha- and Dicer-related genes contain a single dsRNA-binding domain and two tandem RNAse III domains (RIIIDs). In addition, Dicers contain two other conserved sequence motifs: a DExH/DEAH ATPase/RNA helicase domain and a PAZ domain (unique to RNAi genes) (Bernstein et al. 2001a). Ago proteins, which are components of the RNA-induced silencing complex (RISC), contain a PAZ domain and a carboxyl-terminal PIWI domain, which shares a high degree of similarity to the catalytic core of RNase H enzymes (reviewed in Tolia and Joshua-Tor 2007).

The current model for RNAi, with respect to miRNA biogenesis, begins with the conversion of miRNAs into siRNAs by Drosha and Dicer (Bernstein et al. 2001a) (Fig. 1). Drosha and Dicer trimming results in a defined dsRNA containing approx. 17–23 bp of dsRNA and 3′ 2-nt overhangs. These small RNAs (~18–25 nt in size) become incorporated into a RISC that uses the sequence of the siRNAs as a guide either to identify homologous mRNAs (Tuschl et al. 1999; Hammond et al. 2000; Zamore et al. 2000; Nykanen et al. 2001) or, alternately, in some invertebrate systems to identify similar regions in euchromatin (Fig. 1). Depending on the organism and the cellular context, different Ago-associated "effector" complexes either trigger mRNA destruction (i.e., RISC), translational inhibition (Grishok et al. 2001), or transcriptional gene silencing (Hall et al. 2002; Volpe et al. 2002; Zilberman et al.

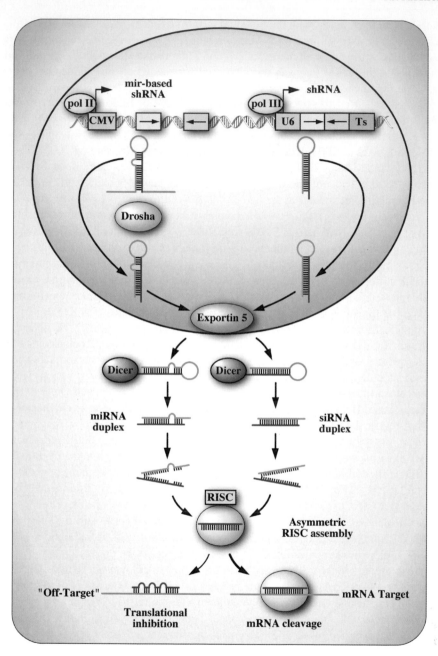

Fig. 1 Post-transcriptional gene silencing in mammals

2003). Recent biochemical and structural determination experiments have revealed several important aspects of how Drosha, Dicer, and Ago enzymes function in the RNAi pathway.

2.1 Drosha

Drosha was first implicated in RNAi through its biochemical activity when it became apparent that many primary miRNA (pri-miRNA) transcripts contain multiple miRNAs that were first trimmed in the nucleus into separate "pre-miRNA" species before Dicer processing. Drosha was found to be responsible for this pri-RNA cropping in human nuclear extracts (Lee et al. 2003b). Drosha is contained within a large (500–650 kDa) nuclear complex dubbed the "microprocessor" (Denli et al. 2004; Gregory et al. 2004; Han et al. 2004), where it interacts with a cofactor, DGCR8/Pasha, which may initiate binding to the pri-miRNA and is essential for its activity (Denli et al. 2004; Gregory et al. 2004; Han et al. 2004; Landthaler et al. 2004). The cleavage of the pri-miRNA is determined by the ssRNA–dsRNA junction at the base of the miRNA hairpin, where Drosha cuts approx. 11 bp, or one dsRNA helical turn, from the base (Han et al. 2006). The resulting "pre-miRNA" is a hairpin containing a 3′ 2-nt overhang. After Drosha cleavage the pre-miRNA then exits the nucleus via transport by exportin-5, which binds the 3′ 2-nt overhang of the pre-miRNA (Yi et al. 2003; Bohnsack et al. 2004; Lund et al. 2004). Drosha is conserved only in animals (Filippov et al. 2000; Wu et al. 2000; Fortin et al. 2002). Although plants express a wide variety of miRNAs, they do not possess a Drosha homolog. Instead this step is carried out by a Dicer homolog (Dicer-like 1) (Kurihara and Watanabe 2004).

2.2 Dicer

Dicers process dsRNA into pieces ranging from 21 to 27 nt. Similar to Drosha, Dicer is capable of cleaving dsRNA as a monomer, owing to tandem RIIIDs. Just how Dicers specify cuts of precise lengths from pre-miRNAs came from the notion that Dicer binds the end of the pre-miRNA and cuts a pre-determined length from the end, which in high eukaryotes is approx. 22 nt, or the average length of a mature miRNA. The end-recognition hypothesis was first presented in Carmell and Hannon (2004). It originated from knowledge of the function of highly conserved (~130 aa) PAZ domains that are found only in Dicer and Ago family members (reviewed in Carmell et al. 2002). Crystal structures of Ago PAZ domains revealed a high degree of similarity with an oligo-binding fold (Song et al. 2003). Additional experimentation demonstrated that PAZ domains would preferentially bind 3′-OH binding of siRNAs (Song et al. 2003b). Thus, the presence of a PAZ domain in Dicer would allow it to coordinate its own activity with that of Drosha's during miRNA maturation.

Consistent with this notion, recombinant human Dicer has been shown to preferentially cut 22nt from the 3′ end of RNA hairpins specifically containing a 2nt 3′ overhang which mimics Drosha's cleavage product (Siolas et al., 2005). Interestingly, a crystal structure of a Dicer from the parasite *Giardia* revealed that the distance between the PAZ and RIIIDs exactly matches the length spanned by the *Giardia* Dicer cleavage product (25 bp of dsRNA) (MacRae et al. 2006). These results suggest that Dicer itself is the molecular ruler that recognizes dsRNA ends and cuts a pre-determined distance from the end.

2.3 Argonaute

Ago family proteins participate in the effector step, where they utilize small RNAs as guides to silence cognate gene targets. Ago family members have at least two highly conserved domains important for their function: PAZ and PIWI domains. The PAZ domain enables binding of the 3′ end of the guide RNA (Song et al. 2003b). The importance of the PIWI domain was revealed by its structure from *Pyrococcus furiosus* (Song et al. 2004). It showed a high degree of similarity to the catalytic core domain of RNase H enzymes, containing a DDH motif. It was found that the presence of these three amino acids determined whether Ago family members possess inherent slicer activity. However, slicer activity is also determined by guide RNA complementarily to an mRNA target. If the guide RNA and the target match perfectly, RISC "slices" the mRNA 10 nt from where the 5′ end of the RNA hybridizes to the target mRNA (Elbashir et al. 2001). If the match is imperfect (as is the case with most miRNAs in higher eukaryotes) several outcomes are possible: inhibition of translational initiation or elongation, de-adenylation, transport to the cytoplasmic "P-body" for nuclease degradation, or a combination of these the three (reviewed in Valencia-Sanchez et al. 2006). In addition to miRNA and siRNA-mediated post-transcriptional gene silencing (PTGS), Agos can also act as effectors for transcriptional gene silencing, where RNAi feeds back to shut off transcription. In these scenarios (best characterized in plants and *Schizosaccharomyces pombe*) particular Ago complexes enter the nucleus and effect chromatin structure, repressive histone modifications, or both (see Irvine et al. 2006).

2.4 Other Players

Drosha, Dicer, and Ago-related proteins are of course not the only participants in the RNAi pathway. Some invertebrate systems contain pathways that amplify and/or transport guide RNA sequences to other parts of the organism. In *C. elegans* and plants, amplification of the dsRNA signal is thought to initially be mediated by RNA-dependent RNA polymerases (RdRP). An RNA degradation product (e.g., a guide RNA) may prime RdRPs along the mRNA template, resulting in the production of dsRNA homologous to sequences 5' (i.e., upstream) of the initially targeted sequence (Sijen et al. 2001). When combined with transport, amplification results in a self-propagating silencing effect throughout the organism. *C. elegans* appears to stand alone among metazoans, however, in the conservation of RdRPs, and thus amplification of RNAi. One possible explanation is that *C. elegans* acquired RdRPs through horizontal gene transfer, for example, from RNA viruses (C. Mello, personal communication). Mammalian and *Drosophila* cells lack any evidence of an amplification step (Schwarz et al. 2002; Stein et al. 2003) and, at least in cultured cells, any indication of transport of gene silencing triggers (P. Paddison, personal observation).

3 Triggers of RNAi in Mammals

The first evidence that dsRNA could evoke gene silencing in mammals came from studies using long dsRNA in mouse oocytes, pre-implantation embryos (Svoboda et al. 2000; Wianny and Zernicka-Goetz 2000), and embryonic cell lines (Billy et al. 2001; Yang et al. 2001; Paddison et al. 2002a). In these contexts, cells lack the prominent antiviral responses found in most somatic cells. Such responses include protein kinase R (PKR) and RNase L pathways, which are triggered by dsRNA exceeding 30 bp and result in nonspecific translational repression and apoptosis (reviewed in Baglioni and Nilsen 1983; Williams 1997; Gil and Esteban 2000). These initial glimpses of gene silencing combined with the strong conservation of key players in the RNAi pathway such as Dicer and Ago (reviewed in Carmell et al. 2002) suggested that silencing phenomena might be available in somatic cell types if the nonspecific dsRNA responses could be circumvented. However, even where nonspecific dsRNA responses are removed from somatic cells, by either viral inhibitors or targeted disruption, long dsRNA still triggers a residual nonspecific repression of gene expression (Abraham et al. 1999; Paddison et al. 2002a).

Another way around these nonspecific dsRNA responses is to simply reduce the size of the dsRNA trigger of RNAi to less than 30 nt to duck the size threshold of PKR and RNase L. In the past 2 years, two short RNA structures have emerged, which provoke sequence-specific gene silencing without activating antiviral responses. These are the siRNA and the shRNA. Both are modeled after biologically active structures in the RNAi pathway: Dicer cleavage products and small temporal RNAs or miRNAs, respectively (Fig. 1).

The first published indication that small dsRNA could trigger RNAi in mammals came from Tuschl and colleagues (Elbashir et al. 2001), who demonstrated that short RNA duplexes resembling the cleavage products of Dicer could trigger sequence-specific silencing in mammalian cell lines (see also Caplen et al. 2001). These siRNAs contain 21 nt of identity to a homologous mRNA target, 19 nt of dsRNA, and a 2-nt 3' overhang. siRNAs presumably bypass the requirement for Dicer and enter the silencing pathway by direct incorporation into Ago-containing complexes. At the same time, as an alternative strategy, several groups developed in vivo expression constructs for small dsRNA triggers in mammalian cells, which resemble endogenously expressed hairpin RNAs (Paddison et al. 2002b; Brummelkamp et al. 2002a; McManus et al. 2002; Paul et al. 2002; Sui et al. 2002; Yu et al. 2002; Zeng et al. 2002). These have been dubbed short hairpin RNAs (shRNAs) since, unlike siRNAs, they have an optimal RNA duplex of 23–29 nt, contain a loop structure that joins both strands of the duplex, and require processing by Dicer to gain admittance to the RNAi pathway.

shRNAs can be categorized by which RNA polymerase is used to drive their expression. In the most popular strategy, simple hairpins containing 19–29 bp of dsRNA are driven from RNA polymerase III promoters [either human or mouse U6-snRNA or human RNase P (H1) RNA promoters] and result in short transcripts of defined length containing 2-nt 3′ overhangs. The latter feature, though unrecognized at first, is likely critical for nuclear export and incorporation into the RNAi pathway through interactions with exportin-5 and Dicer's PAZ domain. In regard to structural elements of the hairpins themselves, there is some in vitro biochemical evidence that suggests that RNaseIII enzymes (e.g., Dicer) might have loop structure or sequence preferences (e.g., Lamontagne et al. 2003). A second shRNA expression strategy utilizes RNA POLII promoters. However, instead of a simple hairpin, these shRNAs are modeled after endogenous miRNAs, which are also expressed from RNA POLII promoters. These miRNA-based shRNAs enter the pathway through Drosha rather than Dicer (Fig. 1). miRNA-based shRNAs have several advantages over simple hairpins. First, they allow tremendous flexibility in the shRNA expression platform, as they can be expressed from any number of well-characterized POLII expression systems (e.g., tet-regulatable or tissue-specific promoters) (Yu et al. 2002; Dickins et al. 2005; Stegmeier et al. 2005; Shin et al. 2006) Second, the exact 22-nt sequence which will be incorporated into RISC via Drosha and Dicer processing is known beforehand. This feature enables the application of rule-based designs using any number of algorithms predicting effective target sequences (Silva et al. 2005).

In addition to expressed shRNAs, chemically and in vitro synthesized shRNAs have been highly effective (Siolas et al. 2005). Chemically synthesized shRNAs containing 25–29 dsRNA and 2-nt 3′ overhangs, in particular, have been more effect than siRNAs containing the same target sequence, working at 5–10× lower concentrations (Siolas et al. 2004; P. Paddison, unpublished results). This added bump in efficiency might be because these RNAi triggers enter the pathway via Dicer processing rather than direct incorporation into RISC.

The main limitation of siRNAs, shRNAs, and transiently transfected shRNA vectors is the inability to evoke stable or inducible gene silencing in mammals. In mammalian cell systems, transient transfection of RNAi triggers, e.g., long dsRNA, siRNAs, or shRNAs, results in a transient effect, lasting 2–7 days due to lack of prominent amplification steps available in other systems. Thus, siRNAs by definition have half-lives and are diluted by cell division and turnover of the RISC complex. However, a number of well-characterized stable expression technologies have now been used in combination with shRNA expression to evoke stable gene silencing in mammals both in vitro and in vivo. Among recent reports, stable RNAi has been demonstrated using random plasmid integration (Brummelkamp et al. 2002a; Paddison et al. 2002b; Carmell et al. 2003), episomal plasmid maintenance (Miyagishi and Taira 2002), and retroviral delivery (Paddison and Hannon 2002; Brummelkamp et al. 2002b; Devroe and Silver 2002; Barton and Medzhitov 2002; Qin et al. 2003; Tiscornia et al. 2003; Hemann et al. 2003). In particular, delivery strategies involving retroviruses, adenovirus, or adeno-associated virus are attractive for exploring RNAi in primary cells, which are particularly difficult to manipulate in vitro.

The ability to trigger RNAi in somatic cells using expressed shRNAs has raised the possibility that these RNAi constructs could be used in animals as dominant transgene suppressors of a target gene. To this end, several groups have demonstrated shRNA-mediated gene silencing in transgenic mice (Carmell et al. 2003; Rubinson et al. 2003), in transplanted mouse hematopoietic stem cells (Hemann et al. 2003; Qin et al. 2003), and in the adult mouse liver (McCaffrey et al. 2002; Song et al. 2003a).

4 Genome-Wide Approaches Using RNAi

The first systematic use of RNAi was in *C. elegans*. Two groups initially used long dsRNA libraries to target all of the predicted *C. elegans* open reading frames (ORFs) on either chromosomes I or III (Fraser et al. 2000; Gönczy et al. 2000). Using time-lapse microscopy to view RNAi-treated embryos from fertilization to the four cell stage, Gönczy and colleagues identified 133 genes from chromosome III that were required for meiosis, pronuclear appearance and migrations, spindle assembly, mitosis, and cytokinesis. Fraser and colleagues found 339 genes from chromosome I that gave rise to identifiable phenotypes such as lethality, visible changes (e.g., in behavior), and sterility. Both screens emphasize the power of RNAi reverse genetics, where phenotypes could immediately be associated with genomic sequences without the tedium of, in this case, positionally cloning mutations. In the past few years, RNAi screens in *C. elegans* have probed phenotypes ranging from genome instability (Pothof et al. 2003) to fat regulation (Ashrafi et al. 2003) to longevity (Lee et al. 2003a).

Cell-based RNAi screens in another invertebrate system, cultured *Drosophila* S2 cells, have served as a counterpoint to whole-animal screens in *C. elegans*. Largely through the efforts of Perrimon's group, genome wide-screens have now been carried out in this system for growth and viability (Boutros et al. 2004), protein secretion (Bard et al. 2006), and modifiers of several signaling pathways, including Erk (Friedman and Perrimon 2006), Hedgehog (Lum et al. 2003; Nybakken et al. 2005), Jak/Stat (Baeg et al. 2005), and Wnt-wingless (DasGupta et al. 2005). Collectively, these studies in invertebrate systems have demonstrated the utility of RNAi in probing gene function in unbiased, systematic ways in both whole organisms and cultured cells.

In cultured human cells, there are now several examples of RNAi screens using either siRNAs or shRNAs. The results from these screens are summarized in

Table 1 Recent large gene-set RNAi screens in human cells

Screen	Cell type	RNAi trigger	Genes targeted	Positive hits	Reference
Apoptosis	HeLa	siRNA	510	>20	Aza-Blanc et al. 2003
Cell survival	HeLa	siRNA	872	73	MacKeigan et al. 2005
p53-Induced cell cycle arrest	Fibroblast	shRNA	7,914	5	Berns et al. 2004
26s proteasome function	293	shRNA	4,873	~100	Paddison et al. 2004b
Cell division	HeLa	esiRNA	5,305	37	Kittler et al. 2004
Transformation	HMEC	shRNA	~9,000	8	Westbrook et al. 2005
Cisplatin sensitization	HeLa	siRNA	~20,000	53	Bartz et al. 2006

esiRNA, endoribonuclease-prepared siRNAs; HMEC, human mammary epithelial cells

Table 1 and included screens probing genes involved in apoptosis (Aza-Blanc et al. 2003), survival (MacKeigan et al. 2005), p53-induced cell cycle arrest (Berns et al. 2004), 26s proteasome function (Paddison et al. 2004), cell division (Kittler et al. 2004), transformation of human mammary epithelial cells (Westbrook et al. 2005), and chemotherapeutic sensitization (Bartz et al. 2006).

In general these screens have demonstrated that RNAi *can* work in mammalian cell systems. However, one important question is why more genome-scale RNAi screens have not been published since 2001–2002 when siRNAs and shRNAs became widely accessible? There are several contributing factors that are worthwhile to consider. These include: (1) the construction/synthesis of affordable genome-wide libraries; (2) the development of RNAi compatible biological assays; and (3) the cost and man-hours involved in infrastructure development for screening.

Several genome-wide siRNAs and shRNAs are currently available from companies such as Dharmacon (siRNAs), Sigma (siRNAs), and Open Biosystems [who distributes shRNAs libraries generated by Cold Spring Harbor Laboratory (CSHL) and the Broad Institute]. However, costs loom large. For example, the arrayed siRNA library used by Linsley and colleagues (Bartz et al. 2006) costs at least US $6,000,000 in today's market (assuming a discounted price of $100 per siRNA). Expressed shRNAs may be a cheaper, renewable alternative (~$200,000–$1,000,000 per genome-wide library) but require additional handling steps (e.g., DNA preps, virus production) that add costs, man-hours, and additional quality-control measures. Additionally, for an RNAi screen to be successful several screen variables must first be explored, including the dynamic range of the biological response, RNAi efficacy, and assay variability. Understanding each of these variables is necessary to define the frequency of false positives and negatives. The most successful RNAi screens to date in mammals were modeled using RNAi-positive controls before moving to the genome-wide scale.

In the near future, one novel RNAi screening strategy will likely supercede other approaches: shRNA barcoding. DNA barcoding strategies have been used with success in *S. cerevisiae* deletion collections to follow individual mutants in complex populations via microarray analysis (Winzeler et al. 1999; Birrell et al. 2001; Giaever et al. 2002). Following this pioneering work in yeast, the CSHL shRNA retroviral libraries have been constructed such that shRNAs are linked to a unique 60-nt DNA barcode so that the fate of shRNAs can be followed during the outgrowth of virally transduced cells (Paddison et al. 2004; Silva et al. 2005). Using microarray analysis to track the shRNA barcodes has already proved to be a powerful approach to follow the biological effects of RNAi in in vitro cell populations (Berns et al. 2004; Paddison et al. 2004; Westbrook et al. 2005).

With respect to the future of RNAi in mammalian systems, applications of genome-wide RNAi libraries in mammals will likely be as varied as those seen in invertebrate systems. Much of the initial work in mammals will likely explore concepts derived from model systems—for example, cell cycle progression, programmed cell death, synthetic lethality (reviewed in Paddison and Hannon 2002). However, the ultimate triumph of RNAi in mammals may be the identification and validation of putative therapeutic targets in cell culture and in vivo rodent models.

5 Off-Target Effects

One issue complicating the use of the RNAi pathway for gene silencing is the production of "off-target" effects. Off-target effects occur when mismatches between the guide RNA and target sequences are tolerated such that both cognate and non-cognate mRNA targets are silenced. These effects arise as a direct result of guide RNA/Ago binding properties, which are determined by the identity of only the first 2–8 nt of the 5' end of the guide strand (Jackson et al. 2003; Haley and Zamore 2004; Birmingham et al. 2006). Thus, this so-called "seed" sequence by its nature allows miRNAs to promiscuously target multiple mRNAs through partial sequence complementarily (Doench et al. 2003). Just so, it also allows siRNAs and shRNAs multiple mRNA targets and creates off-target effects. The strongest evidence for off-target effects comes from genome-wide transcript array analysis of RNAi triggers with different sequences targeting the same gene. Each trigger gives rise to a unique "finger print" of expression patterns that strongly correlate with the sequence of nucleotides 2–8 on the 5' end of the guide strand of an siRNA (Jackson et al. 2003). Thus, any particular RNAi trigger can produce unintended interactions that give rise to desirable or undesirable phenotypes.

If true, does this mean that RNAi screens by their nature will give uninterpretable results? And how are we able to prove specificity for a particular target? From a biological standpoint, while guide RNA "targeting" may be promiscuous, Ago-dependent slicing activity, which will give the most penetrant knockdown, is not. In fact, to achieve efficient target cleavage, complementarily must extend through nucleotide 13 in the guide RNA, if not further (Haley and Zamore 2004). Thus, the higher degree of identity, the more productive the gene silencing. An additional consideration is that miRNAs generally require multiple target sites in a single target to be effective. This could further decrease the possible pool of off-targets in cells. However, from a practical standpoint the easiest way to avoid off-target effects and ensure specificity is to simply demonstrate that multiple RNAi triggers targeting the same gene give rise to the same phenotype. This removes the possibility of off-target effects since the seed sequences of each RNAi trigger will likely be heterologous. Thus, although off-target risks are inherent to using RNAi as a functional genetic tool, they can be dispensed by simply demonstrating that two or more RNAi triggers are effective at both silencing their intended target and eliciting the desired phenotype.

6   RNAi in the Clinic?

RNAi also holds promise for the clinic. Since siRNAs and shRNAs result in sequence-specific gene silencing, in theory they could function as small molecule inhibitors for use in the treatment of human disease. Although delivery is a key issue in general, certain organs such as the liver appear to be readily transfectable by noninvasive techniques in mouse models (see McCaffrey et al. 2002; Song et al. 2003). Moreover, it is conceivable that they could be used in therapies requiring allele-specific or exon-specific targeting events (for example see Brummelkamp et al. 2002b). Intriguingly, the first clinical trials using RNAi-based therapies are currently underway for age-related macular degeneration (Check 2005; McFarland et al. 2004) and respiratory syncytial virus infection (Bitko et al. 2005). In addition, many groups are attempting preclinical development of RNAi-based therapies for other viral diseases (Rossi 2006; Dykxhoorn and Lieberman 2006), neurodegenerative disorders (Raoul et al. 2006), and cancers (Pai et al. 2006).

In vitro, RNAi has proved effective at inhibiting replication of many infection viruses including human immunodeficiency virus (HIV) (Jacque et al. 2002; Lee et al. 2002; Novina et al. 2002), hepatitis C (Kapadia et al. 2003; Randall et al. 2003), rotavirus (Dector et al. 2002), γ-herpesvirus (Jia and Sun 2003), and influenza (Ge et al. 2003). Thus, efficient delivery of siRNAs or shRNA could be used to target viral transcripts directly to reduce viral loads in patients.

Yet another medical application would make use of stably expressed shRNAs. It has been suggested from the study of HIV-resistant populations that removal of the CCR5 and CXCR4 co-receptors may confer resistance to HIV infection (reviewed in Doms and Trono 2000). The use of self-inactivating retroviruses expressing shRNAs targeting these receptors could in theory cure this disease, at least during the early to middle stages when stromal support cells are not ravaged, if shRNAs were incorporated into hematopoietic stem cells ex vivo and then reintroduced into patients.

Given the tremendous potential, it is likely that RNAi will find its way into the clinic in some capacity. Only time will tell whether RNAi represents a "miracle" tool for disease research or merely a step beyond existing antisense technologies.

7   Concluding Remarks

In the last few years the major effect that RNAi has had in invertebrate systems such as *C. elegans* and *Drosophila* is beginning to take hold in mammalian systems through both single gene knockdown experiments and genome-scale screens. In the next decade there will no doubt be both notable successes and failures as we attempt to apply this genetic tool to various biological problems for the first time in academia and industry. Through the introduction of RNAi, mammalian systems have finally gained admittance to the pantheon of model genetic systems.

Acknowledgements This work was supported by the CSHL Fellows Program. PJP thanks Katherine McJunkin of the Watson School of Biological Sciences for reviewing this manuscript.

References

Abraham N, Stojdl DF, Duncan PI, Methot N, Ishii T, Dube M, Vanderhyden BC, Atkins HL, Gray DA, McBurney MW, Koromilas AE, Brown EG, Sonenberg N, Bell JC (1999) Characterization of transgenic mice with targeted disruption of the catalytic domain of the double-stranded RNA-dependent protein kinase, PKR. J Biol Chem 274:5953–5962

Ashrafi K, Chang FY, Watts JL, Fraser AG, Kamath RS, Ahringer J, Ruvkun G (2003) Genome-wide RNAi analysis of Caenorhabditis elegans fat regulatory genes. Nature 421:268–272

Aza-Blanc P, Cooper CL, Wagner K, Batalov S, Deveraux QL, Cooke MP (2003) Identification of modulators of TRAIL-induced apoptosis via RNAi-based phenotypic screening. Mol Cell 12:627–637

Baeg GH, Zhou R, Perrimon N (2005) Genome-wide RNAi analysis of JAK/STAT signaling components in Drosophila. Genes Dev 19:1861–1870

Baglioni C, Nilsen TW (1983) Mechanisms of antiviral action of interferon. Interferon 5:23–42

Bard F, Casano L, Mallabiabarrena A, Wallace E, Saito K, Kitayama H, Guizzunti G, Hu Y, Wendler F, Dasgupta R, Perrimon N, Malhotra V (2006) Functional genomics reveals genes involved in protein secretion and Golgi organization. Nature 439:604–607

Barton GM, Medzhitov R (2002) Retroviral delivery of small interfering RNA into primary cells. Proc Natl Acad Sci U S A 99:14943–14945

Bartz SR, Zhang Z, Burchard J, Imakura M, Martin M, Palmieri A, Needham R, Guo J, Gordon M, Chung N, Warrener P, Jackson AL, Carleton M, Oatley M, Locco L, Santini F, Smith T, Kunapuli P, Ferrer M, Strulovici B, Friend SH, Linsley PS (2006) Small interfering RNA screens reveal enhanced cisplatin cytotoxicity in tumor cells having both BRCA network and TP53 disruptions. Mol Cell Biol 26:9377–9386

Berns K, Hijmans EM, Mullenders J, Brummelkamp TR, Velds A, Heimerikx M, Kerkhoven RM, Madiredjo M, Nijkamp W, Weigelt B, Agami R, Ge W, Cavet G, Linsley PS, Beijersbergen RL, Bernards R (2004) A large-scale RNAi screen in human cells identifies new components of the p53 pathway. Nature 428:431–437

Bernstein E, Caudy AA, Hammond SM, Hannon GJ (2001a) Role for a bidentate ribonuclease in the initiation step of RNA interference. Nature 409:363–366

Bernstein E, Denli AM, Hannon GJ (2001b) The rest is silence. Rna 7:1509–1521

Billy E, Brondani V, Zhang H, Muller U, Filipowicz W (2001) Specific interference with gene expression induced by long, double-stranded RNA in mouse embryonal teratocarcinoma cell lines. Proc Natl Acad Sci U S A 98:14428–14433

Birmingham A, Anderson EM, Reynolds A, Ilsley-Tyree D, Leake D, Fedorov Y, Baskerville S, Maksimova E, Robinson K, Karpilow J, Marshall WS, Khvorova A (2006) 3′ UTR seed matches, but not overall identity, are associated with RNAi off-targets. Nat Methods 3:199–204

Birrell GW, Giaever G, Chu AM, Davis RW, Brown JM (2001) A genome-wide screen in Saccharomyces cerevisiae for genes affecting UV radiation sensitivity. Proc Natl Acad Sci U S A 98:12608–12613

Bitko V, Musiyenko A, Shulyayeva O, Barik S (2005) Inhibition of respiratory viruses by nasally administered siRNA. Nat Med 11:50–55

Bohnsack MT, Czaplinski K, Gorlich D (2004) Exportin 5 is a RanGTP-dependent dsRNA-binding protein that mediates nuclear export of pre-miRNAs. RNA 10:185–191

Boutros M, Kiger AA, Armknecht S, Kerr K, Hild M, Koch B, Haas SA, Paro R, et al (2004) Genome-wide RNAi analysis of growth and viability in Drosophila cells. Nat Med 303:832–835

Brummelkamp TR, Bernards R, Agami R (2002a) A system for stable expression of short interfering RNAs in mammalian cells. Science 296:550–553

Brummelkamp TR, Bernards R, Agami R (2002b) Stable suppression of tumorigenicity by virus-mediated RNA interference. Cancer Cell 2:243–247

Caplen NJ, Parrish S, Imani F, Fire A, Morgan RA (2001) Specific inhibition of gene expression by small double-stranded RNAs in invertebrate and vertebrate systems. Proc Natl Acad Sci U S A 98:9742–9747

Carmell MA, Hannon GJ (2004) RNase III enzymes and the initiation of gene silencing. Nat Struct Mol Biol 11:214–218

Carmell MA, Xuan Z, Zhang MQ, Hannon GJ (2002) The Argonaute family: tentacles that reach into RNAi, developmental control, stem cell maintenance, and tumorigenesis. Genes Dev 16:2733–2742

Carmell MA, Zhang L, Conklin DS, Hannon GJ, Rosenquist TA (2003) Germline transmission of RNAi in mice. Nat Struct Biol 10:91–92

Check E (2005) A crucial test. Nat Med 11:243–244

DasGupta R, Kaykas A, Moon RT, Perrimon N (2005) Functional genomic analysis of the Wnt-wingless signaling pathway. Science 308:826–833

Dector MA, Romero P, Lopez S, Arias CF (2002) Rotavirus gene silencing by small interfering RNAs. EMBO J 3:1175–1180

Denli AM, Tops BB, Plasterk RH, Ketting RF, Hannon GJ (2004) Processing of primary microRNAs by the Microprocessor complex. Nature 432:231–235

Devroe E, Silver PA (2002) Retrovirus-delivered siRNA. BMC Biotechnol 2:15

Dickins RA, Hemann MT, Zilfou JT, Simpson DR, Ibarra I, Hannon GJ, Lowe SW (2005) Probing tumor phenotypes using stable and regulated synthetic microRNA precursors. Nat Genet 37:1289–1295

Doench JG, Petersen CP, Sharp PA (2003) siRNAs can function as miRNAs. Genes Dev 17:438–442

Doms RW, Trono D (2000) The plasma membrane as a combat zone in the HIV battlefield. Genes Dev 14:2677–2688

Dykxhoorn DM, Lieberman J (2006) Silencing viral infection. PLoS Med 3:e242

Edgar R, Wood W (1966) Morphogenesis of bacteriophage T4 in extracts of mutant-infected cells. Proc Natl Acad Sci U S A 55:498–505

Elbashir SM, Harborth J, Lendeckel W, Yalcin A, Weber K, Tuschl T (2001) Duplexes of 21-nucleotide RNAs mediate RNA interference in cultured mammalian cells. Nature 411:494–498

Filippov V, Solovyev V, Filippova M, Gill SS (2000) A novel type of RNase III family proteins in eukaryotes. Gene 245:213–221

Fire A, Xu S, Montgomery MK, Kostas SA, Driver SE, Mello CC (1998) Potent and specific genetic interference by double-stranded RNA in Caenorhabditis elegans. Nature 391:806–811

Fortin KR, Nicholson RH, Nicholson AW (2002) Mouse ribonuclease III. cDNA structure, expression analysis, and chromosomal location. BMC Genomics 3:26

Fraser AG, Kamath RS, Zipperlen P, Martinez-Campos M, Sohrmann M, Ahringer J (2000) Functional genomic analysis of C. elegans chromosome I by systematic RNA interference. Nature 408:325–330

Friedman A, Perrimon N (2006) A functional RNAi screen for regulators of receptor tyrosine kinase and ERK signalling. Nature 444:230–234

Ge Q, McManus MT, Nguyen T, Shen CH, Sharp PA, Eisen HN, Chen J (2003) RNA interference of influenza virus production by directly targeting mRNA for degradation and indirectly inhibiting all viral RNA transcription. Proc Natl Acad Sci U S A 100:2718–2723

Giaever G, Chu AM, Ni L, Connelly C, Riles L, Veronneau S, Dow S, Lucau-Danila A, Anderson K, Andre B, Arkin AP, Astromoff A, El-Bakkoury M, Bangham R, Benito R, Brachat S, Campanaro S, Curtiss M, Davis K, Deutschbauer A, Entian KD, Flaherty P, Foury F, Garfinkel DJ, Gerstein M, Gotte D, Guldener U, Hegemann JH, Hempel S, Herman Z, Jaramillo DF, Kelly DE, Kelly SL, Kotter P, LaBonte D, Lamb DC, Lan N, Liang H, Liao H, Liu L, Luo C, Lussier M, Mao R, Menard P, Ooi SL, Revuelta JL, Roberts CJ, Rose M, Ross-Macdonald P, Scherens B, Schimmack G, Shafer B, Shoemaker DD, Sookhai-Mahadeo S, Storms RK, Strathern JN, Valle G, Voet M, Volckaert G, Wang CY, Ward TR, Wilhelmy J, Winzeler EA, Yang Y, Yen G, Youngman E, Yu K, Bussey H, Boeke JD, Snyder M, Philippsen P, Davis RW, Johnston M (2002) Functional profiling of the Saccharomyces cerevisiae genome. Nature 418:387–391

Gil J, Esteban M (2000) Induction of apoptosis by the dsRNA-dependent protein kinase (PKR): mechanism of action. Apoptosis 5:107–114

Gönczy P, Echeverri C, Oegema K, Coulson A, Jones SJ, Copley RR, Duperon J, Oegema J, Brehm M, Cassin E, Hannak E, Kirkham M, Pichler S, Flohrs K, Goessen A, Leidel S, Alleaume AM, Martin C, Ozlu N, Bork P, Hyman AA (2000) Functional genomic analysis of cell division in C. elegans using RNAi of genes on chromosome III. Nature 408:331–336

Gregory RI, Yan KP, Amuthan G, Chendrimada T, Doratotaj B, Cooch N, Shiekhattar R (2004) The Microprocessor complex mediates the genesis of microRNAs. Nature 432:235–240

Grishok A, Pasquinelli AE, Conte D, Li N, Parrish S, Ha I, Baillie DL, Fire A, Ruvkun G, Mello CC (2001) Genes and mechanisms related to RNA interference regulate expression of the small temporal RNAs that control C. elegans developmental timing. Cell 106:23–34

Ha I, Wightman B, Ruvkun G (1996) A bulged lin-4/lin-14 RNA duplex is sufficient for Caenorhabditis elegans lin-14 temporal gradient formation. Genes Dev 10:3041–3050

Haley B, Zamore PD (2004) Kinetic analysis of the RNAi enzyme complex. Nat Struct Mol Biol 11:599–606

Hall IM, Shankaranarayana GD, Noma K, Ayoub N, Cohen A, Grewal SI (2002) Establishment and maintenance of a heterochromatin domain. Science 297:2232–2237

Hammond SM, Bernstein E, Beach D, Hannon GJ (2000) An RNA-directed nuclease mediates post-transcriptional gene silencing in Drosophila cells. Nature 404:293–296

Han J, Lee Y, Yeom KH, Kim YK, Jin H, Kim VN (2004) The Drosha-DGCR8 complex in primary microRNA processing. Genes Dev 18:3016–3027

Han J, Lee Y, Yeom KH, Nam JW, Heo I, Rhee JK, Sohn SY, Cho Y, Zhang BT, Kim VN (2006) Molecular basis for the recognition of primary microRNAs by the Drosha-DGCR8 complex. Cell 125:887–901

Hannon GJ (2002) RNA interference. Nature 418:244–251

Hartwell LH, Weinert TA (1989) Checkpoints: controls that ensure the order of cell cycle events. Science 246:629–634

Hartwell LH, Culotti J, Pringle JR, Reid BJ (1974) Genetic control of the cell division cycle in yeast. Science 183:46–51

Hemann MT, Fridman JS, Zilfou JT, Hernando E, Paddison PJ, Cordon-Cardo C, Hannon GJ, Lowe SW (2003) An epi-allelic series of p53 hypomorphs created by stable RNAi produces distinct tumor phenotypes in vivo. Nat Genet 33:396–400

Hutvagner G, McLachlan J, Pasquinelli AE, Balint E, Tuschl T, Zamore PD (2001) A cellular function for the RNA-interference enzyme Dicer in the maturation of the let-7 small temporal RNA. Science 293:834–838

Irvine DV, Zaratiegui M, Tolia NH, Goto DB, Chitwood DH, Vaughn MW, Joshua-Tor L, Martienssen RA (2006) Argonaute slicing is required for heterochromatic silencing and spreading. Proc Natl Acad Sci U S A 313:1134–1137

Jackson AL, Bartz SR, Schelter J, Kobayashi SV, Burchard J, Mao M, Li B, Cavet G, Linsley PS (2003) Expression profiling reveals off-target gene regulation by RNAi. Nat Biotechnol 21:635–637

Jacque JM, Triques K, Stevenson M (2002) Modulation of HIV-1 replication by RNA interference. Nature 418:435–438

Jia Q, Sun R (2003) Inhibition of gammaherpesvirus replication by RNA interference. J Virol 77:3301–3306

Kapadia SB, Brideau-Andersen A, Chisari FV (2003) Interference of hepatitis C virus RNA replication by short interfering RNAs. Proc Natl Acad Sci U S A 100:2014–2018

Ketting RF, Fischer SE, Bernstein E, Sijen T, Hannon GJ, Plasterk RH (2001) Dicer functions in RNA interference and in synthesis of small RNA involved in developmental timing in C. elegans. Genes Dev 15:2654–2659

Kittler R, Putz G, Pelletier L, Poser I, Heninger AK, Drechsel D, Fischer S, Konstantinova I, Habermann B, Grabner H, Yaspo ML, Himmelbauer H, Korn B, Neugebauer K, Pisabarro MT, Buchholz F (2004) An endoribonuclease-prepared siRNA screen in human cells identifies genes essential for cell division. Nature 432:1036–1040

Knight SW, Bass BL (2001) A role for the RNase III enzyme DCR-1 in RNA interference and germ line development in Caenorhabditis elegans. Science 293:2269–2271

Kurihara Y, Watanabe Y (2004) Arabidopsis micro-RNA biogenesis through Dicer-like 1 protein functions. Proc Natl Acad Sci U S A 101:12753–12758

Lagos-Quintana M, Rauhut R, Lendeckel W, Tuschl T (2001) Identification of novel genes coding for small expressed RNAs. Science 294:853–858

Lamontagne B, Ghazal G, Lebars I, Yoshizawa S, Fourmy D, Elela SA (2003) Sequence dependence of substrate recognition and cleavage by yeast RNase III. J Mol Biol 327:985–1000

Landthaler M, Yalcin A, Tuschl T (2004) The human DiGeorge syndrome critical region gene 8 and its D. melanogaster homolog are required for miRNA biogenesis. Curr Biol 14:2162–2167

Lau NC, Lim LP, Weinstein EG, Bartel DP (2001) An abundant class of tiny RNAs with probable regulatory roles in Caenorhabditis elegans. Science 294:858–862

Lee NS, Dohjima T, Bauer G, Li H, Li MJ, Ehsani A, Salvaterra P, Rossi J (2002) Expression of small interfering RNAs targeted against HIV-1 rev transcripts in human cells. Nat Biotechnol 20:500–505

Lee RC, Ambros V (2001) An extensive class of small RNAs in Caenorhabditis elegans. Science 294:862–864

Lee RC, Feinbaum RL, Ambros V (1993) The C. elegans heterochronic gene lin-4 encodes small RNAs with antisense complementarity to lin-14. Cell 75:843–854

Lee SS, Lee RY, Fraser AG, Kamath RS, Ahringer J, Ruvkun G (2003a) A systematic RNAi screen identifies a critical role for mitochondria in C. elegans longevity. Nat Genet 33:40–48

Lee Y, Ahn C, Han J, Choi H, Kim J, Yim J, Lee J, Provost P, Radmark O, Kim S, Kim VN (2003b) The nuclear RNase III Drosha initiates microRNA processing. Nature 425:41

Lum L, Yao S, Mozer B, Rovescalli A, Von Kessler D, Nirenberg M, Beachy PA (2003) Identification of Hedgehog pathway components by RNAi in Drosophila cultured cells. Science 299:2039–2045

Lund E, Guttinger S, Calado A, Dahlberg JE, Kutay U (2004) Nuclear export of microRNA precursors. Science 303:95–98

MacKeigan JP, Murphy LO, Blenis J (2005) Sensitized RNAi screen of human kinases and phosphatases identifies new regulators of apoptosis and chemoresistance. Nat Cell Biol 7:591–600

MacRae IJ, Zhou K, Li F, Repic A, Brooks AN, Cande WZ, Adams PD, Doudna JA (2006) Structural basis for double-stranded RNA processing by Dicer. Science 311:195–198

McCaffrey AP, Meuse L, Pham TT, Conklin DS, Hannon GJ, Kay MA (2002) RNA interference in adult mice. Nature 418:38–39

McFarland TJ, Zhang Y, Appukuttan B, Stout JT (2004) Gene therapy for proliferative ocular diseases. Expert Opin Biol Ther 4:1053–1058

McManus MT, Haines BB, Dillon CP, Whitehurst CE, van Parijs L, Chen J, Sharp PA (2002) Small interfering RNA-mediated gene silencing in T lymphocytes. J Immunol 169:5754–5760

Miyagishi M, Taira K (2002) U6 promoter driven siRNAs with four uridine 3′ overhangs efficiently suppress targeted gene expression in mammalian cells. Nat Biotechnol 20:497–500

Mourelatos Z, Dostie J, Paushkin S, Sharma A, Charroux B, Abel L, Rappsilber J, Mann M, Dreyfuss G (2002) miRNPs: a novel class of ribonucleoproteins containing numerous microRNAs. Genes Dev 16:720–728

Novina CD, Murray MF, Dykxhoorn DM, Beresford PJ, Riess J, Lee SK, Collman RG, Lieberman J, Shankar P, Sharp PA (2002) siRNA-directed inhibition of HIV-1 infection. Nat Med 8:681–686

Nybakken K, Vokes SA, Lin TY, McMahon AP, Perrimon N (2005) A genome-wide RNA interference screen in Drosophila melanogaster cells for new components of the Hh signaling pathway. Nat Genet 37:1323–1332

Nykanen A, Haley B, Zamore PD (2001) ATP requirements and small interfering RNA structure in the RNA interference pathway. Cell 107:309–321

Paddison PJ, Hannon GJ (2002) RNA interference: the new somatic cell genetics? Cancer Cell 2:17–23

Paddison PJ, Caudy AA, Hannon GJ (2002a) Stable suppression of gene expression in mammalian cells by RNAi. Proc Natl Acad Sci U S A 99:1443–1448

Paddison PJ, Caudy AA, Bernstein E, Hannon GJ, Conklin DS (2002b) Short hairpin RNAs (shRNAs) induce sequence-specific silencing in mammalian cells. Genes Dev 16:948–958

Paddison PJ, Silva JM, Conklin DS, Schlabach M, Li M, Aruleba S, Balija V, O'Shaughnessy A, Gnoj L, Scobie K, Chang K, Westbrook T, Cleary M, Sachidanandam R, McCombie WR, Elledge SJ, Hannon GJ (2004) A resource for large-scale RNA-interference-based screens in mammals. Nature 428:427–431

Pai SI, Lin YY, Macaes B, Meneshian A, Hung CF, Wu TC (2006) Prospects of RNA interference therapy for cancer. Gene Ther 13:464–477

Pasquinelli AE, Reinhart BJ, Slack F, Martindale MQ, Kuroda MI, Maller B, Hayward DC, Ball EE, Degnan B, Muller P, Spring J, Srinivasan A, Fishman M, Finnerty J, Corbo J, Levine M, Leahy P, Davidson E, Ruvkun G (2000) Conservation of the sequence and temporal expression of let-7 heterochronic regulatory RNA. Nature 2000 408:86–89

Paul CP, Good PD, Winer I, Engelke DR (2002) Effective expression of small interfering RNA in human cells. Nat Biotechnol 20:505–508

Pothof J, van Haaften G, Thijssen K, Kamath RS, Fraser AG, Ahringer J, Plasterk RH, Tijsterman M (2003) Identification of genes that protect the C. elegans genome against mutations by genome-wide RNAi. Genes Dev 17:443–448

Qin XF, An DS, Chen IS, Baltimore D (2003) Inhibiting HIV-1 infection in human T cells by lentiviral-mediated delivery of small interfering RNA against CCR5. Proc Natl Acad Sci U S A 100:183–188

Randall G, Grakoui A, Rice CM (2003) Clearance of replicating hepatitis C virus replicon RNAs in cell culture by small interfering RNAs. Proc Natl Acad Sci U S A 100:235–240

Raoul C, Barker SD, Aebischer P (2006) Viral-based modeling and correction of neurodegenerative diseases by RNA interference. Gene Ther 13:487–495

Reinhart BJ, Slack FJ, Basson M, Pasquinelli AE, Bettinger JC, Rougvie AE, Horvitz HR, Ruvkun G (2000) The 21-nucleotide let-7 RNA regulates developmental timing in Caenorhabditis elegans. Nature 403:901–906

Rossi JJ (2006) RNAi as a treatment for HIV-1 infection. Biotechniques 40:s25–s29

Rubinson DA, Dillon CP, Kwiatkowski AV, Sievers C, Yang L, Kopinja J, Zhang M, McManus MT, Gertler FB, Scott ML, Van Parijs L (2003) A lentivirus-based system to functionally silence genes in primary mammalian cells, stem cells and transgenic mice by RNA interference. Nat Genet 33:401–406

Schwarz DS, Hutvagner G, Haley B, Zamore PD (2002) Evidence that siRNAs function as guides, not primers, in the Drosophila and human RNAi pathways. Mol Cell 10:537–548

Shin KJ, Wall EA, Zavzavadjian JR, Santat LA, Liu J, Hwang JI, Rebres R, Roach T, Seaman W, Simon MI, Fraser ID (2006) A single lentiviral vector platform for microRNA-based conditional RNA interference and coordinated transgene expression. Proc Natl Acad Sci U S A 103:13759–13764

Sijen T, Fleenor J, Simmer F, Thijssen KL, Parrish S, Timmons L, Plasterk RH, Fire A (2001) On the role of RNA amplification in dsRNA-triggered gene silencing. Cell 107:465–476

Silva JM, Li MZ, Chang K, Ge W, Golding MC, Rickles RJ, Siolas D, Hu G, Paddison PJ, Schlabach MR, Sheth N, Bradshaw J, Burchard J, Kulkarni A, Cavet G, Sachidanandam R, McCombie WR, Cleary MA, Elledge SJ, Hannon GJ (2005) Second-generation shRNA libraries covering the mouse and human genomes. Nat Genet 37:1281–1288

Siolas D, Lerner C, Burchard J, Ge W, Linsley PS, Paddison PJ, Hannon GJ, Cleary MA (2005) Synthetic shRNAs as potent RNAi triggers. Nat Biotechnol 23:227–231

Slack FJ, Basson M, Liu Z, Ambros V, Horvitz HR, Ruvkun G (2000) The lin-41 RBCC gene acts in the C. elegans heterochronic pathway between the let-7 regulatory RNA and the LIN-29 transcription factor. Mol Cell 5:659–669

Song E, Lee SK, Wang J, Ince N, Ouyang N, Min J, Chen J, Shankar P, Lieberman J (2003a) RNA interference targeting Fas protects mice from fulminant hepatitis. Nat Med 9:347–351

Song JJ, Liu J, Tolia NH, Schneiderman J, Smith SK, Martienssen RA, Hannon GJ, Joshua-Tor L (2003b) The crystal structure of the Argonaute2 PAZ domain reveals an RNA binding motif in RNAi effector complexes. Nat Struct Biol 10:1026–1032

Song JJ, Smith SK, Hannon GJ, Joshua-Tor L (2004) Crystal structure of Argonaute and its implications for RISC slicer activity. Science 305:1434–1437

Stegmeier F, Hu G, Rickles RJ, Hannon GJ, Elledge SJ (2005) A lentiviral microRNA-based system for single-copy polymerase II-regulated RNA interference in mammalian cells. Proc Natl Acad Sci U S A 102:13212–13217

Stein P, Svoboda P, Anger M, Schultz RM (2003) RNAi: mammalian oocytes do it without RNA-dependent RNA polymerase. RNA 9:187–192

Sui G, Soohoo C, Affar el B, Gay F, Shi Y, Forrester WC, Shi Y (2002) A DNA vector-based RNAi technology to suppress gene expression in mammalian cells. Proc Natl Acad Sci U S A 99:5515–5520

Svoboda P, Stein P, Hayashi H, Schultz RM (2000) Selective reduction of dormant maternal mRNAs in mouse oocytes by RNA interference. Development 127:4147–4156

Tiscornia G, Singer O, Ikawa M, Verma IM (2003) A general method for gene knockdown in mice by using lentiviral vectors expressing small interfering RNA. Proc Natl Acad Sci U S A 100:1844–1848

Tolia NH, Joshua-Tor L (2007) Slicer and the argonautes. Nat Chem Biol 3:36–43

Tuschl T, Zamore PD, Lehmann R, Bartel DP, Sharp PA (1999) Targeted mRNA degradation by double-stranded RNA in vitro. Genes Dev 13:3191–3197

Valencia-Sanchez MA, Liu J, Hannon GJ, Parker R (2006) Control of translation and mRNA degradation by miRNAs and siRNAs. Genes Dev 20:515–524

Volpe TA, Kidner C, Hall IM, Teng G, Grewal SI, Martienssen RA (2002) Regulation of heterochromatic silencing and histone H3 lysine-9 methylation by RNAi. Science 297:1833–1837

Westbrook TF, Martin ES, Schlabach MR, Leng Y, Liang AC, Feng B, Zhao JJ, Roberts TM, Mandel G, Hannon GJ, Depinho RA, Chin L, Elledge SJ (2005) A genetic screen for candidate tumor suppressors identifies REST. Cell 121:837–848

Wianny F, Zernicka-Goetz M (2000) Specific interference with gene function by double-stranded RNA in early mouse development. Nat Cell Biol 2:70–75

Wightman B, Ha I, Ruvkun G (1993) Posttranscriptional regulation of the heterochronic gene lin-14 by lin-4 mediates temporal pattern formation in C. elegans. Cell 75:855–862

Williams BR (1997) Role of the double-stranded RNA-activated protein kinase (PKR) in cell regulation. Biochem Soc Trans 25:509–513

Winzeler EA, Shoemaker DD, Astromoff A, Liang H, Anderson K, Andre B, Bangham R, Benito R, Boeke JD, Bussey H, Chu AM, Connelly C, Davis K, Dietrich F, Dow SW, El Bakkoury M, Foury F, Friend SH, Gentalen E, Giaever G, Hegemann JH, Jones T, Laub M, Liao H, Liebundguth N, Lockhart DJ, Lucau-Danila A, Lussier M, M'Rabet N, Menard P, Mittmann M, Pai C, Rebischung C, Revuelta JL, Riles L, Roberts CJ, Ross-MacDonald P, Scherens B, Snyder M, Sookhai-Mahadeo S, Storms RK, Veronneau S, Voet M, Volckaert G, Ward TR, Wysocki R, Yen GS, Yu K, Zimmermann K, Philippsen P, Johnston M, Davis RW (1999) Functional characterization of the S. cerevisiae genome by gene deletion and parallel analysis. Science 285:901

Wu H, Xu H, Miraglia LJ, Crooke ST (2000) Human RNase III is a 160-kDa protein involved in preribosomal RNA processing. J Biol Chem 275:36957–36965

Yang S, Tutton S, Pierce E, Yoon K (2001) Specific double-stranded RNA interference in undifferentiated mouse embryonic stem cells. Mol Cell Biol 21:7807–7816

Yi R, Qin Y, Macara IG, Cullen BR (2003) Exportin-5 mediates the nuclear export of pre-microRNAs and short hairpin RNAs. Genes Dev 17:3011–3016

Yu JY, DeRuiter SL, Turner DL (2002) RNA interference by expression of short-interfering RNAs and hairpin RNAs in mammalian cells. Proc Natl Acad Sci U S A 99:6047–6052

Zamore PD, Haley B (2005) Ribo-gnome: the big world of small RNAs. Science 309:1519–1524

Zamore PD, Tuschl T, Sharp PA, Bartel DP (2000) RNAi: double-stranded RNA directs the ATP-dependent cleavage of mRNA at 21 to 23 nucleotide intervals. Cell 101:25–33

Zeng Y, Wagner EJ, Cullen BR (2002) Both natural and designed micro RNAs can inhibit the expression of cognate mRNAs when expressed in human cells. Mol Cell 9:1327–1333

Zilberman D, Cao X, Jacobsen SE (2003) Argonaute4 control of locus-specific siRNA accumulation and DNA and histone methylation. Science 299:716–719

RNAi Pathway in *C. elegans*: The Argonautes and Collaborators

Marie-Eve L. Boisvert and Martin J. Simard(✉)

Abstract   Since Dr. Sidney Brenner first used it as an animal model system, the round worm *Caenorhabditis elegans* has significantly contributed to our understanding of important biological processes. Among them, the discovery in the 1990s of new gene silencing pathways orchestrated by tiny non-coding RNAs created a new field of research in biology. In this review, we will discuss the key players of the RNAi pathways in *C. elegans* and particularly the Argonaute genes, an impressive gene family of 27 members important in many aspects of these pathways.

1   A Tiny Worm Shed Light on New Gene Regulation Mechanisms

At 1 mm long, transparent, and eating bacteria, the roundworm *Caenorhabditis elegans* had always lived in the underworld until the animal was brought to the laboratory bench by Dr. Sydney Brenner in 1974. Now that we have a complete

Martin J. Simard
Laval University Cancer Research Center, Hôtel-Dieu de Québec (CHUQ),
Québec City, Québec G1R 2J6, Canada
Martin.Simard@crhdq.ulaval.ca

P.J. Paddison and P.K. Vogt (eds.), *RNA Interference.*
Current Topics in Microbiology and Immunology 320.
© Springer-Verlag Berlin Heidelberg 2008

sequenced genome and the knowledge of the lineage of every single cell of its body, the nematode *C. elegans* is definitely a powerful animal model. Using this animal, the seminal discoveries made in the 1990s created a new field of research in biology: gene silencing mediated by small non-coding RNAs.

Using genetic screens to identify essential genes important for the precise developmental timing of the nematode, Dr. Victor Ambros's lab had stumbled on a unique locus that does not encoded for any protein; it was the first microRNA, *lin-4* (Lee et al. 1993). A few years later, Dr. Gary Ruvkun's group identified the second microRNA, *let-7*, that also regulated the developmental cues of *C. elegans* (Reinhart et al. 2000). Once they realized that the *let-7* microRNA is conserved throughout evolution (Pasquinelli et al. 2000), many groups hunted for microRNAs in various species and identified many of these small RNA species in worm, fly, and human (Lee and Ambros 2001; Lagos-Quintana et al. 2001; Lau et al. 2001). It was then clear that microRNAs are extremely important for cell homeostasis in many species (see Chap. 12, this volume).

Originally, worm geneticists used the RNA interference or RNAi as a magic tool to efficiently knock down gene expression (Guo and Kemphues 1995; Rocheleau et al. 1997). In 1998, collaborative work from the groups led by Drs. Fire and Mello elucidated how RNAi actually worked; they discovered that the double-stranded RNA molecule triggers specific gene silencing in *C. elegans* (Fire et al. 1998). The double-stranded RNA trigger can be applied to worms in different ways: by (1) injecting them into the body cavities; (2) endogenously expressing in cells; (3) soaking the worm in liquid containing double-stranded RNA (dsRNA) molecules; and (4) feeding the animals with bacteria expressing dsRNA (Fig. 1).

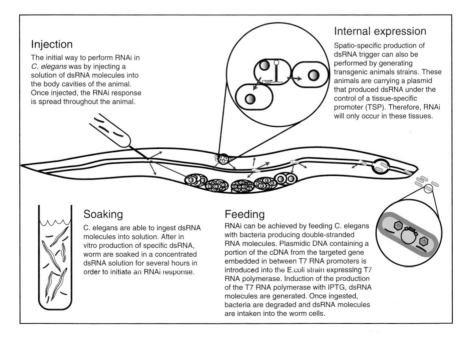

Fig. 1 The various methods to exogenously initiate RNAi in *Caenorhabditis elegans*

Besides the extremely important contribution of RNAi as a tool to study gene function in *C. elegans* and in many other species, it has been recently discovered that the RNAi pathway is also important in animals in nature. In a molecular process called endogenous RNAi, dsRNA molecules produced in *C. elegans* lead to the formation of two classes of small non-coding RNAs: endogenous siRNAs and tiny non-coding RNAs or tncRNAs (Ambros et al. 2003).

The extensive study of these various small non-coding RNA-mediated gene-silencing pathways has uncovered many cellular factors playing important roles in these processes. In this chapter we will discuss the key players of the RNAi pathways (Table 1) and particularly the Argonaute genes, an impressive gene family in *C. elegans* that is important in many aspects of these pathways.

2   The Argonautes: The Heroes of RNAi Pathways

Originally, their quest was to find the Golden Fleece. About 50 ancient Greek heroes, sailing on their ship the Argo, were heading to Colchis. Today, we find in the human and fruit fly genome 5 gene analogs that are the namesakes of these ancient warriors; there are 10 in *Arabidopsis thaliana*, only 1 in *Schizosaccharomyces pombe*, and not less than 27 in *Caenorhabditis elegans* (see Fig. 3 in Yigit et al. 2006). The association of Argonaute proteins with small non-coding RNAs generates the core of the RNA-induced silencing complex (RISC), the central element of all RNA silencing pathways (reviewed in Carmell et al. 2002). The Argonaute proteins contain two signature domains, PAZ (PIWI/Argonaute/Zwille) and Piwi. These RNA binding domains interact with the 3′ and 5′ overhangs of the small single-stranded RNA guides and leave internal nucleotides available for base-pairing (Ma et al. 2005; Parker et al. 2005). The PIWI domain contains a catalytic region called "DDH" (two aspartate residues and one histidine residue), a motif analogous to the catalytic motif of the RNase H family (Song et al. 2004). A mutation of any of these residues in human Ago2 abolished slicer activity (Liu et al. 2004; Rivas et al. 2005). Thus, the Argonaute binds to both ends of the small non-coding RNA which then pairs with the target mRNA. Finally, the Argonaute is presumed to "slice" the poor mRNA (nicely reviewed in Song and Joshua-Tor 2006).

We found Argonaute genes in all organisms that are able to specifically silence genes using the small RNA-guided strategy. It is quite intriguing that the *C. elegans* genome contains 27 members of this gene family. Why is there as many distinct Argonaute proteins in *C. elegans*, and less than 10 in the other species?

2.1   The "First-Line" Argonautes

The Argonaute protein RDE-1 (for RNA interference-deficient) was the first Argonaute implicated in the RNAi pathway (Tabara et al. 1999). Early genetic studies have shown that RDE-1 is required for the initial steps of the RNAi pathway

Table 1 Cellular components of the RNAi pathways in *C. elegans*. The Argonautes ALG–1 and ALG–2 are marked with an asterisk because they are not involved in the RNAi pathway per se but are instead essential for the microRNA pathway. The Argonaute ALG–1 has also been shown recently to be involved in transcriptional silencing of transgenes in soma cells (Grishok et al. 2005). The Argonaute PPW–2 was initially identified as an important factor for transposon silencing (Vastenhouw et al. 2003). *smg–2* and a subset of *smg* genes have been proposed to be important for the persistence of RNAi (Domeier et al. 2000). Hypothetical functions are in italics

Name	Family	RNAi	Function
CSR–1 (chromosome segregation and RNAi)	Argonaute	Endo	Germline RNAi/chromosome segregation
ERGO–1 (endogenous RNAi-deficient Argonaute)	Argonaute	Endo	Interaction with the *endo*-siRNA
PPW–1 (PAZ/PIWI-related protein)	Argonaute	Exo/endo?	Interaction with secondary siRNA ?
PPW–2 (PAZ/PIWI-related protein)	Argonaute	?	Interaction with secondary siRNA?/transposon silencing in germ line
PRG–1 PIWI-related Gene)	Argonaute	Endo	Germline proliferation and maintenance/gonadogenesis
RDE–1 (RNA interference-deficient)	Argonaute	Exo	Interaction with the primary siRNA, formation of the RISC complex
SAGO–1 (synthetic secondary-siRNA defective AGO)	Argonaute	Exo/endo	Interaction with secondary siRNA
SAGO–2 (synthetic secondary-siRNA defective AGO)	Argonaute	Exo/endo	Interaction with secondary siRNA
*ALG–1 (Argonaute-like gene)	Argonaute	–	Formation of miRISC with miRNA/implication in transcriptional silencing
*ALG–2 (Argonaute-like gene)	Argonaute	–	In complex with ALG–1, interaction with microRNAs
RDE–4 (RNA interference-deficient)	dsRNA binding protein	Exo	Interaction with trigger dsRNA/*may present primary siRNA to DCR–1*
DRH–1 (Dicer-related helicase)	Helicase	Exo	*May give an accessible conformation to dsRNA for DCR complex*
DRH–2 (Dicer-related helicase)	Helicase	Exo	*May give an accessible conformation to dsRNA for DCR complex*
DRH–3 (Dicer-related helicase)	Helicase	Endo	*May give an accessible conformation to dsRNA for DCR complex*

Table 1 (continued)

Name	Family	RNAi	Function
MUT–14 (mutator)	Helicase	Exo	Transposon silencing into germ line/*permit the novo RNA synthesis by RdRPs*
SMG–2 (suppressor with morphological effect on genitalia)	Helicase	Exo	*May be important for the persistence of RNAi*
RDE–3 (RNA interference-deficient)	Polymerase b-nucleotidyl-transferase	Exo/endo?	*May polyadenylate the 3′ end of cleavage product, and recruit RdRP*
EGO–1 (enhancer of glp–1)	RNA-dependent RNA polymerase	Exo	Polymerization of secondary siRNA precursor for exo-RNAi in germinal cells
RRF–1 (RdRP family)	RNA-dependent RNA polymerase	Exo	Polymerization of secondary siRNA precursor for exo-RNAi in somatic cells
RRF–2 (RdRP family)	RNA-dependent RNA polymerase	?	?
RRF–3 (RdRP family)	RNA-dependent RNA polymerase	Endo	Polymerization of secondary siRNA precursor for endo-RNAi in somatic cells
PIR–1 (RNA phosphatase homolog)	RNA phosphatase	Exo/endo	Implicated in the processing of secondary siRNAs
			May remove 5′ β- and γ-phosphate of secondary siRNAs
DCR–1 (Dicer related)	RNase III	Exo/endo	Cleavage of dsRNA and miRNA precursor into siRNA and miRNA
SID–1 (systemic RNA interference-deficient)	Transmembrane protein	Exo	Systemic transmission of dsRNA and transmission to progeny
MUT–7/MUT–8/MUT–15 (mutator)	?	Exo/endo?	Transposon silencing into germline

in *C. elegans* (Grishok et al. 2000). Since several structural and functional studies from different systems suggested that members of the Argonaute protein family are key components of the RISC (Liu et al. 2004; Meister et al. 2004; Song et al. 2004), biochemical tools have been developed to address whether or not RDE-1 is the key component of the RISC complex in worms. By feeding animals with a dsRNA trigger that targets a very small region on the mRNA and using a 2'-*O*-methylated RNA affinity matrix that retains the small non-coding RNA-protein complex (Hutvágner et al. 2004), it has been shown that the RDE-1 proteins interact with both sense and antisense small RNA strands generated by the cleavage of the dsRNA trigger by the RNase III enzyme Dicer (Yigit et al. 2006). These observations then suggested that (1) RDE-1 takes up duty downstream of the systemic transport of the dsRNA trigger into animal tissues and (2) dsRNA trigger processing into a single strand forms the RISC complex. It has also been shown in a mutant strain unable to produce secondary small interfering RNAs (siRNAs) (described below) that the interaction of RDE-1 with small RNA is not altered, suggesting that the downstream steps of the RNAi pathway in *C. elegans* are not important for the binding of RDE-1 and for the production of siRNAs generated by the dsRNA processing (called primary siRNAs). Other experiments confirmed that RDE-1 interacts only with the primary siRNAs, and not with the secondary siRNAs, thus characterizing RDE-1 as a primary Argonaute (Yigit et al. 2006). When a dsRNA trigger is introduced into *C. elegans*, it is transformed in a primary siRNA by the endonuclease Dicer (DCR-1 in worm) and then interacts with RDE-1 to form the RISC complex (Fig. 2). To date, it is not yet known if the RDE-1 Argonaute protein is able to cleave directly the mRNA target, as reported for the Argonaute found in the RISC complex of *Drosophila* and human (Hammond et al. 2001; Liu et al. 2004; Meister et al. 2004). Sequence alignments of PIWI domains of Argonaute proteins from many species demonstrated that RDE-1 possesses the catalytic residues essential for the RISC activity (Tolia and Joshua-Tor 2007), suggesting that RDE-1 may have the molecular capacity to induce endonucleolytic cleavage of targeted mRNA. Future exhaustive biochemical studies on RDE-1 and other Argonaute proteins of *C. elegans* will certainly shed light on their molecular activities.

In parallel, the *endo*-RNAi pathway in *C. elegans* also requires a primary Argonaute protein. The study of Argonaute genes has revealed that the R09A1.1 gene is most likely the alter ego of *rde-1* for the RNA silencing pathway induced by endogenously produced dsRNA molecules (Yigit et al. 2006). The R09A1.1 mutant strain displayed (1) an enhanced sensitivity to exogenously induced RNAi as previously observed in animals defective in *endo*-RNAi components (Duchaine et al. 2006; Kennedy et al. 2004; Lee et al. 2006; Simmer et al. 2002) and (2) a level of endogenous siRNAs that was significantly increased, as also observed for other components of the *endo*-RNAi pathway (Duchaine et al. 2006; Lee et al. 2006). For these reasons, the R09A1.1 gene (renamed *ergo-1* for endogenous RNAi-deficient Argonaute mutant) is considered to play a similar role as RDE-1 protein, and thus for the *endo*-RNAi pathway in *C. elegans*.

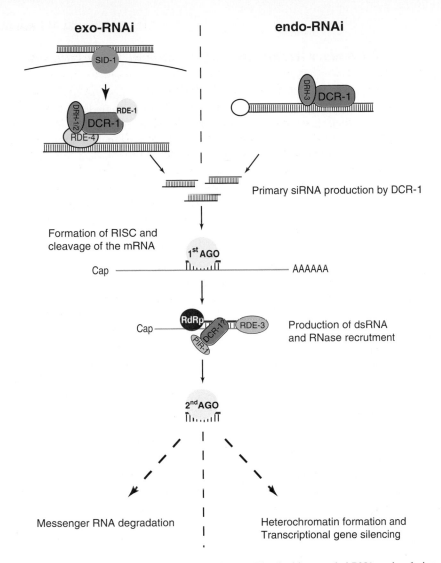

Fig. 2 Models for the RNAi pathways in *C. elegans*. The double-stranded RNA molecule introduced artificially into the animal enters the *exo*-RNAi pathway and will be processed by Dicer (DCR-1) to generate primary siRNAs. The *endo*-RNAi pathway is initiated by double-stranded RNA (dsRNA) duplexes produced by either bi-directional transcription of a specific part of the genome (i.e., centromeric regions) or by the hairpin dsRNA structures formed by the transcription of the X chromosome cluster and tiny non-coding RNA precursors. In each pathway, specific DCR-1 complexes will recognize dsRNA triggers. Once primary siRNAs are produced, they associate with the primary Argonaute (1st AGO): RDE-1 for the *exo*-RNAi pathway and potentially ERGO-1 and CSR-1 for the *endo*-RNAi pathway. After the endonucleolytic cleavage of the messenger RNA, RDE-3 will stabilize the 5′ end cleavage products to favor the polymerization of the antisense strand by the RNA-dependent RNA polymerases (RdRPs). The nascent dsRNA will be then cleaved by an RNase (most likely DCR-1) to generate the secondary siRNAs. These small RNA species will be bound by secondary Argonautes (2nd AGO), and thus downstream biochemical steps will lead to complete gene silencing. The recycling of the RDE-1 complex (not illustrated) may be required to maintain the RNAi response (for further details see Yigit et al. 2006). The *dashed arrows* indicate speculative elements of the model

2.2   The Secondary Argonautes: Merging both RNAi Pathways

Since RDE-1 is only associated with primary siRNAs, it became possible that other members of the family of Argonaute genes could bind the secondary siRNAs and be important for the RNAi pathways. Once the exogenous- or endogenous-supplied dsRNA molecules have initiated their respective RNAi pathway, RDE-1/small RNA and ERGO-1/small RNA complexes bind their mRNA targets and start the production of another class of small RNAs; the secondary siRNAs (Fig. 2). The exhaustive analysis of the Argonaute gene family has uncovered a new group of Argonaute genes important for RNAi pathways in *C. elegans*. Among them, the *ppw-1* gene is important for the germline RNAi; *sago-1* and *sago-2* are required for proper somatic RNAi; and the F58G1.1 gene contributes to both germline and somatic *exo*-RNAi (Yigit et al. 2006). A mutant strain carrying loss-of-function alleles of all the previous genes (called MAGO strain) is completely resistant to both germline and somatic *exo*-RNAi and is also defective in the production of endogenous siRNAs. Rescue experiments have demonstrated that RDE-1, as well as SAGO-1, SAGO-2, and PPW-1, have qualitatively distinct activities in the *exo*-RNAi pathway and that the expression of either SAGO-1 or SAGO-2 can rescue the RNAi deficiency as well as reestablish the level of endogenous siRNAs in the MAGO strain (Yigit et al. 2006). Therefore, SAGO-1, SAGO-2, and PPW-1 became excellent candidates to bind secondary siRNAs in both RNAi pathways. Using immunoprecipitation assays it has been observed that both SAGO-1 and SAGO-2 Argonaute proteins bind secondary siRNAs and endogenous siRNAs, suggesting that this subgroup of Argonaute proteins (called secondary Argonautes) may lead to a competition between the *exo*-RNAi and the *endo*-RNAi pathways. In contrast to RDE-1 and ERGO-1, SAGO-1, SAGO-2, and PPW-1 PIWI domains lack the three amino acids residues important for endonuclease activity. Thus, it is proposed that these secondary siRNAs would require other cellular factors to control the fate of targeted mRNAs.

2.3   Implication of Argonaute Genes in C. elegans Development and Viability

Among the small RNA-mediated silencing pathways found in metazoans, the microRNA pathway clearly plays a crucial role in the control of developmental cues and cell differentiation (Bartel 2004). As observed for the RNAi pathways, the microRNA pathway also requires Argonaute to abrogate protein synthesis.

In mammals, all four members of the Argonaute gene family are able to bind microRNAs (Meister et al. 2004). In contrast, Ago1 is the only Argonaute protein implicated in the microRNA pathway in *Drosophila melanogaster* (Okamura et al. 2004). Similarly, among the 27 members of the Argonaute gene family found in *C. elegans*, only *alg-1* and *alg-2* have been strictly associated with the microRNA pathway so far. The alteration of *alg-1* and *alg-2* gene expression leads to severe developmental phenotypes (Grishok et al. 2001). In fact, phenotypes observed are identical to the ones generated by the loss-of-function of the *let-7* microRNA, a small RNA essential for the larvae-to-adult transition (Reinhart et al. 2000). In addition, the knockdown of both *alg-1* and *alg-2* generated diminution of *let-7* and *lin-4* microRNA levels and an accumulation of their respective microRNA precursors (Grishok et al. 2001). Biochemical approaches have demonstrated that ALG-1 and ALG-2 are associated with the *let-7* microRNA in vivo (Hutvágner et al. 2004), and our recent observations indicate they are interacting with many, if not all, *C. elegans* microRNAs (E.L. Rondeau, E. A. Miska and M.J. Simard., unpublished data). For the microRNA pathway, ALG-1 and ALG-2 therefore play a similar role to RDE-1 and ERGO-1 in the *exo-* and *endo*-RNAi pathways respectively.

We also found members essential for animal viability within the *C. elegans* Argonaute gene family. A knockdown of *csr-1* demonstrated its role in chromosome segregation; the *csr-1* loss-of function allele showed partially resistance to germline RNAi, and most of the animals were sterile (Yigit et al. 2006). The Argonaute *csr-1* thus belongs to a new gene class whose members exhibit loss-of-function phenotypes with defects in both chromosome segregation and RNAi. Another member of the Argonaute gene family, *prg-1*, when disrupted displayed a reduced brood size and a temperature-sensitive sterile phenotype (Yigit et al. 2006). It is suggested that the Argonaute PRG-1 is essential for germline proliferation and maintenance, and even for the proper gonadogenesis (Cox et al. 1998).

3 The Argonautes Are Not Alone

The *C. elegans* Argonaute proteins are clearly key players in the RNA silencing pathways. However, the RNAi pathway also necessitates other cellular factors for many biochemical aspects such as generating primary siRNAs from dsRNA molecules and maintaining the silencing response.

3.1 RDE-4: A Partner of RDE-1

In the initial genetic screen performed to identify genes essential for the RNA interference pathway in *C. elegans*, along with *rde-1* mutant alleles, two other strains carrying lesions on the right arm of chromosome III have been isolated in an unknown gene that they named *rde-4* (Tabara et al. 1999). Clever genetic studies demonstrated that *rde-4* along with *rde-1* is required at the initial steps of the RNAi pathway (Grishok et al. 2000), and biochemical studies showed that *rde-4* mutant has a reduced level of siRNAs (Parrish and Fire 2001; Tabara et al. 2002). Because of its dsRNA binding motif, RDE-4 binds preferentially to long dsRNA molecules but not siRNAs (Tabara et al. 2002). RDE-4 interacts with RDE-1 as well as DCR-1,

DRH-1, and DRH-2 (Dicer related helicase), cellular factors all required for RNAi (Tabara et al. 2002). These observations led to suggestions that the role for RDE-4 is to recognize the entering dsRNA trigger and to present it to DCR-1 for processing (Tabara et al. 2002).

3.2   Dicer and Friends

The RNaseIII enzyme Dicer was first associated with the production of siRNAs from studies performed in cultured *Drosophila* cells (Hammond et al. 2000). In *C. elegans*, *dcr-1* has been shown to be required for *lin-4* and *let-7* microRNA production (Grishok et al. 2001), for *exo*-RNAi (Grishok et al. 2001; Knight and Bass 2001), and for germline development (Knight and Bass 2001). The requirement of *Dicer* in the initiation of RNAi was initially suggested in fly (Bernstein et al. 2001) and in *C. elegans* by its interaction with RDE-4 (Tabara et al. 2002). It has been also reported that DCR-1 enzyme activity is essential for the *endo*-RNAi pathway (Ambros et al. 2003).

The Dicer-related helicase genes *drh-1*, *drh-2*, and *drh-3* are found in complex with the DCR-1 complex (Duchaine et al. 2006). This *C. elegans* gene family shares a helicase domain that is similar to the one found in DCR-1 (Tabara et al. 2002). In contrast with *drh-1* and *drh-2*, both essential for *exo*-RNAi (Tabara et al. 2002), *drh-3* is an essential gene for animal viability and appears to be important for the *endo*-RNAi pathway (Duchaine et al. 2006). The interaction of DRH-1 and DRH-2 proteins with RDE-4 (Tabara et al. 2002) and the nature of their conserved domain suggest that they may contribute to make the dsRNA trigger molecule accessible to the DCR-1 complex.

A particular class of genes, the enhancer of RNAi or *eri* genes, has also been found as DCR-1 interactors (Duchaine et al. 2006). The first member of this gene family *eri-1* was identified in a genetic screen designed to isolate mutants able to increase the sensitivity to dsRNA molecules (Kennedy et al. 2004). The animal carrying a mutation in *eri-1* accumulates more siRNAs than wildtype animals and is hypersensitive to *exo*-RNAi (Kennedy et al. 2004). Biochemical assays demonstrated that *C. elegans* ERI-1 protein and its human ortholog degrade siRNAs in vitro (Kennedy et al. 2004). From these studies, it has been suggested that ERI-1 siRNase activity attenuates the RNAi response. The two other members of these gene family, *eri-3* and *eri-5*, that have been identified in the DCR-1 complex also display hypersensitivity to *exo*-RNAi when their gene products are inactive (Duchaine et al. 2006). It also been observed that the presence of ERI-3 and ERI-5 is required for the interaction between ERI-1 and DCR-1 (Duchaine et al. 2006). The accumulation of *endo*-siRNAs and tncRNAs requires the ERI proteins, suggesting an important role for the *eri* gene family in the *endo*-RNAi pathway in *C. elegans* (Duchaine et al. 2006). Consistent with this idea, a study has recently demonstrated that *eri-1* mutant animals displayed a low amount of *endo*-siRNAs and an increased level of *exo*-siRNAs (Lee et al. 2006). These observations suggest that the *exo*- and *endo*-RNAi silencing pathways compete for specific groups of proteins important to both RNAi pathways in *C. elegans*, and in the absence of ERI-1, these proteins are only associated with the *exo*-RNAi pathway that thus lead to a hypersensitivity to exogenously provided dsRNA. Further studies need to be accomplished to elucidate the exact role of the *eri* gene family.

Among the DCR-1 interactors, *pir-1*, an RNA phosphatase, is an essential gene required for *exo*-RNAi. The *pir-1* mutant displays developmental defect as observed in the *drh-3* mutant (Duchaine et al. 2006). When *pir-1* mutant animals are exposed to dsRNA, 120-nucleotide-long dsRNA species that bear the sequence of the trigger dsRNA as well as sequences upstream of the trigger accumulate in the animals (Duchaine et al. 2006). These dsRNA molecules are produced by the RNA-dependent RNA polymerase (see the following section) and are the precursors of the secondary siRNAs. Thus, DCR-1 (or the effector protein) seems unable to process the secondary siRNAs without PIR-1 activity. PIR-1 is a member of the RNA phosphatase family highly conserved throughout evolution (Duchaine et al. 2006). The vertebrate PIR-1 homolog is able to remove the $5'$ γ- and β-phosphates from RNA triphosphate substrates (Deshpande et al. 1999; Yuan et al. 1998). Recent evidence supports that RNA-dependent polymerases could produce dsRNA substrates with $5'$ triphosphates (Pak and Fire 2007; Sijen et al. 2007), and then PIR-1 could generate the $5'$ monophosphate products that would be recognized by a DCR-1 complex and/or an Argonaute (Duchaine et al. 2006).

3.3   RNA-Dependent RNA Polymerases and Secondary siRNAs

One of the amazing features of the *exo*-RNAi in *C. elegans* is that a unique delivery of dsRNA trigger can induce gene silencing in all cells of the animal's body-with the exception of neurons-even in subsequent generations of the injected animal (Fire et al. 1998; Grishok et al. 2000). This phenomenon has led to speculation that it should have some kind of amplification of the interfering agent. The amplification process has been rapidly supported with the discovery of a new set of genes, the RNA-dependent RNA polymerases (RdRPs), essential for the RNAi-mediated silencing in fungi, nematodes, and plants (Cogoni and Macino 1999; Dalmay et al. 2000; Mourrain et al. 2000; Smardon et al. 2000). Four members of the RdRP gene family are found in the *C. elegans* genome: *ego-1*, *rrf-1*, *rrf-2*, and *rrf-3*. The EGO-1 gene is essential for germline development, and the loss-of-function mutant is highly resistant to RNAi targeting germline-specific genes (Smardon et al. 2000). On the other hand, it has been shown that the RdRP protein RRF-1 is essential only for RNAi targeting somatic genes (Sijen et al. 2001). They also observed that RRF-1 (and most likely EGO-1 in germline tissues) is important to the production of secondary siRNAs (Sijen et al. 2001). Thus, EGO-1 is required for germline-specific *exo*-RNAi while RRF-1 is essential for the somatic *exo*-RNAi pathway. In contrast to *ego-1* and *rrf-1* mutants, a deletion of *rrf-3* does not reduce the sensitivity to *exo*-RNAi in germline and soma tissues, but instead leads to a hypersensitivity for *exo*-RNAi (Sijen et al. 2001; Simmer et al. 2002). It has also been observed that RRF-3 interacts with the DCR-1 complex (Duchaine et al. 2006) and *rrf-3* mutant animals have a decreased level of *endo*-siRNAs and an increased level of *exo*-siRNAs, as observed in the *eri-1* mutant strain (Lee et al. 2006). Therefore, these observations suggest that RRF-3 and ERI-1 are both associated with the *endo*-RNAi pathway in *C. elegans*.

The production of the secondary siRNAs by RdRPs required for RNAi pathways in *C. elegans* is still not well understood. The discovery of RDE-3, a member of the polymerase β-nucleotidyltransferase superfamily, has suggested that the stabilization of the targeted mRNA by the polyadenylation of the 3′ end of cleavage product may favor the recruitment of RdRP to produce secondary siRNAs (Chen et al. 2005). Recently, it has been reported that secondary siRNA production does not necessitate the use of primary siRNAs as a primer for specific amplification (Pak and Fire 2007; Sijen et al. 2007). In addition, the authors also observed in these studies that the secondary siRNAs carry di- or triphosphates at their 5′ end (Pak and Fire 2007; Sijen et al. 2007). This distinctive mark may explain how secondary siRNAs can be recognized by the secondary Argonautes, with the help of the phosphatase PIR-1 (described in the previous section).

4 RNAi Important to Maintain Genome Integrity: A Primitive Immune System in *C. elegans*?

In most *C. elegans* strains, transposition of the Tc1 transposon happens in somatic cells, but transposon shuffling is completely silenced in the germline. Many genes essential for transposon silencing, called the mutators, are also important for the RNAi pathway (Ketting et al. 1999; Ketting and Plasterk 2000; Tabara et al. 1999; Tijsterman et al. 2002; Vastenhouw et al. 2003). The common requirement of these specific genes in both silencing processes strongly points to the important role played by the *exo*-RNAi pathway in maintaining the genome integrity of future generations (for review see Vastenhouw and Plasterk 2004).

The *exo*-RNAi system in worms may also be important to protect against external intruders. The nematode *C. elegans* shares with plants the capacity of spreading the exogenously dsRNA-mediated RNAi response from cell to cell and to subsequent generations. It has even been observed recently that the RNAi response can still be detected after 80 generations (Vastenhouw et al. 2006). The transmembrane protein systemic RNA interference defective (SID)-1 is essential for the systemic transmission in *C. elegans* (Winston et al. 2002). It is suggest that SID-1 is likely to form a channel for the passive transport of dsRNA into cells, while having an active retention of the dsRNA (Feinberg and Hunter 2003). There is no homolog of the SID-1 gene in *Drosophila*, consistent with the absence of systemic RNAi in this organism. However, there are homologous proteins in mammals, where systematic RNAi has not been yet demonstrated.

In plants, the RNAi pathway serves as an antiviral mechanism. Spreading of the silencing signal throughout the plant ensures that, when the plant is later exposed to same virus, it will be resistant to further infection. Although it has yet not been clearly demonstrated, the *exo*-RNAi pathway in worms may represent a primitive immune system for the animal. Recent studies have shown that the Argonaute RDE-1 is required for a potential antiviral silencing triggered by viral replication (Lu et al. 2005), and in vitro studies demonstrate the importance of the *exo*-RNAi components for antiviral defense in *C. elegans* (Wilkins et al. 2005).

5 Closing Remarks

If the origin of the RNAi system in *C. elegans* is not totally clear, one thing nevertheless is sure: the worm has become a simple and powerful tool for understanding a new role of small non-coding RNAs. Future biochemical studies and new innovative genetic screens made with the tiny worm will contribute to our unraveling of the whole truth about the small RNA phenomenon.

Acknowledgements We would like to thank Dr. Jean-Yves Masson and members of the laboratory for comments on the manuscript. This work has been funded by the Canadian Institutes of Health Research (MOP-81186). M.E.L.B. is supported by a fellowship from the Natural Sciences and Engineering Research Council of Canada (NSERC) and M.J.S. holds a Junior 1 scholarship from the Fonds en Recherche de la Santé du Québec (FRSQ).

References

Ambros V, Lee RC, Lavanway A, Williams PT, Jewell D (2003) MicroRNAs and other tiny endogenous RNAs in C. elegans. Curr Biol 13:807-818

Bartel DP (2004) MicroRNAs: genomics, biogenesis, mechanism, and function. Cell 116:281-297

Bernstein E, Caudy AA, Hammond SM, Hannon GJ (2001) Role for a bidentate ribonuclease in the initiation step of RNA interference. Nature 409:363-366

Carmell MA, Xuan Z, Zhang MQ, Hannon GJ (2002) The Argonaute family: tentacles that reach into RNAi, developmental control, stem cell maintenance, and tumorigenesis. Genes Dev 16:2733-2742

Chen CC, Simard MJ, Tabara H, Brownell DR, McCollough JA, Mello CC (2005) A member of the polymerase beta nucleotidyltransferase superfamily is required for RNA interference in C. elegans. Curr Biol 15:378-383

Cogoni C, Macino G (1999) Gene silencing in Neurospora crassa requires a protein homologous to RNA-dependent RNA polymerase. Nature 399:166-169

Cox DN, Chao A, Baker J, Chang L, Qiao D, Lin H (1998) A novel class of evolutionarily conserved genes defined by piwi are essential for stem cell self-renewal. Genes Dev 12:3715-3727

Dalmay T, Hamilton A, Rudd S, Angell S, Baulcombe DC (2000) An RNA-dependent RNA polymerase gene in Arabidopsis is required for posttranscriptional gene silencing mediated by a transgene but not by a virus. Cell 101:543-553

Deshpande T, Takagi T, Hao L, Buratowski S, Charbonneau H (1999) Human PIR1 of the protein-tyrosine phosphatase superfamily has RNA 5 -triphosphatase and diphosphatase activities. J Biol Chem 274:16590-16594

Domeier ME, Morse DP, Knight SW, Portereiko M, Bass BL, Mango SE (2000) A link between RNA interference and nonsense-mediated decay in Caenorhabditis elegans. Science 289:1928-1931

Duchaine TF, Wohlschlegel JA, Kennedy S, Bei Y, Conte D Jr, Pang K, Brownell DR, Harding S, Mitani S, Ruvkun G, et al (2006) Functional proteomics reveals the biochemical niche of C. elegans DCR-1 in multiple small-RNA-mediated pathways. Cell 124:343-354

Feinberg EH, Hunter CP (2003) Transport of dsRNA into cells by the transmembrane protein SID-1. Science 301:1545-1547

Fire A, Xu S, Montgomery MK, Kostas SA, Driver SE, Mello CC (1998) Potent and specific genetic interference by double-stranded RNA in Caenorhabditis elegans. Nature 391:806-811

Grishok A, Tabara H, Mello CC (2000) Genetic requirements for inheritance of RNAi in C. elegans. Science 287:2494-2497

Grishok A, Pasquinelli AE, Conte D, Li N, Parrish S, Ha I, Baillie DL, Fire A, Ruvkun G, Mello CC (2001) Genes and mechanisms related to RNA interference regulate expression of the small temporal RNAs that control C. elegans developmental timing. Cell 106:23-34

Grishok A, Sinskey JL, Sharp PA (2005) Transcriptional silencing of a transgene by RNAi in the soma of C. elegans. Genes Dev 19:683-696

Guo S, Kemphues KJ (1995) par-1, a gene required for establishing polarity in C. elegans embryos, encodes a putative Ser/Thr kinase that is asymmetrically distributed. Cell 81:611-620

Hammond SM, Bernstein E, Beach D, Hannon GJ (2000) An RNA-directed nuclease mediates post-transcriptional gene silencing in Drosophila cells. Nature 404:293-296

Hammond SM, Boettcher S, Caudy AA, Kobayashi R, Hannon GJ (2001) Argonaute2, a link between genetic and biochemical analyses of RNAi. Science 293:1146-1150

Hutvágner G, Simard MJ, Mello CC, Zamore PD (2004) Sequence-specific inhibition of small RNA function. PLoS Biol 2:E98

Kennedy S, Wang D, Ruvkun G (2004) A conserved siRNA-degrading RNase negatively regulates RNA interference in C. elegans. Nature 427:645-649

Ketting RF, Plasterk RH (2000) A genetic link between co-suppression and RNA interference in C. elegans. Nature 404:296-298

Ketting RF, Haverkamp TH, van Luenen HG, Plasterk RH (1999) Mut-7 of C. elegans, required for transposon silencing and RNA interference, is a homolog of Werner syndrome helicase and RNaseD. Cell 99:133-141

Knight SW, Bass BL (2001) A role for the RNase III enzyme DCR-1 in RNA interference and germ line development in Caenorhabditis elegans. Science 293:2269-2271

Lagos-Quintana M, Rauhut R, Lendeckel W, Tuschl T (2001) Identification of novel genes coding for small expressed RNAs. Science 294:853-858

Lau NC, Lim LP, Weinstein EG, Bartel DP (2001) An abundant class of tiny RNAs with probable regulatory roles in Caenorhabditis elegans. Science 294:858-862

Lee RC, Ambros V (2001) An extensive class of small RNAs in Caenorhabditis elegans. Science 294:862-864

Lee RC, Feinbaum RL, Ambros V (1993) The C. elegans heterochronic gene lin-4 encodes small RNAs with antisense complementarity to lin-14. Cell 75:843-854

Lee RC, Hammell CM, Ambros V (2006) Interacting endogenous and exogenous RNAi pathways in Caenorhabditis elegans. Rna 12:589-597

Liu J, Carmell MA, Rivas FV, Marsden CG, Thomson JM, Song JJ, Hammond SM, Joshua-Tor L, Hannon GJ (2004) Argonaute2 is the catalytic engine of mammalian RNAi. Science 305:1437-1441

Lu R, Maduro M, Li F, Li HW, Broitman-Maduro G, Li WX, Ding SW (2005) Animal virus replication and RNAi-mediated antiviral silencing in Caenorhabditis elegans. Nature 436:1040-1043

Ma JB, Yuan YR, Meister G, Pei Y, Tuschl T, Patel DJ (2005) Structural basis for 5′-end-specific recognition of guide RNA by the A. fulgidus Piwi protein. Nature 434:666-670

Meister G, Landthaler M, Patkaniowska A, Dorsett Y, Teng G, Tuschl T (2004) Human Argonaute2 mediates RNA cleavage targeted by miRNAs and siRNAs. Mol Cell 15:185-197

Mourrain P, Beclin C, Elmayan T, Feuerbach F, Godon C, Morel JB, Jouette D, Lacombe AM, Nikic S, Picault N, et al (2000) Arabidopsis SGS2 and SGS3 genes are required for posttranscriptional gene silencing and natural virus resistance. Cell 101:533-542

Okamura K, Ishizuka A, Siomi H, Siomi MC (2004) Distinct roles for Argonaute proteins in small RNA-directed RNA cleavage pathways. Genes Dev 18:1655-1666

Pak J, Fire A (2007) Distinct populations of primary and secondary effectors during RNAi in C. elegans. Science 315:241-244

Parker JS, Roe SM, Barford D (2005) Structural insights into mRNA recognition from a PIWI domain-siRNA guide complex. Nature 434:663-666

Parrish S, Fire A (2001) Distinct roles for RDE-1 and RDE-4 during RNA interference in Caenorhabditis elegans. Rna 7:1397-1402

Pasquinelli AE, Reinhart BJ, Slack F, Martindale MQ, Kuroda MI, Maller B, Hayward DC, Ball EE, Degnan B, Muller P, et al (2000) Conservation of the sequence and temporal expression of let-7 heterochronic regulatory RNA. Nature 408:86-89

Reinhart BJ, Slack FJ, Basson M, Pasquinelli AE, Bettinger JC, Rougvie AE, Horvitz HR, Ruvkun G (2000) The 21-nucleotide let-7 RNA regulates developmental timing in Caenorhabditis elegans. Nature 403:901-906

Rivas FV, Tolia NH, Song JJ, Aragon JP, Liu J, Hannon GJ, Joshua-Tor L (2005) Purified Argonaute2 and an siRNA form recombinant human RISC. Nat Struct Mol Biol 12:340-349

Rocheleau CE, Downs WD, Lin R, Wittmann C, Bei Y, Cha YH, Ali M, Priess JR, Mello CC (1997) Wnt signaling and an APC-related gene specify endoderm in early C. elegans embryos. Cell 90:707-716

Sijen T, Fleenor J, Simmer F, Thijssen KL, Parrish S, Timmons L, Plasterk RH, Fire A (2001) On the role of RNA amplification in dsRNA-triggered gene silencing. Cell 107:465-476

Sijen T, Steiner FA, Thijssen KL, Plasterk RH (2007) Secondary siRNAs result from unprimed RNA synthesis and form a distinct class. Science 315:244-247

Simmer F, Tijsterman M, Parrish S, Koushika SP, Nonet ML, Fire A, Ahringer J, Plasterk RH (2002) Loss of the putative RNA-directed RNA polymerase RRF-3 makes C. elegans hypersensitive to RNAi. Curr Biol 12:1317-1319

Smardon A, Spoerke JM, Stacey SC, Klein ME, Mackin N, Maine EM (2000) EGO-1 is related to RNA-directed RNA polymerase and functions in germ-line development and RNA interference in C. elegans. Curr Biol 10:169-178

Song JJ, Joshua-Tor L (2006) Argonaute and RNA-getting into the groove. Curr Opin Struct Biol 16:5-11

Song JJ, Smith SK, Hannon GJ, Joshua-Tor L (2004) Crystal structure of Argonaute and its implications for RISC slicer activity. Science 305:1434-1437

Tabara H, Sarkissian M, Kelly WG, Fleenor J, Grishok A, Timmons L, Fire A, Mello CC (1999) The rde-1 gene, RNA interference, and transposon silencing in C. elegans. Cell 99:123-132

Tabara H, Yigit E, Siomi H, Mello CC (2002) The dsRNA binding protein RDE-4 interacts with RDE-1, DCR-1, and a DExH-box helicase to direct RNAi in C. elegans. Cell 109:861-871

Tijsterman M, Ketting RF, Okihara KL, Sijen T, Plasterk RH (2002) RNA helicase MUT-14-dependent gene silencing triggered in C. elegans by short antisense RNAs. Science 295:694-697

Tolia NH, Joshua-Tor L (2007) Slicer and the argonautes. Nat Chem Biol 3:36-43

Vastenhouw NL, Plasterk RH (2004) RNAi protects the Caenorhabditis elegans germline against transposition. Trends Genet 20:314-319

Vastenhouw NL, Fischer SE, Robert VJ, Thijssen KL, Fraser AG, Kamath RS, Ahringer J, Plasterk RH (2003) A genome-wide screen identifies 27 genes involved in transposon silencing in C. elegans. Curr Biol 13:1311-1316

Vastenhouw NL, Brunschwig K, Okihara KL, Muller F, Tijsterman M, Plasterk RH (2006) Gene expression: long-term gene silencing by RNAi. Nature 442:882

Wilkins C, Dishongh R, Moore SC, Whitt MA, Chow M, Machaca K (2005) RNA interference is an antiviral defence mechanism in Caenorhabditis elegans. Nature 436:1044-1047

Winston WM, Molodowitch C, Hunter CP (2002) Systemic RNAi in C. elegans requires the putative transmembrane protein SID-1. Science 295:2456-2459

Yigit E, Batista PJ, Bei Y, Pang KM, Chen CC, Tolia NH, Joshua-Tor L, Mitani S, Simard MJ, Mello CC (2006) Analysis of the C. elegans Argonaute family reveals that distinct Argonautes act sequentially during RNAi. Cell 127:747-757

Yuan Y, Li DM, Sun H (1998) PIR1, a novel phosphatase that exhibits high affinity to RNA ribonucleoprotein complexes. J Biol Chem 273:20347-20353

Genetics and Biochemistry of RNAi in *Drosophila*

Harsh H. Kavi, Harvey Fernandez, Weiwu Xie, and James A. Birchler(✉)

Abstract RNA interference (RNAi) is the technique employing double-stranded RNA to target the destruction of homologous messenger RNAs. It has gained wide usage in genetics. While having the potential for many practical applications, it is a reflection of a much broader spectrum of small RNA-mediated processes in the cell. The RNAi machinery was originally perceived as a defense mechanism against viruses and transposons. While this is certainly

James A. Birchler
Division of Biological Sciences, University of Missouri, Tucker Hall,
Columbia, MO 65211, USA
BirchlerJ@Missouri.edu

P.J. Paddison and P.K. Vogt (eds.), *RNA Interference.*
Current Topics in Microbiology and Immunology 320.
© Springer-Verlag Berlin Heidelberg 2008

true, small RNAs have now been implicated in many other aspects of cell biology. Here we review the current knowledge of the biochemistry of RNAi in *Drosophila* and the involvement of small RNAs in RNAi, transposon silencing, virus defense, transgene silencing, pairing-sensitive silencing, telomere function, chromatin insulator activity, nucleolar stability, and heterochromatin formation.

The discovery of the role of RNA molecules in the degradation of mRNA transcripts leading to decreased gene expression resulted in a paradigm shift in the field of molecular biology. Transgene silencing was first discovered in plant cells (Matzke et al. 1989; van der Krol et al. 1990; Napoli et al. 1990) and can occur on both the transcriptional and posttranscriptional levels, but both involve short RNA moieties in their mechanism. RNA interference (RNAi) is a type of gene silencing mechanism in which a double-stranded RNA (dsRNA) molecule directs the specific degradation of the corresponding mRNA (target RNA). The technique of RNAi was first discovered in *Caenorhabditis elegans* in 1994 (Guo and Kemphues 1994). Later the active component was found to be a dsRNA (Fire et al. 1998). In subsequent years, it has been found to occur in diverse eukaryotes such as *Drosophila*, *Schizosaccharomyces pombe*, *Dictyostelium*, *Neurospora*, plants, mice, humans, and many other organisms (Baulcombe 2004; Hall et al. 2003; Kennerdell and Carthew 2000; Paddison et al. 2002). It is possible that RNAi is a reflection of a much broader spectrum of small RNA functions in the cell as described below.

It is believed that RNAi evolved as a means of protection against viruses and against aberrant transposition by transposable elements in the genome (Kalmykova et al. 2005; Sijen and Plasterk 2003). However recent discoveries of the involvement of small RNAs in many other processes might suggest that these defense mechanisms, while obviously important, might actually be derivative processes rather than evolutionarily basal in origin. The RNAi genes also play an important role in the maintenance of centromeric heterochromatin (Volpe et al. 2002; Pal-Bhadra et al. 2004b) and germline stem cell division (Kennerdell et al. 2002). As a technique, RNAi can also be used as a tool for gene silencing studies and for developing (potentially) therapeutic agents (Jacque et al. 2002).

The trigger for all RNAi-related mechanisms known to date is a dsRNA molecule. This molecule can be introduced artificially or synthesized endogenously, for example, from heterochromatic repeats. The most potent source of artificial dsRNA is a sequence of about 500–700 bp cloned as inverted repeats, which is transcribed to give hairpin-loop dsRNA (Hannon and Conklin 2004). This dsRNA is then cleaved by specialized enzymes and assembled into a multiprotein complex. This results in specific cleavage of the target mRNA by virtue of complementarity between the small RNA (from the trigger) and the target mRNA. A series of genetic, biochemical, and structural studies have identified the different components of the RNAi machinery in *Drosophila* and also elucidated many mechanistic steps as described below (Fig. 1).

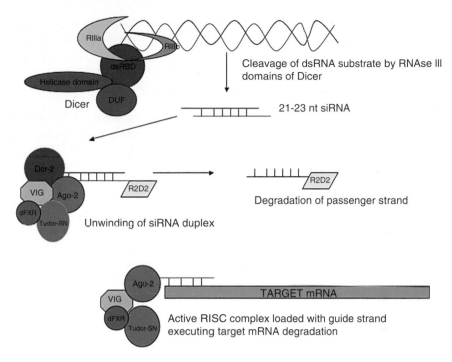

Fig. 1 Overview of the RNAi mechanism. The trigger for RNAi is the presence of a dsRNA molecule, which is cleaved by the ribonuclease enzyme Dicer. The cleavage is carried out by the two ribonuclease domains (RIIIa/RIIIb). The resulting duplex of 21- to 23-nt small interfering RNA (siRNA) is then loaded onto a multiprotein complex, RNAi-induced silencing complex (RISC). The RISC (80S) consists of Ago2, vasa intronic gene (*VIG*), dFXR1, and potentially other associated proteins and is loaded with the guide strand bearing complementarity with the target mRNA

1 Dicer: RNAi Initiation

Dicer is a ribonuclease III type of enzyme bearing characteristic structural features, which serves a crucial role in the RNAi mechanism (Bernstein et al. 2001). It acts upon the trigger dsRNA molecule to cleave it into small RNA molecules. The molecular weight of Dicer is predicted to be about 200 kDa. The structure of the human and *Drosophila* Dicer has been relatively well studied. Dicer orthologs and paralogs have been found in all organisms capable of performing RNAi; for example, *Drosophila* has two paralogs of Dicer, *dcr-1* and *dcr-2;* plants typically have four Dicer paralogs (*dcl-1*, *-2*, *-3*, and *-4*) while humans have only one Dicer gene (Zhang et al. 2002).

The common structural characteristics of all Dicer proteins studied to date includes a C-terminal dsRNA binding domain, two RNase III domains, a PAZ domain, a domain of unknown function (DUF-283), and an N-terminal DEXH-box helicase domain (Zhang et al. 2004). Dicer acts on dsRNA or aberrant RNAs arising from at least some of the highly repetitive regions of the genome, cleaves them into short RNAs of about 21–23 nucleotides (nt) in length, which then enter the RNAi pathway. Recent studies have implicated Dicer in the downstream steps after small interfering RNA (siRNA) production such as the RNAi-induced silencing complex (RISC) assembly, as discussed later.

X-ray structure studies of the human Dicer revealed some clues about the different structural domains present. It is proposed, based on these studies, that Dicer forms an intramolecular dimer such that the longer RIIIa domain and the smaller RIIIb domain come together to form a single catalytically active dsRNA processing center (Zhang et al. 2004). The RNase III domains in addition to being the catalytically active center also participate in various protein–protein interactions that are important for the overall efficiency of the RNAi process. The RNase III domains interact with the PIWI domains of the Argonaute (Ago) proteins (Tahbaz et al. 2004). The PAZ domain is involved in the recognition of 3′ overhang ends of the dsRNA substrate and, together with the RIIIa domain, is believed to be involved in determining the distance between the substrate terminus and the cleavage site. This in turn might be responsible for generating the characteristic length of 21–23 nt of siRNA. In a mutant with an absence of a dsRNA binding domain, Dicer is more dependant on dsRNA substrate molecules with overhangs at the terminal position. The wildtype enzyme cleaves both blunt and terminal overhang substrates with more or less equal efficiency. A study performed using human Dicer demonstrated that certain structural features of the dsRNA substrate significantly affects the catalytic efficiency (Vermeulen et al. 2005). The composition of nucleotide sequences at the 3′ overhang of substrate termini is important for the efficiency of Dicer action with certain combinations of nucleotides in the terminal positions being favored over the other. The length of the nucleotides at the 3′ end of the dsRNA substrate when increased beyond 3 nt significantly compromised the cleavage of the substrate by Dicer.

The *Drosophila* genome encodes two Dicer paralogs (Lee et al. 2004): (1) *dicer-1* is primarily involved in the biogenesis of microRNA (miRNA) (a class of regulatory small RNA molecules with important roles in development). *dcr-1* lacks the helicase domain and does not affect siRNA generation. (2) *dicer-2* is primarily involved in the generation of siRNA and lacks the PAZ domain. The *Drosophila* Dicer cleaves the dsRNA substrate from the termini in an ATP-dependent manner. Deletion of *dcr-2* does not affect miRNA biogenesis. It has been shown recently that *dcr-2* has an important role in RISC assembly and selection of bona fide siRNA. It is believed that the PAZ domain might have a potential role in miRNA biogenesis based on the fact that PAZ-less Dicers (for example, *dcr-2* and Dicer orthologs in *S. pombe*) cannot process miRNA.

In the case of flies, a second distinct type of ribonuclease III also exists known as Drosha, which is involved in the generation of precursor miRNA molecules (Han et al. 2004). R2D2 has been identified as a binding partner of Dicer-2 as discussed in Sect. 13. Dicer-1 has also been shown to bind to the dsRNA binding protein known as loquacious (loqs), which plays a role in germline stem cell development (Forstemann et al. 2005).

In addition to playing a vital role in the RNAi mechanism, Dicer has been involved in other important biological processes. For example, Dicer knockouts in vertebrate and mouse embryonic stem cells have a defective heterochromatin structure near the centromeres, in addition to the accumulation of aberrant transcripts from this region (Kanellopoulou et al. 2005). Dicer has also been shown to be involved in the intergenic transcription from the human beta-globin gene region (Haussecker and Proudfoot 2005).

2   siRNA: Structure and Its Impact on RNAi

Dicer acts on a dsRNA structure to produce siRNA, which is the hallmark of RNA-based silencing mechanisms. The structural integrity of the siRNA molecule is important for the efficiency of the RNAi process. The two strands of the siRNA duplex have different thermodynamic stabilities at their ends, a property that is exploited to identify the bona fide single strand of the siRNA. The unwinding of siRNA generates the "guide strand," which is incorporated into the RISC, and binds to the specific target mRNA by virtue of its sequence complementarity. The other strand of the duplex generated during unwinding is called the "passenger strand," which is eventually destroyed. Thus, the siRNA has to interact with a number of proteins involved in the RNAi machinery from its stage of generation to the final step of target mRNA recognition. It is therefore crucial that the siRNA has the favorable helical structure and functional groups not only to promote its incorporation into RISC but also enhance the entire RNAi mechanism.

The siRNAs generated in *Drosophila* are about 21–23 nt in length with a characteristic $5'$-PO_4 group and a $3'$-OH group with 2-nt overhangs at the $3'$ ends (Elbashir et al. 2001a, b). These functional groups are indicative of the ribonuclease III catalytic activity to which Dicer belongs. The sense strand of the siRNA duplex is relatively more tolerant to chemical modifications than the antisense strand. In addition, mutations in the central part of the sense strand and toward the $3'$ end (in an siRNA duplex) have a relatively severe effect on the RNAi efficiency compared to those mutations toward the $5'$ end of the sense strand (Amarzguioui et al. 2003).

This finding is in agreement with the antisense strand playing an important part in sense-target RNA degradation. The length of the overhangs at the $3'$ end also has a significant impact on the RNAi process, with an increase or decrease in the number of nucleotides at the $3'$ end decreasing the efficiency of the mechanism. Attempts to replace the $5'$-PO_4 with bulky groups such as $2'$-O-methyl groups result in a severely compromised ability of the siRNA duplex to initiate RNAi in vivo. This and several other observations have highlighted the importance of the $5'$-PO_4 group.

The presence of the $5'$-PO_4 group stabilizes the RISC and is important for RISC fidelity in determining the correct cleavage site on the target RNA. In the absence of the $5'$-PO_4 group, the siRNA slides along the RISC, providing alternative scissile phosphate groups on the target for cleavage (Rivas et al. 2005). An siRNA duplex lacking both or one $5'$-PO_4 group cannot initiate RNAi in vivo. This reflects the importance of the 5′-PO$_4$ group in the various protein–protein interactions taking place during RNAi machinery assembly. The presence of the 3′-OH group is important but not absolutely essential as mutations in this end are relatively well tolerated. In order to increase the effectiveness of siRNAs as a therapeutic tool, several attempts have been made to modify the sugar backbone to increase the in vivo stability of siRNA. These experiments revealed that the presence of the 2′-OH group of the sugar backbone can be replaced by 2′-fluoro phosphorothioate and 2′-O methyl groups to give nuclease resistant siRNA without drastically affecting their target RNA cleavage capability. However, complete substitution of the antisense strand or along the entire duplex with 2′-O-methyl groups entirely abolished the RNAi mechanism. In a recent study it was shown that substitution of the entire sense strand of a 20-bp blunt-ended siRNA duplex resulted in efficient target RNA cleavage (Kraynack and Baker 2005). These types of substitutions result in selective incorporation of the antisense strand in the RISC, thus curtailing off-target side effects arising while using siRNA. Similarly, replacement of the sugar backbone of the 5′ terminal nucleotide with 2′-deoxyribose sugar results in selective reduction of the entry of its cognate strand into RISC. These modifications of the functional groups are economical and should be addressed while using synthetic siRNAs for in vivo studies. It has also been shown that chemical modifications that distort the A-form of the helical structure between the siRNA and target RNA severely affect RNAi (Chiu and Rana 2003).

miRNAs are a unique type of small RNAs that perform a vital role during the development of an organism. Unlike siRNA, miRNAs are partially complementary to their message. They do not cleave their target molecules but rather suppress translation from the target mRNA. However, experiments have shown that an siRNA can function as a miRNA by translational repression if its sequence is partially complementary to the target mRNA (Doench et al. 2003). Thus, the degree of complementarity between the small RNA and its target mRNA decides whether the target is silenced by the miRNA or siRNA pathway.

3   Argonaute Proteins: Structure and Function

The Ago gene family is a conserved class of highly basic proteins found in all organisms with a functional RNA silencing machinery. Besides playing a role in RNA silencing they perform other vital biological functions such as germline stem cell development, nuclear division, and centromeric heterochromatin formation during early embryogenesis in *Drosophila* (Deshpande et al. 2005). Ago2-null mice are embryonic lethal, highlighting their biological role in development. Structural studies of Ago proteins, especially Ago2, have contributed to the unraveling of mechanistic steps involved in RNA silencing and a greater understanding of its biological role (Parker et al. 2005). The Ago proteins have a characteristic PAZ domain of about 130 amino acids and a C-terminal PIWI domain of about 300 amino acids. The PAZ domain is a RNA binding motif and plays a role in binding the 2-nt overhangs at the 3′ end of the single-stranded siRNA, while the C-terminal PIWI domain is involved in the interaction with the ribonuclease domain of the Dicer protein as well as in the binding of the 5′-PO$_4$ end of the single-stranded siRNA as revealed by the crystal structure of AGO2 from *Pyrococcus furiosus*. A major challenge in studying the crystal structure of Ago proteins from higher metazoan cells that exhibit RNA silencing is the availability and expression of large quantities of AGO proteins. Hence, structural biologists have resorted to the purification and characterization of AGO crystal structure from prokaryotes in which related proteins exist.

The role of Ago2 as the "catalytic engine" has been demonstrated by interpreting the crystal structure data from the human T-293 cell line (Liu et al. 2004). The important observation from this study was that the PAZ domain has conserved aromatic residues, which form the oligonucleotide binding fold, helping in binding the 3′ end of the siRNA. The PIWI domain has a structure similar to RNase H and binds the 5′-PO$_4$ group of the guide strand of the siRNA. The mutations of the residues in the PIWI domain (which are similar in the RNase H catalytic center) abolish the target cleavage ability, thus increasingly pointing toward Ago2 as the "slicer" in human cells. RNase H produces cleavage products with 5′-PO$_4$ and 3′-OH and also requires metal ions for its activity; these properties are shared by the RISC enzyme. The crystal structure of *Aquifex aeolicus* Ago2 identifies a highly basic pocket adjacent to the PIWI domain called the mid-domain (Ma et al. 2005). It was shown that the 5′-PO$_4$ end of guide siRNA is embedded in this pocket containing basic amino acids. An interesting feature of AGO proteins from prokaryotes is their affinity for single-stranded DNA (ssDNA) unlike their homologs in higher metazoan cells, which preferentially bind ssRNA. The crystal structure studies from these two prokaryotes further revealed a catalytic triad of the three amino acids Asp-Asp-His (DDH motif), which is involved in the cleavage of the target mRNA. In addition, human Ago2 (hAgo2) structure revealed the presence of a QH (Arg-His) catalytic motif. The amino acid replacements in either of these two domains to their corresponding residues found in hAgo1 or hAgo3 abolished the catalytic activity of the mutant Ago2. It is postulated that the characteristic "slicer" activity is not conditioned by hAgo1 or hAgo3 because they lack these DDH and QH domains.

4 *Drosophila* AGO Proteins: Unique Features and Crucial Role in RNAi

Biochemical and genetic studies performed in *Drosophila* have strongly implicated Dm*Ago2* to be involved in target mRNA degradation by the siRNA pathway (Okamura et al. 2004). The deletion of Dm*Ago2* had no effect on the miRNA-mediated gene-silencing pathway. The results also showed that deletion of Dm*Ago1* severely compromises the ability to perform translational repression of target genes via miRNA. The defects in the RNAi pathway exhibited by the Dm*Ago2* mutants were recapitulated by the *dcr-2* mutants, thus pointing toward the cooperation between Dm*Ago2* and *dcr-2*.

A series of biochemical experiments performed with *Drosophila* embryo lysates has generated a wealth of information about the RNAi mechanism in *Drosophila* and the crucial role played by DmAGO proteins (Matranga et al. 2005; Miyoshi et al. 2005). Peptide and nucleotide sequence analysis revealed that DmAgo1 closely resembles hAgo2. This comparison was further validated by biochemical experiments showing that DmAgo1 has the "slicer" activity by virtue of its association with the guide strand siRNA, thereby mediating cleavage of the target mRNA. In vitro studies using recombinant full-length DmAgo1 and its various truncated forms showed that the PAZ domain is dispensable for target cleavage, while the PIWI domain and the amino acids in the adjacent domain are the chief determinants of the "slicer" activity. It is entirely possible that, in vivo, the PAZ domain might be enhancing the RNAi mechanism by virtue of different protein–protein interactions. Thus, in *Drosophila* both AGO1 and AGO2 have the catalytic activity to cleave the target mRNA. It may be speculated that certain miRNA crucial to development are perfectly complementary to their targets. This in turn further explains the presence of the catalytic PIWI domain, which can cleave the target via the specific miRNA instead of translational suppression (as observed with imperfectly base paired miRNA).

These experiments unraveled a heretofore unknown step in the RNAi pathway, namely, the degradation of the "passenger strand" in the siRNA duplex. The study revealed that AGO2, by virtue of its catalytic activity, cleaves the passenger strand while still part of the siRNA duplex; this observation implicates AGO2 in the unwinding of the siRNA duplex. The passenger strand modified with 2′-*O*-methyl modifications (which makes it resistant to nucleases) abolished the RISC assembly. Thus, cleavage of the passenger strand by AGO2 is important for RISC assembly. This experiment also showed the presence of a new species of siRNA in the AGO2–RISC assembly: a double-stranded siRNA with a nick present on the passenger strand. *Ago2* mutants did not cleave the passenger strand, which further explains the importance of the passenger strand cleavage. In the case of miRNAs, which are not perfectly base-paired in the miRNA duplex, substitution of the passenger strand with nuclease-resistant functional groups (thus, the passenger strand is resistant to cleavage) did not have any significant effect on the RISC assembly. It is thus postulated that in the case of the miRNA passenger strand, which imperfectly binds to its natural guide strand because of the presence of imperfect complementarity between them, cleavage of the former does not take place. As a result, a "bypass mechanism" is accelerated that obviates the need for AGO2-mediated cleavage/unwinding of the miRNA duplex. Thus, unlike in plants and humans, in the case of *Drosophila*, both AGO1 and AGO2 have the catalytic centers to mediate target RNA cleavage via siRNA. The inability to cleave the passenger strand in the siRNA duplex might be another possible explanation for the lack of catalytic ability in hAgo1 and hAgo3, which can bind siRNA/miRNA, but cannot cleave the target RNA.

In the case of Arabidopsis, the "slicer" activity resides in AGO1, whose PIWI domain shows conserved acidic residues similar to the hAgo2 and RNase H catalytic fold (Baumberger and Baulcombe 2005). It seems from these biochemical data that distinct types of small RNAs associate with a unique Ago protein to be assembled in a distinct effector complex. These small RNAs in turn are processed by different Dicers. For example, in the case of plants, AGO4 associates with 24-nt siRNAs to bring about chromatin modifications. These 24-nt siRNA are processed by *DCR4*. On the other hand, AGO1 associates with miRNA and *trans*-acting siRNA (synthesized by *dcr1*). The "Dicer channeling hypothesis" is a possible explanation for these diversifications (Baumberger and Baulcombe 2005). This hypothesis is further bolstered by the involvement of Dicer in the RISC assembly and the interactions between the PAZ domain of AGO and the ribonuclease domain of Dicer.

The *Drosophila* genome encodes three additional Ago gene family members involved in RNAi. *piwi* and *aubergine* are important for oogenesis and germline stem cell differentiation (Kennerdell et al. 2002). Mutations in these two genes affect heterochromatin structure and certain aspects of the cosuppression mechanism in flies (Pal-Bhadra et al. 2002, 2004). *aubergine* affects siRNA-mediated homology-dependent gene silencing of the *Stellate* locus, which is important for maintenance of male fertility (Aravin et al. 2001). The *aub* mutants are also defective for RISC assembly, and hence its gene product is required for the formation of the active RISC as discussed in the following section. The role of DmAgo3 is involved with repeat-associated short interfering RNAs (rasiRNA) (Gunawardane et al. 2007) as are other family members in the RNA silencing mechanisms, which are as yet not fully understood.

5   RISC Assembly

RISC is a multiprotein complex reported to be in the range of 200 to 500 kDa. Several in vitro experiments have been performed using minimal RISC containing only the AGO "slicer" and the guide strand of siRNA; these complexes are in the range of 150 to 200 kDa. It is postulated that the various protein components found in vivo in the RISC might play an important role in assembly, target cleavage, formation of a distinct effector complex, or all of the above. Biochemical purification of the *Drosophila* embryonic lysate has led to the identification of the following components: (1) Ago2, (2) dFXR (*Drosophila* ortholog of fragile X mental retardation protein), (3) VIG (vasa intronic gene), (4) Tudor-SN (a nuclease with a tudor domain and bearing five nuclease domains homologous to the *Staphylococcus* nuclease domain), (5) R2D2 (a dsRNA binding protein with two dsRNA binding domains), (6) Aubergine (an Ago family protein), (7) Armitage–RNA helicase, and potentially other unidentified factors. RISC is an endonuclease as revealed by the biochemical characterization of its $5'$-PO_4 and $3'$-OH cleavage products, which are of equal length. Thus, RISC is a $5'$-phosphomonoester producing RNA endonuclease (Meister et al. 2004). RISC can cleave a target as small as 15 nt in length. Mutations or mismatches in the central part of the substrate that pairs with the 13-nt central part of the guide siRNA significantly compromises the target cleavage. RISC containing the 5'-PO$_4$ guide siRNA cleaves the target RNA at the 10th and 11th nucleotide across the guide siRNA measured from its 5'-PO$_4$ end. In other words, the cleavage site on the target RNA lies between the 11th and 12th nucleotide, where the 1st nucleotide on the target base pairs with the 21st nucleotide on the siRNA guide strand. RISC requires Mg^{2+} for its catalytic activity; addition of ethylenediaminetetraacetate (EDTA) reduces the target RNA cleavage (Schwarz et al. 2004).

It is believed that the two nonbridging oxygens of the scissile phosphodiester bond between the 11th and 12th nucleotide on the target RNA may be a ligand for Mg^{2+}. The substitution of the ribose sugar of the target (substrate) with bulky moieties such as 2'-O-methyl groups severely decreased the target cleavage; however, substitution of the ribose with 2'-deoxy modification did not affect target cleavage significantly. This result highlights the fact that the limiting step in the case of RISC is not the rate of chemical cleavage but rather steric hindrance, conformational transitions associated with active site residues, or both.

6   RISC Assembly Pathway and Target mRNA Cleavage

Recent biochemical experiments performed using *Drosophila* embryo extracts has indicated that the assembly of active siRNA loaded RISC takes place in a step-wise manner (Fig. 2). During these steps many different proteins together with the thermodynamic properties of the siRNA duplex play a crucial role in the selection of bona fide siRNA "guide strand," which enters the RISC. The siRNA duplex, which has been synthesized chemically, has different thermodynamic stabilities at either end. The concerted action of Dcr2–R2D2 ensures that the strand whose 5' end is near the relatively thermodynamically unstable end of the siRNA duplex enters the RISC (Tomari et al. 2004b). R2D2 binds to the 5' end of the strand, which lies near the more thermodynamically stable end; this strand is referred to as the "passenger strand." As discussed previously, this strand is then cleaved by Ago2 and finally discarded. Dcr-2 by virtue of its PAZ domain and dsRNA binding domain remains associated with the stable end at its 3' end. This strand is known as the "passenger strand."

This experiment revealed a dual role for Dicer wherein it generates siRNA as well as delivers it to the RISC, thus stabilizing the siRNA bound to RISC. This action is consistent with the view that *dcr-2*-null embryos do not show significant RNAi when injected with siRNA duplex, suggesting a downstream role for Dicer in effective channeling of an siRNA to the RISC. Similarly, *r2d2* mutant embryos show defective RNAi and fail to develop normally (Liu et al. 2003). In the case of siRNA generated in vivo the rules of thermodynamic asymmetry might conflict with the direction of dsRNA processing by Dicer, i.e., the thermodynamically stable end might be nearest to the dsRNA binding domain of Dicer (3'-end of this stable end is bound to the PAZ domain of Dicer); hence it should enter RISC. However,

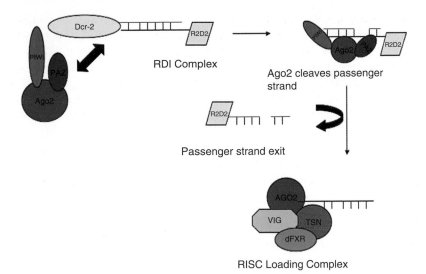

RDI Complex

Ago2 cleaves passenger strand

Passenger strand exit

RISC Loading Complex

Fig. 2 RISC loading complex. The asymmetric siRNA molecule is bound by Dcr2 and R2D2, which sense the thermodynamic stability at both ends of the siRNA duplex (see text for details). This initial complex is known as R2D2–Dcr2 initiator complex (RDI)/R1 complex. Dcr2 is eventually exchanged with Ago2, which by virtue of its PIWI domain cleaves the passenger strand. This results in the formation of an active RISC loading complex (RLC)/complex A. The RLC bears the guide strand and cleaves the complementary target mRNA presumably due to the endonucleolytic property of the Ago2 PIWI domain (see text for details)

if it does, then it violates the rule of thermodynamic asymmetry, which favors the entry of the unstable end.

The first step in the RISC assembly is the binding of the R2D2–Dicer-2 heterodimer to the siRNA duplex. This complex is now known as RDI (R2D2–Dicer-2 initiator) complex (also known as R1). Both proteins are required for loading siRNA into RISC and both dsRNA binding domains of R2D2 are required (Liu et al. 2006). Recent in vitro experiments with *Drosophila* embryo extracts showed that when the recombinant RDI complex is subjected to pulse-chase with wildtype extract, it alone can initiate the formation of holo-RISC (active RISC) (Pham and Sontheimer 2005). The formation of this complex is ATP independent. It has been shown that two transient complexes, i.e., complex B and the R2 complex, also exist as a precursors to the holo-RISC formation (Pham et al. 2004; Sontheimer 2005; Sontheimer and Carthew 2004). Recent evidence indicates that the R2 complex is similar to another complex known as the RLC (RISC loading complex). In the RLC, siRNA is unwound with the help of AGO2, which cleaves the passenger strand bound by R2D2 and is thus discarded. *ago2* mutants are defective in RISC assembly and cannot initiate transition from R2/RLC to the holo-RISC complex similar to *aubergine* and *armitage* mutants (Tomari et al. 2004a). This paves the way for the guide strand entry into the holo-RISC. This holo-RISC, in addition to the siRNA, contains other additional proteins such as Tudor-SN, dFXR, etc., which presumably aid in the formation of holo-RISC (Ishizuka et al. 2002). The catalytic activity of the RNAi machinery resides in this 80S holo-RISC. This study further revealed the importance of the $5'$-PO_4 group, which needs to be present on both strands of the siRNA duplex. Absence of both $5'$-PO_4 results in failure of the duplex to initiate RNAi, while presence of one of the groups can initiate the formation of early complexes such as RDI and R2 but not holo-RISC. It is believed that $5'$-PO_4 groups are recognized at multiple steps in the RISC assembly. The siRNA duplex containing only one $5'$-PO_4 is required for the recognition by R2D2; this explains the formation of the RDI complex with the use of these duplexes. However, the second $5'$-PO_4 might be required for the recognition by AGO2 based upon its role in unwinding the siRNA duplex and crystal structure data, indicating that the PIWI domain of AGO2 binds $5'$-PO_4. As discussed earlier, mutations in the PIWI domain residues abolish the catalytic activity of AGO2. The $2'$-hydroxyl group (of the ribose sugar) of the $5'$-terminal nucleotide, when substituted with a $2'$-deoxyribose, results in selective entry of this modified strand into RISC. It is possible that this modified strand has less affinity for R2D2 or more affinity for some other downstream components, which result in its selective incorporation into the RISC, resulting in degradation of the cognate strand in the siRNA duplex.

This modification can be used to reduce off-target silencing effects for gene silencing studies using artificial siRNA. The active RISC is directed to its target RNA via the guide strand, which then results in selective degradation of the target mediated by Ago2. The specificity is conferred by the guide siRNA, which is complementary to the target. The accessibility of the target is important for efficient cleavage because target RNA adopting a complex secondary/hairpin structure hinders cleavage by RISC.

The site of target mRNA is believed generally to be in the cytoplasm. However, there are some reports that RNAi can occur in the nucleus. Studies performed with mammalian and HeLa cell lines indicate that P bodies/GW bodies are the sites of target mRNA degradation (Coller and Parker 2004). This observation fits well with earlier reports showing that P bodies (GW bodies) are enriched with decapping enzymes, proteins involved with degradation of mRNA and translation inhibitory proteins. Green fluorescent protein (GFP)-labeled Ago2 proteins were shown to be colocalized with GW182 (RNA binding protein in P/GW bodies). Disruption of GW182 protein resulted in ablation of GW bodies and inhibition of RNAi. It was also shown that transfected siRNA also localized to the GW bodies (Jakymiw et al. 2005). Similarly, mutations that affect only the translocation of Ago2 to the GW bodies resulted in inhibition of RNAi. It has been proposed that Ago2/RISC shuttles between cytoplasm and P bodies (Liu et al. 2005a; Liu et al. 2005b). At the same time there exists an equilibrium between proteins that promote translation and those that prevent it. Both these pools compete for binding to the mRNA. When the Ago2-RISC binds to their target mRNA, this equilibrium is shifted, and possibly this complex is now exported into the P bodies for degradation of the target mRNA.

7 Kinetics of RISC: Consolidating the Structural and Biochemical Data

The *Drosophila* RISC behaves as a classical Michaelis–Menten enzyme in the presence of ATP (Haley and Zamore 2004); ATP enhances multiple rounds of cleavage of the target substrate (multiple turnover reaction where target RNA was in excess). In conditions of excessive RISC enzyme (single turnover reaction), ATP does not have any significant impact on the rate of target cleavage. The nucleotides at the 5′ end of the guide siRNA contribute to the K_m of the RISC, i.e., affinity for binding to the target RNA and mutations in this region are tolerated to a lesser extent when compared to those in the 3′ end. The nucleotides in the center and the 3′ end determine the K_{cat} (catalytic efficiency) of the RISC and have a negligible role in binding to the target RNA molecule. The 3′ end is bound to the PAZ domain of AGO2 to prevent its binding to the target mRNA. The amount of energy required to bind this end of the siRNA to the target will be offset by the amount of energy spent in releasing the 3′ end of the siRNA from the PAZ domain. These energetics will naturally affect the catalytic efficiency more than the K_m of the enzyme. Thus, nucleotides at the 3′ end are important for target cleavage but not for binding of the target. It was also shown in these kinetic studies that the identity of the scissile phosphodiester bond, i.e., 11th and 12th nucleotides on the target mRNA, is possibly identified by a protein loaded on the siRNA during the RISC assembly.

In the case of *Drosophila*, unlike plants and worms, there is an absence of transitive silencing, namely, the extension of siRNA production beyond the targeted region. Also there is no evidence for systemic silencing, the spreading of silencing from cell to cell, in *Drosophila*. Zamore and co-workers note that siRNAs act as guides and not "primers," thus arguing against the prevalence of systemic silencing in *Drosophila* (Schwarz et al. 2002). Their argument is bolstered by the fact that the genome of *Drosophila* contains no ortholog of RNA-dependent RNA polymerase (RdRP). They also note that the 3′-OH group of the siRNA guide strand is not essential for RNAi, an observation that goes against the "primer" model, which would be required for systemic silencing. On the other hand, Patterson and his colleagues propose that siRNAs function as primers and not "guides," thus arguing in favor of the presence of systemic silencing in *Drosophila* (Lipardi et al. 2001). This group claims that the 3′-OH is essential for RNAi; RdRp uses this end for amplification of the siRNA strand thus amplifying the trigger. It may be possible that there can be some other molecule than RdRp that fosters systemic silencing.

Yet another interesting avenue that needs to be explored in more detail is the connection between different RNAi components and their possible role in chromatin modifications. A relationship between transgene silencing and poly(A) tail maintenance has been proposed (Siomi et al. 2005). It was observed that depletion of AGO2 but not AGO1 leads to stabilization of transgenes and shortening of poly(A) tails (Siomi et al. 2005). In the case of *Arabidopsis*, mutations in the *xrn4* gene resulted in enhanced RNAi. XRN4 is a decapping enzyme (5′-3′ exonuclease activity) whose depletion might be causing aberrant decapped transcripts to get accumulated, thus exposing them to the RNAi machinery for degradation (Gazzani et al. 2004). The relationship between RNAi and other cellular processes involved in transcription such as mRNA stability, poly(A) tail maintenance, and probably nonsense-mediated decay (NMD) pathways need to be explored in more detail.

8 Transcriptional Gene Silencing in Relation to the Polycomb Complex and RNAi

The origins of the study of RNA silencing trace to studies of transgene silencing in plant species (Matzke et al. 1989; Napoli et al. 1990; van der Krol et al. 1990). Multiple transgenes introduced into an individual would silence each other and the endogenous homologous locus. A related phenomenon was recognized in *Drosophila* during the study of *white-Alcohol dehydrogenase* (*w-Adh*) promoter–reporter constructs (Pal-Bhadra et al. 1997). This construct was produced to examine *trans*-acting modifiers of the *white* eye color gene (Rabinow et al. 1991). When present as a single copy, expression was good; but it decreased dramatically when each insertion was homozygous, exhibiting the phenomenon of pairing-sensitive silencing. The observation of note, however, was that as the copy number was increased in the genome, whether paired or not, the total expression of *Adh* messenger RNA was reduced with increasing dosage of the encoding transgene. Several lines of evidence indicated that the endogenous *Adh* gene was also included in the silencing pool. Numerous genetic modifier systems were tested for an effect on this phenomenon with the finding that Polycomb group (PcG) mutations would ameliorate the silencing. Indeed antibodies to PcG proteins were found to colocalize with the silenced transgenes, but not with single insertions with high expression.

Interestingly, when the *w-Adh* transgenes were crossed to the exact reciprocal transgene carrying the regulatory portion of the *Adh* gene and the structural part of the *white* (*Adh-w*), the latter was silenced despite the lack of direct homology between the two transgenes (Pal-Bhadra et al. 1999). This enigma was resolved when it was realized that the *w-Adh* transgene silenced the endogenous *Adh* gene, which must in turn transfer the silencing signal to *Adh-w* via the homologous regulatory regions. This scenario was shown to occur by deleting the endogenous *Adh* gene from the genome with the result that the silencing interaction was eliminated. However, the silencing could be re-established by introducing a full-length *Adh* transgene in the absence of the endogenous copy. When deletion constructs were then reintroduced into the genome, the 5′ enhancer sequences were found to be those that are required for the transfer of silencing to *Adh-w*. The target *Adh-w* transgene also accumulates the PC complex when silenced.

The involvement of the Polycomb complex implicated a transcriptional level silencing, which was confirmed by run-on transcription assays (Pal-Bhadra et al. 2002). In contrast, a dosage series from 1 to 10 copies of full-length *Adh* transgenes departs from linearity after 5 copies, and this silencing is posttranscriptional. The flies with the silenced copies accumulate siRNAs homologous to the *Adh* gene.

The reason why the two types of transgenes exhibit a difference in terms of transcriptional versus posttranscriptional silencing is unknown. Despite this difference, both types of silencing are reversed by mutations in the Ago family genes *piwi* (Pal-Bhadra et al. 2002) and *aubergine* (Birchler et al. 2003a). This finding indicated that the RNAi machinery was involved with both posttranscriptional and transcriptional silencing.

As noted above, the *w-Adh* transgene exhibits pairing-sensitive silencing. This phenomenon refers to the situation in which paired transgenes in *Drosophila*, which exhibits somatic pairing of homologs, have less expression than a single unpaired copy (Kassis et al. 1991). The first example involved an *engrailed-white* transgene. The *engrailed* sequences that mediate the pairing-sensitive silencing surround the Polycomb response element (PRE). To test for an involvement of the "RNAi" genes in pairing sensitive silencing, various mutations in the pathway were tested for an impact on *engrailed-white* pairing-sensitive silencing (Pal-Bhadra et al. 2004a). The *piwi* and *homeless* mutations caused an increase in the silencing of *engrailed-white* when two copies were paired, but had no impact on the expression of an unpaired copy. These results indicate that the RNAi genes affect the pairing-sensitive silencing process itself.

Indeed, it appears that the RNA silencing genes are involved in various aspects of pairing-sensitive silencing and long-range contacts exhibited by PREs. Bantignies et al. (2003) found that the *Fab-7* PRE from the bithorax complex (BX-C), which regulates expression of the homeotic gene *Abdominal-B* (*Abd-B*), affected interchromosomal interactions. Interestingly, these interactions were heritable from one generation to the next. Transgenes with a 3.6-kb *Fab-7* fragment inserted upstream of *lacZ* or *mini-white* reporters were used in their experiments. One insertion (Fab-X) was adjacent to and upstream of the *scalloped* (*sd*) wing morphology gene, which was silenced. This silencing was temperature sensitive and pairing sensitive, being present in almost all homozygous female flies grown at 29°C, while absent in heterozygous females or hemizygous males. Mutations in any one of the Polycomb group genes attenuated this silencing.

The repression of *sd* requires the endogenous *Fab-7* element. A transgenic line with a deletion of the endogenous *Fab-7* resulted in a restoration of eye color and a greatly suppressed *sd* mutant wing phenotype. The repression of *sd* expression was also shown to be present at all stages of development, exhibiting an increased effect as development progressed. Using FISH analysis of embryos, it was found that the chromosomal region with the transgenic *Fab-7* element displayed associations across the genome with the endogenous *Fab-7*. This association was dependent on the presence of both the transgene and the endogenous locus and was also dependent on the presence of a functional copy of the Polycomb-like gene (*Pcl*). Transcription of the transgene had no effect on this pairing, but the frequency of pairing increased as development proceeded. The associations of the endogenous *Fab-7* with different copies of the transgene occurred independently of location of the latter. The pairing of *Fab-7* elements was analyzed to determine which characteristics of the BX-C were necessary by deleting the endogenous element, which relieved the *sd* silencing. Its replacement with a second transgenic element re-establishes this silencing.

Previous work had demonstrated that *Fab-7* elements were epigenetically marked for both the silenced as well as the de-repressed states when transmitted through female meiosis. The de-repression of *mini-white* expression resulting from deletion of endogenous *Fab-7* (as noted above) was transmitted through meiosis for at least five generations when flies were maintained at 18°C. This de-repression was demonstrated to be reversible by transferring the flies to 29°C to lay eggs, which was done to boost PcG levels. This silencing was retained in subsequent generations upon return to 18°C. The same observations were reported when *sd* expression was analyzed. This meiotic inheritance of *sd* de-repression was concomitant with loss of long-range pairing of *Fab-7* elements, indicating that these interactions involving the PcG proteins are heritable through cell division.

In subsequent work, the role of the RNA silencing genes was investigated (Grimaud et al. 2006). The mutations *dcr-2*, *aub*, and *piwi* reverse silencing of the *mini-white* reporter gene in *Fab-7* homozygous flies, suggesting an involvement of RNA silencing processes. Indeed, the multiple transgene copies of *Fab-7* generate homologous 21- to 23-nt siRNAs. These small RNAs were reduced in quantity in the *piwi* and *dcr-2* mutants. Similarly, fluorescent in situ hybridization (FISH) experiments revealed that associations of Polycomb proteins with the transgenes was also diminished. However, loss of Polycomb proteins at the *Fab-7* transgene did not correlate with global loss of Polycomb binding at other endogenous loci. The experiments also revealed that RNA silencing participates in the maintenance of long-distance interactions between *Fab-7* sequences during development and that this role can be uncoupled from its function of PcG protein recruitment to *Fab-7*. The RNAi components, mainly *dcr-2* and *piwi*, colocalize with PcG nuclear bodies. The RNA silencing gene products are responsible for the contacts between the PREs of endogenous loci of homeobox genes such as the *Antennapedia* and *Bithorax-C* loci. The contacts between these loci were compromised in the *piwi* and *dcr-2* mutant backgrounds.

The collective studies indicate a role for the RNAi machinery in at least some aspects of Polycomb complex establishment on silenced elements. Their function for endogenous PC accumulation is less clear, but the nuclear interactions of endogenous genes are in fact affected by their mutation. Further work will be required to understand the role of small RNAs in Polycomb functions and intranuclear interactions.

9   RNAi and Transposable Element Expression

It has been recognized for some time that transposable elements (TEs) had to be silenced in order to prevent destruction of the host organism. However, the mechanism by which the repression of the elements is achieved by the host was largely unclear until the RNAi mechanism was recognized as a defense against parasitic sequences such as viruses and TEs. Evidence is accumulating that RNAi is generally involved in TE silencing in the *Drosophila* genome. First, elements with multiple copies existing in the genome, e.g., the non-long-term terminal repeat (non-LTR) retrotransposon I, are silenced by homology-dependent cosuppression. Second, mutations of the components of the RNA silencing pathway, namely *piwi, aubergine, homeless*, and others, have been shown to increase the transposition activity of many elements in the germline. Third, certain transposons are evidently involved in antisense RNA transcription, which consequently induces dsRNA and triggers small RNA generation and gene silencing. Lastly, comprehensive investigation of small RNAs in *Drosophila* cells detected siRNA or rasiRNA (repeat associated siRNA, 24–26 nt) corresponding to many known transposons, thus suggesting RNA-based mechanisms are commonly used for repressing transposition.

10 Cosuppression and I Factor Repression

The I factor was identified as the element responsible for one type of hybrid dysgenesis in *Drosophila melanogaster* (Picard 1976). Hybrid dysgenesis is a syndrome composed of high mutation rate, chromosomal abnormalities, and sterility in the offspring following hybridization between different strains. When the males of an I inducer strain, which contain potential active I factors, is crossed to females of a sensitive strain that is devoid of the element (the reactive strain), a burst of transposition of the element occurs in the daughters' ovaries, resulting in multiple new insertions of the I element and female sterility. However, in the reciprocal cross, sterility is usually not observed. Because the I factor in the inducer strain is inactivated, the inactive state was thought be able to pass from the eggs to the next generation but not through the sperm. In fact, this maternal effect can persist for generations, but will gradually decrease in the absence of the I factor in the genome. The element can also remain active in the dysgenic germline for a few generations until the number in a genome reaches 10–15 copies. This copy number threshold may trigger the inactivation of the element (reviewed by Bucheton et al. 2002).

Northern blot analysis detected full-length I transcription in the dysgenic female germline but not in other tissues, correlating to the tissue-specific high rate of transposition (Chaboissier et al. 1990). The 186-nt 5'-untranslated region (UTR) sequence is characterized as containing an internal RNA polymerase II (polII) promoter (McLean et al. 1993). When the sequence was fused to a chloramphenicol acetyltransferase (CAT) reporter, the reporter gene showed higher expression limited to the ovaries of the reactive strain, confirming the tissue-specific promoter function. The expression of this fusion was inhibited in an I strain (inducer), suggesting the promoter region could also mediate silencing of the I factor (McLean et al. 1993). Continued work demonstrated that increasing the copy number of the 5'-UTR—of which two or three tandem copies were fused to CAT and transformed into the I reactive strains—decreased CAT activity in the ovaries. Additionally, dysgenesis was decreased when the strains were crossed to an inducer male containing one copy of functional I factor. These data suggested the repression of the element is dependent on the copy number of the short 5′-UTR in the genome (Chaboissier et al. 1998).

Later it was found, however, that the copy number of a homologous sequence is responsible for the suppression effect and the 5′-UTR region is not particularly needed (Jensen et al. 1999a, b; Malinsky et al. 2000; Robin et al. 2003). When the heat shock promoter is used, the fragments of coding region can introduce repression of the element even with only one copy; the increased dosage strengthens the effect. The effect depends on the transcription of the transgenes, but not on the translated proteins because transgenes with frame-shifted or prematurely terminated reading frames were still effective (Jensen et al. 1999b). Different sequences from the I element are effective and the combinations were additive. Intriguingly, expression of the sense or the antisense fragments is equally efficient (Jensen et al. 1999a; Malinsky et al. 2000). Therefore, it is strongly implicated that a dsRNA and cosuppression-like mechanism are involved with the silencing of the I element.

A distinction between cosuppression and I element silencing is that the latter is maternal and long-term. Interestingly, the I repression caused by homologous transgenes driven by the heat shock promoter showed both effects (Jensen et al. 1999a). The repression effect is only transmitted maternally but lost upon one generation of paternal transmission. The long-term effect is also observed in this case. First, the repression is positively correlated with the generation number for which the transgene is present. With higher copy number of the transgenes, fewer generations are needed to reach a saturated repression. Second, the repression is observed after at least one generation of maternal transmission without the transgenes being present in the genome. A simple RNAi-based explanation for maternal effect would be the existence of siRNAs for the I factor, which would be transferred from the egg cytoplasm to the offspring but absent in the sperm. In this scenario, however, supporting evidence is needed to understand how the siRNA survives through generations without the source DNA. The involvement of RNAi is supported by the observation that *aubergine* and *homeless* were shown to be required, but siRNA of I has yet to be identified (Vagin et al. 2004).

11   Heterochromatin and P Element Control

The P element is a DNA transposon responsible for another type of hybrid dysgenesis (Bingham et al. 1981, 1982; Rubin et al. 1982). A regular P inducer strain (or P strain) contains 50–60 copies of the element, among which about one-third are functional (O'Hare et al. 1992). The proteins derived from the element-encoded transposases originating from alternative splicing or truncated copies are thought to inhibit transposition in somatic tissue (Rio et al. 1986; Black et al. 1987). In the germline, the P element can transpose in both sexes. Nevertheless, investigating how repression is established, maintained, and transmitted in a P strain appears more difficult than in an I strain in which a smaller copy number of transposons is involved. Fortunately, simplified P strains were isolated in which only one or two copies present in telomeric regions exhibited suppression of dysgenesis comparable to 20–30 copies scattered in euchromatin (Ronsseray et al. 1991; Simmons et al. 2004).

In the telomeric P strains, the elements are inserted to telomere associated sequences (TAS) repeats of the X chromosome (Ronsseray et al. 1996; Stuart et al. 2002). The *white* transgene inserted at the same region shows variegation, indicating these chromosomal domains are heterochromatic and the P elements tend to be silenced (Karpen and Spradling 1992). Expression analysis confirmed this expectation (Roche et al. 1995). HP1 is an essential component of heterochromatin and is required for variegation effects. Mutation of this gene impairs the silencing effect of the telomeric P strain (Ronsseray et al. 1996; Haley et al. 2005). This observation suggests the heterochromatic state is integral for the silencing.

The P element is also the most commonly used transgene vector in *Drosophila*. Transgenes carrying a reporter gene such as *lacZ*, driven by various promoters, can be silenced by regular or telomeric P strains (Lemaitre et al. 1993; Ronsseray et al. 2003). This phenomenon is referred to as the *trans*-silencing effect (TSE). When a transgene was inserted in the telomeric TAS repeats, TSE is observed for a euchromatic transgene with the same length of the 5′ P sequence and the same reporter gene despite different promoters and distances from the P sequences. TSE was demonstrated to be dependent on homology, with a minimal requirement either from the vector or the reporter gene itself, and characterized by a maternal effect (Ronsseray et al. 2003). The data imply that an RNA-mediated cosuppression is involved similar to the I factor silencing. Accordingly, expression of sense or antisense RNAs can lead to partial P repression (Simmons et al. 1996). The transgenes do not repress dysgenic sterility, but interestingly, combined with a natural regulatory P element, show the repression effect (Ronsseray et al. 1998). This observation might be explained by cosuppression in which two genes sharing no homology can be silenced via an intermediate that shares homology with both genes as described above (Pal-Bhadra et al. 1999). TSE can only be initiated by P itself or a P transgene in a telomeric or other heterochromatin-like region, implying its requirement of a heterochromatic state (Ronsseray et al. 2003).

The evidence that the germline RNAi component gene *aubergine* is essential for telomeric P repression (Reiss et al. 2004) suggests that RNA silencing is involved. The siRNA might be used for establishing the silenced state *in trans* to homologous euchromatic P element or transgenes; thus, silencing might occur transcriptionally via chromatin modifications. Nevertheless, how the heterochromatin state facilitates the production of homologous siRNA as well as the relationship of TSE to standard P element silencing under nondysgenic circumstances remains to be understood.

12   Hybrid Dysgenesis in *D. virilis*

In *D. virilis* an unusual form of hybrid dysgenesis occurs in that many types of transposable elements are mobilized in crosses between certain strains (Lozovskaya et al. 1990). The types of elements mobilized are both DNA and retroelements. One type of retroelement, Penelope, appears to play a critical role in the process. Blumenstiel and Hartl (2005) discovered siRNAs homologous to Penelope in the strain carrying this element, but not in the other strain involved with dysgenic crosses. During the process of dysgenesis, these siRNAs were diminished. Thus, it was postulated that the presence of the siRNAs could serve to repress the expression of Penelope in nondysgenic circumstances and that the maternal effect for repression of elements typical of dysgenesis might be mediated by siRNAs transmitted through the female germline. The role of the other mobilized elements and how specifically Penelope can trigger dysgenesis remain unknown. Recent studies in mice have identified a novel class of small RNAs known as *piwi* interacting RNAs (piRNAs), which are about 26–31 nt in length. The piRNAs interact with MIWI protein (mouse homolog of PIWI) and are believed to play an important role in spermatogenesis (Girard et al. 2006).

13   siRNAs Homologous to Transposable Elements and Viruses

Aravin et al. (2003) isolated and cloned small RNAs from *Drosophila* at different developmental stages and from testes. About one-third of the clones with sequences that were likely RNase III (for example, Dicer-1 and Dicer-2) cleavage products were homologous to repeat sequences including TEs, satellite and microsatellite DNA, and others. The cloned rasiRNAs from 38 different elements cover 40% of all known TEs in the genome. Among those, the most frequently present rasiRNAs were for roo, an LTR retrotransposon with the highest abundance in the genome (Kaminker et al. 2002). The data imply a general role for siRNA-based silencing in controlling expression and hence transposition. The rasiRNAs were largely 24–26 nt in length, implying that they may be used for transcriptional silencing rather than posttranscriptional silencing, which typically use RNAs 21–23 bp in length (Hamilton et al. 2002; Llave et al. 2002; Mette et al. 2002). P or I siRNAs were not found in the collection because the laboratory strain used did not contain these elements.

   This study also identified likely siRNAs to a virus—Drosophila C virus (DCV)—that commonly infects flies in nature and the laboratory. It causes no obvious symptoms but reduces lifespan (Aravin et al. 2003). Antiviral siRNAs were shown previously in S2 cultured cells challenged with flock house virus (FHV) (Li et al. 2002). FHV encodes a virulence gene, B2, that counteracts RNAi by binding dsRNA and blocking Dicer-mediated cleavage (Galiana-Arnoux et al. 2006). The production of the viral siRNA requires AGO2 (Li et al. 2002) as well as Dicer-2 (Galiana-Arnoux et al. 2006) function. B2 was shown to decrease the siRNA level. B2 can also suppress RNAi silencing in plants, indicating conserved RNAi mechanisms from plants to insects. Wang et al. (2006) and Galiana-Arnoux et al. (2006) demonstrated a role for RNAi in viral immunity in adult flies.

14   Germinal Versus Somatic Silencing

RNAi mutations will alter the expression of TE. For retrotransposons *mdg1*, *1731*, and the *F* element, the expression in the testes and ovaries was shown to be increased in the *homeless* mutants (Aravin et al. 2001). Subsequently, the results were confirmed by in situ hybridization—*homeless* and *piwi* caused accumulation of the LTR elements *mdg1*, *1731*, and *copia* transcripts in nurse cells of the ovaries but not in the oocyte (Kalmykova et al. 2005). On the other hand, in the developing oocyte, mutants of *aubergine*, *homeless*, *armitage*, and *vasa* increase the expression of the non-LTR *HeT-A* and I elements (Vagin et al. 2004). This study was the first to show that *vasa* is involved in controlling transposon expression. The *vasa* gene encodes an RNA helicase as do *homeless* and *armitage*. It is not known if this helicase could be an RNAi component, but its intron-encoded *VIG* (vasa intronic gene) has been demonstrated biochemically to be part of the RISC (Caudy et al. 2002, 2003). The *vasa* mutant remains intact for *VIG*.

Interestingly, in the conditions mentioned above, *copia* is only activated in the germline but not in somatic cells. It was shown that the *copia* LTR driven marker gene *lacZ* was usually repressed in germinal cells but activated when *piwi* and *homeless* functions were missing (Vagin et al. 2004; Kalmykova et al. 2005).

The rasiRNAs are primarily antisense to various transposons (Vagin et al. 2006). Their structure is such that they are unlikely to be formed by Dicer in that they lack $2'$ $3'$ hydroxyl termini, which are characteristic of siRNA and miRNAs. Also, they are 24–30 bp in length, which also is not characteristic of Dicer action. The germline appears to use this system for the regulation of transposons. The *piwi* and *aub* mutations eliminate the rasiRNA formation of the *Suppressor of Stellate*, whereas *Ago2*, which is primarily involved with siRNA formation, has no effect. Various transposons are upregulated in the germline in mutant backgrounds for *armi*, *aub*, *piwi*, and *hls*, but not in *loq*, *dcr-2*, *R2D2*, or *Ago2*. Interestingly, *dicer-1* mutations caused a downregulation of many transposon families in the germline. Because *dicer-1* is generally thought to be involved with miRNA formation, this finding raises the possibility of interactions among small RNA processing mechanisms.

In further studies, *homeless*, *armi*, *dfmr*, and *piwi* were examined in germline tissue for their effects on transposons (Klenow et al. 2007). Major effects were not found in somatic cells. In *hls* ovaries rasiRNAs were reduced. The rasiRNAs homologous to transposons were found to be mainly antisense for the roo transposon, but other sense and antisense small RNAs were present for copia and I elements. Only sense rasiRNAs were found for the telomeric Het-A. The mutations *hls* and *armi* changed the histone H3 methylation signature of the transposons to one that is more typical of actively transcribed genes.

The finding of these germline processes sparked an interest in the small RNAs that bind to the PIWI family proteins. PIWI-associated RNAs were cloned and sequenced (Saito et al. 2006). There were no miRNAs—but mainly rasiRNAs homologous to transposons—present. The PIWI protein was also demonstrated to have Slicer activity in this study with both rasiRNAs and siRNAs. Further studies of small RNAs bound to PIWI and AUB found that they were mostly antisense to transposons (Brennecke et al. 2007) whereas the otherwise less-characterized protein, AGO3, contains sense small RNAs homologous to transposons. Of the thousands of PIWI-associated small RNAs cloned and sequenced, most were found only once, indicating their diversity. A cluster of them is coincident with the *flamenco* locus, which had previously been shown to control the gypsy, Idefix, and ZAM transposons. The *flamenco* locus appears to consist of an array of transposons sequences that might be transcribed into a continuous RNA. Another cluster corresponded to the telomere-associated sequences on the X chromosome. When the *flamenco* mutation was present, there was a reduction in the PIWI-associated RNAs. Of the *flamenco* originating RNAs, 94% of them associated with PIWI. Apparently, the transcript of the *flamenco* locus is cleaved to small RNAs that can then act to target homologous transposon transcripts originating from any location in the genome. Disruption of the *flamenco* "locus" eliminates this control.

The PIWI, AUB, and AGO3 proteins form one clade of the AGO proteins, while AGO1 and AGO2 constitute the other. The PIWI protein is mainly nuclear and found in the germline, but also in the somatic cells of the ovary (Gunawardane et al. 2007; Brennecke et al. 2007). AUB and AGO3 are mainly cytoplasmic in their cellular localization (Gunawardane et al. 2007; Brennecke et al. 2007). The small RNAs found associated with AGO3 were mainly sense strands of transposons (Gunawardane et al. 2007; Brennecke et al. 2007). The small RNAs found with the PIWI clade proteins have complements with partners whose 5' end is 10 nt away (Gunawardane et al. 2007; Brennecke et al. 2007). AGO3- and AUB-associated RNAs have the best complementarity, with lesser amounts found between those RNAs associated with AGO3 and PIWI. These authors (Brennecke et al. 2007) thus propose that the AGO3 sense strands and AUB/PIWI antisense strands seek each other and cleave transcripts from active transposons. Transcripts from clusters of transposon sequences such as *flamenco* and RNA from transposons feed off of each other in the generation of small RNAs, presumably via a posttranscriptional mechanism, although this does not easily explain the chromatin changes found on transposons in germline tissue of *piwi* and *hls* mutants (Klenov et al. 2007).

Another gene found to affect transposon activity in the germline is *cutoff* (*cuff*) (Chen et al. 2007). The *cuff* mutation was first recognized as a female sterile that produced embryos with ventralization. The mutant germline deregulates the telomeric Het-A element 800-fold and the TART element 20-fold. The *cuff* mutants do not affect the rasiRNAs from the roo elements, so it is thought that *cuff* acts in later stages of silencing than the production of small RNAs.

Two other mutations found to upregulate HeT-A and TART, as well as the *Suppressor of Stellate* repeats, are the *zucchini* (*zuc*) and *squash* (*squ*) loci (Pane et al. 2007). The *zuc* mutants have a 1,000-fold upregulation of HeT-A and a 15-fold upregulation of TART. The *squ* mutants only upregulate HeT-A. The *zuc* gene encodes a phospholipase-D/nuclease family member and *squ* encodes a predicted RNase HII, whose family members degrade RNA in RNA–DNA hybrids. The products of both *zuc* and *squ* physically interact with Aub and are required for rasiRNA formation in the germline. An examination of the rasiRNAs for roo and Su(Stellate) in *zuc*, *aub*, and *hls* demonstrated their elimination. The *squ* mutation, however, reduced their quantities but did not eliminate them. Thus, Zuc might be a candidate nuclease for rasiRNA 3′ end formation and Aub might be responsible for producing rasiRNA 5′ ends. Because Squ does not eliminate rasiRNAs, it might act later in the silencing process.

In addition to transposons, satellite repeat clusters were examined for the impact of the RNAi genes on their expression in the germline (Usakin et al. 2007). A 359-bp tandem array of the 1.688 satellite is present on the X chromosome in the centromeric region. Other versions with a unit length of 260 and 361 bp are present in the heterochromatin of chromosome arm 2L. These repeats are transcribed in ovaries and testes. In mutant *hls* testes there was no effect, but an upregulation was found in mutant ovaries. For the satellite sequences, both sense and antisense siRNAs are found in contrast to the rasiRNAs for transposons described above. A greater occupancy of the transcription factor, TAF1, was found on the satellites in the mutant background, suggesting transcriptional level control.

The above studies of germline transposon control raise the question of how these elements are repressed in somatic tissues. It is known that many alleles of the *white* (*w*) eye-color gene have a variety of phenotypes due to transposable element insertions. By attempting to understand how the inserted TEs regulate the *w* phenotype, many modifier loci were found to affect this regulation. Some of the modifiers appear to regulate a wide range of the TE insertion alleles (Rabinow et al. 1993; Csink et al. 1994; Frolov and Birchler 1998). One of these genes, *Lip* (*Rm62*), is required for RNAi in S2 cells (Ishizuka et al. 2002). Further investigation of these genes may provide evidence that RNAi is also used for somatic TE silencing. Given that *aubergine* and *piwi* are predominantly expressed in the germline and the early embryo (Williams and Rubin 2002), different RNAi components for somatic tissues may be expected, although both *aubergine* and *piwi* exhibit mutant effects in somatic cells (Pal-Bhadra et al. 2002, 2004b; Birchler et al. 2003a; Haynes et al. 2006). It is currently unknown whether these effects are established in embryos and epigenetically maintained during development or whether an active somatic function is provided by these genes.

15　Length Maintenance of the Telomeres

HeT-A and *TART* are the non-LTR retrotransposons that comprise the *Drosophila* telomeres and are used for maintaining telomere length. By in situ hybridization, RNAi mutants were shown to increase the expression of both elements in the ovaries with different patterns: HeT-A is activated in oocyte and nurse cells, but TART transcription occurs substantially in the nurse cells at late stages (Savitsky et al. 2006). Northern analysis of siRNAs confirmed that those homologous to the elements are eliminated in the ovaries of flies in heteroallelic *homeless* mutants. Interestingly, dosage effects of the RNAi mutants (heterozygotes vs homozygotes) were detected and distinguish TART from HeT-A. To characterize the transposition of elements, attachment of the elements to a truncated X chromosome, which then stabilizes it, was significantly increased in the RNAi mutants. In the heterozygous mutants of *hls* and *aub*, TART is predominantly attached to the broken ends. On the other hand, in the homozygotes of *hls*, attachment of HeT-A is predominant over that of TART. Accordingly, TART transcripts and siRNA were shown to be at an intermediate level with one mutant allele of *hls*. HeT-A is only affected in the homozygous mutants.

16   Transposons Regulate Neighboring Genes by RNAi

Transcription originating from TE promoters may extend to a neighboring gene and cause RNAi silencing of this gene. This type of regulation was shown for the *Stellate (Ste)-Suppressor of Stellate [Su(Ste)]* interaction (Aravin et al. 2001). *Su(Ste)* is a male-specific gene located on the Y chromosome and comprises tandem repeats. Each *Su(Ste)* repeat is homologous to *Ste* with regions sharing 90% identity. *Ste* is located on the X chromosomes and is silenced in males by *Su(Ste)*. This downregulation is essential for male fertility (reviewed in Tulin et al. 1997). Sense and antisense RNA for *Su(Ste)* were shown to exist in the testes. The transcriptional initiation site of the antisense RNA was identified in a nearby copy of the transposon *hoppel* (also called *1360*). siRNA was detected matching the overlapping region of the sense and antisense RNAs. A reporter transgene *Ste-lacZ* with a *Ste* sequence as short as 134 bp was silenced in the testes by *Su(Ste)*. The *homeless* and *aubergine* mutations relieved the silencing of the transgene and *Ste* itself (Aravin et al. 2001). A recently identified gene, *loquacious (loqs)*, has also been implicated in this regulation. The *loqs* protein binds to Dicer-1 and has three dsRNA binding domains. It plays an important role in miRNA biogenesis (Forstemann et al. 2005).

17   RNAi Interactions with Heterochromatin,
    RNA Editing, and DNA Repair

The importance of RNAi to the formation and maintenance of heterochromatin was first discovered in fission yeast (Volpe et al. 2002). The deletion of the RNAi genes *argonaute*, *dicer*, and *RNA-dependent RNA polymerase* caused the de-repression of transgenes located at centromeres, which were otherwise silenced by the heterochromatic environment. Histone methylation patterns were also affected; methylation of histone 3 at lysine 9 (H3-mK9) is a heterochromatic marker, while H3-mK4 is preferentially associated with expressed genes. Both of these modifications were altered in the mutants. Wildtype cells have both modifications located at centromeric repeats; however, the mutants had an increase in H3-mK4 and a decrease in H3-mK9. This link between RNAi and heterochromatin was further validated by the report of isolation of siRNAs derived from centromeric repeats (Reinhart and Bartel 2002), including a specific repeat—the dh repeat—that Volpe et al. (2002) had shown to display increased transcription in the RNAi mutants. The mechanisms involving the interactions between the RNAi machinery and heterochromatin were further dissected with the discovery of a complex termed RNA-induced initiation of transcriptional gene silencing (RITS), which was shown to be required for heterochromatin formation (Verdel et al. 2004). RITS contained three proteins including *Ago1*, as well as siRNAs generated by Dicer, which were responsible for the localization of the complex to heterochromatic domains. It was later shown that Ago1 interacts with RNA polymerase II, and that mutation of this polymerase leads to loss of pericentric siRNAs, heterochromatic histone modifications, and transcriptional silencing (Kato et al. 2005; Schramke et al. 2005). These results illustrated the importance of transcription to heterochromatin modification.

The roles of the RNA silencing machinery in heterochromatin formation in *Drosophila* have not yet been elucidated to the same extent as fission yeast; however, some progress has been made (Fig. 3). Three genes involved in RNAi in *Drosophila*: *aubergine* (*aub*), *piwi*, and *homeless* (*hls*), and their effects on heterochromatin have been reported (Pal-Bhadra et al. 2004b). The expression of a transgene in pericentric heterochromatin on the fourth chromosome, which caused a variegated phenotype, was de-repressed in the mutants for these three genes. Similarly, tandem repeats of a *white* transgene causing variegated expression showed a suppression of silencing when mutants of *piwi* and *hls* were introduced.

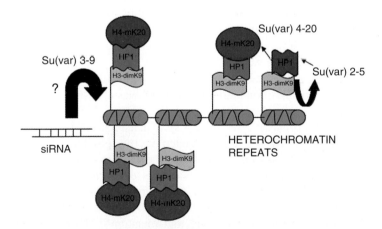

Fig. 3 RNAi-mediated heterochromatin assembly. The heterochromatin structure, such as that found near the centromeres, is composed of a large number of repeated sequences. It is postulated that transcription through these repeats results in production of aberrant RNAs that enter the RNAi machinery to produce siRNAs. The siRNAs might possibly recruit Su(var)3-9 (histone methyl transferase), which brings about H3-mK9 modification at the repeats. This particular histone modification then serves as a docking site for heterochromatin protein 1(HP1). This modification is followed by the activity of Su(var)4-20, which methylates H4 at K20. These modifications in turn maintain the compact structure at the heterochromatic repeats

In order to examine the effects of these RNAi mutations on heterochromatin structure, the staining of polytene chromosomes for heterochromatin protein 1 (HP1), and the chromatin modification with which it interacts, H3-mK9, were carried out. It was found that *hls* mutants had a partial redistribution of HP1, concurrent with a reduction in H3-mK9. There was also a partial loss of H3-mK9 in the *piwi* and *aub* mutants, although not as pronounced as in the *hls* mutant. These results suggested that the RNAi machinery is involved in the targeting of histone modifications and the associated gene silencing.

The RNAi gene *Ago2* was examined for its role in centromeric heterochromatin assembly and chromosome function (Deshpande et al. 2005) to determine whether its mutation has a detrimental effect on these processes as has been found in fission yeast (Volpe et al. 2002, 2003). Centromeric heterochromatin in *Drosophila* contains a centromere-specific histone called centromeric identifier (CID). Immunostaining for this protein was used to show that mutants of *Ago2* had weak staining for CID compared to wildtype and defective migration of chromosomes during anaphase, illustrating the importance of this RNAi protein in centromeric heterochromatin assembly and function. In the centric heterochromatin flanking the centromeres, there was abnormal staining of HP1 in the *Ago2* mutants compared to wildtype, as well as differences in H3-mK9 staining. It was also demonstrated that there was some suppression of variegated expression of transgenes inserted into the pericentric heterochromatin in the *Ago2* mutants.

The product of the *Lighten up* (*Lip*) gene is another example of a possible link between the RNAi apparatus and heterochromatin formation (Csink et al. 1994). When the *Lip* gene was mutated, there was an increase in the number of retrotransposon transcripts, as well as a suppression of position-effect variegation (PEV). The *Lip* gene (which is also called *Rm62* or *Dmp68*) was later shown to encode a dsRNA helicase that is present in a complex containing the *Drosophila* homolog of fragile X protein as well as AGO2 (Ishizuka et al. 2002). When the function of *Lip/Dmp68* gene was knocked down, there was an inhibition of RNAi of a GFP reporter. Furthermore, the complex containing Lip/Dmp68 was also shown to interact with Dicer.

A study of the formation and spreading of heterochromatin domains on the fourth chromosome of *Drosophila* implicated the transposable element *1360* as a determinant in this process (Sun et al. 2004). The *white* eye color gene was used as a reporter, and was inserted at many sites on the fourth chromosome, which contains interspersed heterochromatic and euchromatic regions. Through deletion mapping, it was deduced that proximity to the *1360* element determined whether there was silencing of the reporter, and that mutation of HP1 de-repressed this silencing. The *1360* element initiated the heterochromatic domains; they spread for approximately 10 kb. It was suggested that targeting of the heterochromatic regions was carried out by the RNAi apparatus.

In further studies of the impact of the *1360* element, Haynes et al. (2006) found siRNAs of both sense and antisense in the size range of 23 bp in length. Using Dicer-1 and Dicer-2 knockdowns in Kc tissue culture cells, *1360* is upregulated. A miniwhite reporter transgene was produced that contained a *1360* element that could be conditionally removed. Transgenes near heterochromatin exhibited silencing that was relieved by mutations in *piwi*, *aub*, and *hls*. Removal of the *1360* element from the transgene resulted in less silencing. However, the RNAi mutations still had an impact on the silencing mechanism even in the absence of the *1360* element.

Another protein that has been shown to have a role in heterochromatin function, which could involve the RNAi apparatus, is the multi-KH-domain protein DDP1 (Drosophila dodeca-satellite binding protein 1). The KH domain is a motif that allows single-stranded nucleic acid binding. DDP1 has been shown to bind single stranded nucleic acids, as well as colocalizing with HP1 to pericentric heterochromatin (Cortes et al. 1999). These authors proposed that the DNA binding activity of DDP1 combined with its association with HP1 might indicate its involvement in heterochromatin formation through binding at specific sites and recruiting additional proteins. Subsequent work by this group further characterized the functions of DDP1 by examining the effects of mutation of the *ddp1* gene (Huertas et al. 2004). Mutations in *ddp1* were suppressors of PEV, indicating a role in heterochromatin function, which was additionally supported by the observations that the mutants also had a strong reduction in H3-mK9 and HP1 deposition at the chromocenter of polytene chromosomes. These results, combined with the numerous roles that multi-KH-domain containing proteins have been shown to have in RNA-related processes (Kruse et al. 1998; Kruse et al. 2000; Li et al. 2003), were suggested by the authors as evidence for a role of DDP1 in mediating the RNA-directed formation of heterochromatin.

The proposal that DDP1 had a role in heterochromatin function in association with the RNAi machinery was supported by subsequent work conducted using the mammalian homolog of DDP1, vigilin (Wang et al. 2005). These authors found that the vigilin protein associated with proteins that bound to promiscuously edited dsRNA molecules catalyzed by adenosine deaminases (ADARs). ADARs convert adenosines to inosines through hydrolytic deamination (DeCerbo and Carmichael 2005). Since inosine is recognized by ribosomes as guanosine, only missense rather than nonsense codons are introduced. Site-specific editing by ADARs therefore results in alternate transcripts being generated that have functions in different metabolic processes (DeCerbo and Carmichael 2005). Another type of editing carried out by ADARs called hyper- or promiscuous editing involves perfect dsRNA duplexes of at least 25–30 bp, but preferably more than 100 bp in length, and of which up to 50% of the adenosines are edited. Their previous study had identified proteins binding to promiscuously edited RNA (I-RNA) (Zhang and Carmichael 2001); however, one protein was not identified, which was subsequently found to be vigilin (Wang et al. 2005). Once vigilin was discovered, they determined whether it acted similarly to DDP1 and showed that it also bound to heterochromatin similarly to DDP1. This binding of vigilin to both promiscuously edited RNA molecules as well as being involved in heterochromatin function highlights the interaction between the two processes of RNAi and RNA editing.

It had previously been shown that RNAi is affected by promiscuous editing in vitro (Scadden and Smith 2001), which is understandable considering the requirement for complementarity between the target and the "effector" RNA molecules. These authors used *Drosophila* cell extracts to demonstrate this antagonism between the two processes. These results were subsequently supported in vivo by Tonkin and colleagues studying *C. elegans* (Tonkin et al. 2002). They generated mutations for the two ADAR genes, *adr-1* and *adr-2*, that are present in this species, and showed that transgene expression was silenced in these animals, in contrast to wildtype. In the wildtype animals, formation of putative dsRNA, which would cause silencing, would be targeted for deamination by the ADARs, inhibiting this process; however, in the ADAR mutants this reaction would not occur. Tonkin and Bass later showed that an aberrant phenotype induced by mutation of the two ADAR genes was corrected by concomitant mutation of a gene involved in RNAi, illustrating the possibility that ADARs could regulate dsRNA molecules entering the RNAi pathway (Tonkin and Bass 2003). It was also shown that mammalian ADAR1 and -2 bind to siRNAs in vitro without editing them, and affect the ability of exogenously introduced siRNAs to reduce expression of target genes in cells through RNAi (Yang et al. 2005). While these studies illustrate the concept that each process can negatively regulate the other, the recent report that the RISC subunit Tudor can bind to hyper-edited dsRNA and facilitate its cleavage clouds this picture (Scadden 2005). It does, however, reinforce the idea that the two processes are linked.

To garner further information on how vigilin might work, Wang et al. (2005) sought to identify other proteins that might interact with it. One of the proteins that co-purified with vigilin from I-RNA affinity chromatography was found to be Ku86, which is a subunit of the DNA repair protein DNA-dependent protein kinase (DNA-PK). This finding was another example showing that DNA repair proteins are involved in heterochromatin function, and provides a link between RNAi and DNA repair. The DNA-PK protein is crucial for repair of DNA double strand breaks (Thacker and Zdzienicka 2004), and human Ku70, another subunit of DNA-PK, has been shown to interact with HP1 (Song et al. 2001).

Another example of a protein with dual functions in both DNA repair and heterochromatin formation is ataxia-telangiectasia mutated (ATM), a DNA damage sensor, which in mammalian cells is one of the kinases responsible for the phosphorylation-dependent activation of p53, a tumor suppressor central to the DNA damage response. The *Drosophila* ortholog dATM has also been shown to be involved in responding to DNA damage (Song et al. 2004). Furthermore, it has been demonstrated to be required for the correct localization of HP1 to telomeres (Oikemus et al. 2004). The silencing of a *white* reporter gene after placement near telomeric heterochromatin was partially alleviated in *atm* mutants. A protein complex called MRN (consisting of Mre11, Rad50, and Nbs1) has been shown to be required for ATM activation by DNA damage in mammalian cells (Uziel et al. 2003). When polytene chromosomes were immunostained for HP1 and heterochromatin protein 1/ORC-associated protein (HOAP) in *mre11* and *rad50* mutants, there was a large reduction in their localization to telomeres (Ciapponi et al. 2004).

The Parp [poly(ADP-ribose) polymerase] proteins 1 and 2 are both involved in the immediate response to DNA damage in mammalian cells (Ame et al. 2004). There is one *Parp* gene in *Drosophila*, which in addition to its role in DNA repair has been found to be necessary for the organization of heterochromatin structure, among other functions, during development (Tulin et al. 2002). The *Drosophila* ribosomal protein P0, which is an apurinic/apyrimidinic endonuclease with possible roles in DNA repair, was reported also to be a suppressor of PEV (Frolov and Birchler 1998). There are numerous other genes providing links between DNA repair and heterochromatin function, including (1) *BRU1* in *Arabidopsis* (Takeda et al. 2004) (2) *chromatin assembly factor (CAF-1)*, of which the protein product acts in concert with proliferating cell nuclear antigen (PCNA) in DNA repair (Green and Almouzni 2003) but also interacts with HP1 (Quivy et al. 2004) and (3) the *Mut-9* and *Mut-11* genes in *Chlamydomonas reinhardtii*, which are involved in transcriptional silencing but when mutated lead to increased DNA damage sensitivity (Jeong Br et al. 2002).

18 Role of RNAi Genes with Chromatin Insulators

Chromatin insulators act to separate euchromatin and heterochromatin as well as to block enhancer activity. The gypsy insulator is typically associated with proteins encoded by three genes, *Suppressor of Hairy wing*, *mod(mdg4)*, and *CP190*. Lei and Corces (2006) studied the association of proteins with the chromatin insulator component, CP190. An interacting protein was found to be *Lip*, whose association was RNA dependent. This finding initiated a study of RNAi genes on insulator function. *Lip* causes an improvement of insulator activity, while *piwi* and *aub* reduce insulator function. In multiple mutant combinations, *piwi* and *aub* were found to be epistatic to *Lip* for their impact on insulators. These findings suggest a role of small RNAs in insulator activity, although the nature of such RNAs has yet to be studied.

19 Stability of the Nucleolus

The nucleolus (NOR) is the site of ribosomal RNA (rDNA) synthesis in the nucleus. Several RNAi mutations (*dcr-2*, *Ago-2*, *aub*, *piwi*, *spn-E*) were found to cause multiple nucleoli (Peng and Karpen 2007) thus implicating the normal function as necessary for the proper organization of the NOR. The *dicer-2* mutation was found to reduce the H3-mK9 methyl marks in the rDNA. These initial results suggest a role of the RNAi genes in the normal establishment of the nucleolus.

20 Silencing Interactions with the MSL Complex

The male-specific lethal (MSL) complex is composed of a group of proteins and nontranslated RNAs that associate with many sites on the X-chromosome in male *Drosophila*. Among the proteins in this complex is a histone acetylase, MOF (males absent on the first), which has been shown to be able to target acetylation to a reporter gene in yeast causing increased expression (Akhtar and Becker 2000). The increased presence of MOF on the male X has therefore led to the proposal that the consequent increased acetylation on the X-chromosome causes dosage compensation. However, mutation of *mof* does not eliminate dosage compensation for the majority of genes tested (Bhadra et al. 1999; Pal-Bhadra et al. 2005). In addition, mutation studies on different components of the MSL complex demonstrated that the abnormal acetylation of autosomal genes by MOF due to a release from the X causes a concomitant increase in expression (Bhadra et al. 1999, 2000; Pal-Bhadra et al. 2005). These results, as well as the greater than twofold increase in expression of the MOF-targeted reporter in yeast (Akhtar and Becker 2000), suggest that the MSL complex has a counteractive effect on the hyperacetylation of the male X chromosome, so as to allow a twofold increase in expression to occur rather than an overexpression (Bhadra et al. 1999; Birchler et al. 2003b; Pal-Bhadra et al. 2005).

The genes for the two noncoding RNAs in the complex, *roX1* (RNA on the X chromosome) and *roX2* have been shown to attract the binding of the MSL complex, which then appears to spread into adjacent chromatin (Kelley et al. 1999). A *roX1* transgene with the *mini-white* gene was inserted into different autosomal locations and a number of transgenic lines showed sex-specific expression patterns of the reporter (Kelley and Kuroda 2003). In these lines *white* expression was absent in females; however, males showed expression patterns very similar to PEV, suggesting a spreading of the MSL complex in this sex to affect the silencing. This result suggests that in males the MSL complex is able to suppress the silencing, presumably itself a result of histone methylation that was conferred upon the reporter in females. The suppression of the silencing in males could be analogous to the proposed counteractive effect of histone acetylation of the complex on the male X chromosome. The mechanisms involved in this suppression of the effects of histone modifications are as yet unknown; however, it has recently been shown that the X chromosome of male flies is enriched for HP1, suggesting a possible interaction with the MSL complex (de Wit et al. 2005). A conditional depletion of HP1 levels results in a global increase in the histone modifications associated with active chromatin, illustrating the repressive effects of HP1 (Liu et al. 2005). Furthermore, the bloated X chromosome phenotype in mutants for *Su(var)3-7*, encoding a binding partner of HP1, was rescued in mutants for *maleless* (*mle*, a component of the MSL complex), suggesting an interaction of this repressive complex with the MSL complex (Spierer et al. 2005).

Another study by Zhang et al. (2006) also supports the possible interaction of the MSL complex with heterochromatin by examining the effects of the reduction of the levels of JIL-1 kinase, which has various roles in chromosome structure (Deng et al. 2005; Wang et al. 2001) as well as being enriched on the male X by the MSL complex. It was shown that *jil-1* mutants had an increased spreading of the heterochromatic markers HP1 and H3-mK9 (without a change in their overall levels), which provides further evidence for the proposition that the MSL complex is repressing the effects of the silent chromatin reported by Kelley and Kuroda (2003). These collective observations introduce the interesting scenario that HP1

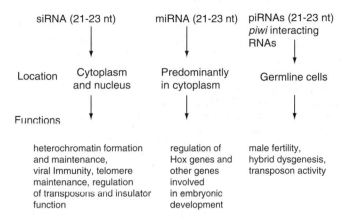

Fig. 4 Summary of RNAi functions in genome regulation

and its other binding partners might play a role in the proposed histone modification-associated repressive functions of the MSL complex; however, the precise mechanisms will require further study.

21 Concluding Remarks

The RNAi machinery likely plays a natural role as a defense mechanism against transposable element mobilization and virus infection. However, emerging data provide growing evidence that the RNAi genes are also involved in establishing chromosomal domains such as centric heterochromatin, telomeric heterochromatin, chromatin insulators, nucleolar stability, and long-range interactions among interstitial silenced loci (Fig. 4). The full spectrum of the roles of small RNAs and the RNA silencing machinery in the cell continues to unfold.

Acknowledgements Work on these topics has been supported in our laboratory by NSF grants MCB 0211376, MCB 0641204 and NIH grant R01 GM068042.

References

Akhtar A, Becker PB (2000) Activation of transcription through histone H4 acetylation by MOF, an acetyltransferase essential for dosage compensation in Drosophila. Mol Cell 5:367–375
Amarzguioui M, Holen T, Babaie E, Prydz H (2003) Tolerance for mutations and chemical modifications in a siRNA. Nucleic Acids Res 31:589–595
Ame JC, Spenlehauer C, de Murcia G (2004) The PARP superfamily. Bioessays 26:882–893

Aravin AA, Naumova NM, Tulin AV, Vagin VV, Rozovsky YM, Gvozdev VA (2001) Double-stranded RNA-mediated silencing of genomic tandem repeats and transposable elements in the D. melanogaster germline. Curr Biol 11:1017–1027

Aravin AA, Lagos-Quintana M, Yalcin A, Zavolan M, Marks D, Snyder B, Gaasterland T, Meyer J, Tuschl T (2003) The small RNA profile during Drosophila melanogaster development. Dev Cell 5:337–350

Bantignies F, Grimaud C, Lavrov S, Gabut M, Cavalli G (2003) Inheritance of Polycomb-dependent chromosomal interactions in Drosophila. Genes Dev 17:2406–2420

Baulcombe D (2004) RNA silencing in plants. Nature 431:356–363

Baumberger N, Baulcombe DC (2005) Arabidopsis Argonaute1 is an RNA Slicer that selectively recruits microRNAs and short interfering RNAs. Proc Natl Acad Sci USA 102:11928–11933

Bernstein E, Caudy AA, Hammond SM, Hannon GJ (2001) Role for a bidentate ribonuclease in the initiation step of RNA interference. Nature 409:363–366

Bhadra U, Pal-Bhadra M, Birchler JA (1999) Role of the male specific lethal (msl) genes in modifying the effects of sex chromosomal dosage in Drosophila. Genetics 152:249–268

Bhadra U, Pal-Bhadra M, Birchler JA (2000) Histone acetylation and gene expression analysis of sex lethal mutants in Drosophila. Genetics 155:753–763

Bingham PM, Levis R, Rubin GM (1981) Cloning of DNA sequences from the white locus of D. melanogaster by a novel and general method. Cell 25:693–704

Bingham PM, Kidwell MG, Rubin GM (1982) The molecular basis of P-M hybrid dysgenesis: the role of the P element, a P-strain-specific transposon family. Cell 29:995–1004

Birchler JA, Pal-Bhadra M, Bhadra U (2003a) Transgene cosuppression in animals. In: Hannon G (ed) RNAi: a guide to gene silencing. Cold Spring Harbor Press, Cold Spring Harbor, pp 23–42

Birchler JA, Pal-Bhadra M, Bhadra U (2003b) Dosage dependent gene regulation and the compensation of the X chromosome in Drosophila males. Genetica 117:179–190

Black DM, Jackson MS, Kidwell MG, Dover GA (1987) KP elements repress P-induced hybrid dysgenesis in Drosophila melanogaster. EMBO J 6:4125–4135

Blumenstiel JP, Hartl DL (2005) Evidence for maternally transmitted small interfering RNA in the repression of transposition in Drosophila virilis. Proc Natl Acad Sci USA 102:15965–15970

Brennecke J, Aravin AA, Stark A, Dus M, Kellis M, Sachidanandam R, Hannon GJ (2007) Discrete small RNA-generating loci as master regulators of transposon activity in Drosophila. Cell 128:1089–1103

Bucheton A, Busseau I, Teninges D (2002) I element in Drosophila melanogaster. In: Craig NL, Craigie R, Gellert M, Lambowitz AM (eds) Mobile DNA II. ASM Press, Washington DC, pp 796–812

Caudy AA, Myers M, Hannon GJ, Hammond SM (2002) Fragile X-related protein and VIG associate with the RNA interference machinery. Genes Dev 16:2491–2496

Caudy AA, Ketting RF, Hammond SM, Denli AM, Bathoorn AM, Tops BB, Silva JM, Myers MM, Hannon GJ, Plasterk RH (2003) A micrococcal nuclease homologue in RNAi effector complexes. Nature 425:411–414

Chaboissier MC, Busseau I, Prosser J, Finnegan DJ, Bucheton A (1990) Identification of a potential RNA intermediate for transposition of the LINE-like element I factor in Drosophila melanogaster. EMBO J 9:3557–3563

Chaboissier MC, Bucheton A, Finnegan DJ (1998) Copy number control of a transposable element, the I factor, a LINE-like element in Drosophila. Proc Natl Acad Sci USA 95:11781–11785

Chen Y, Pane A, Schupbach T (2007) Cutoff and aubergine mutations result in retrotransposon upregulation and checkpoint activation in Drosophila. Curr Biol 17:1–6

Chiu YL, Rana TM (2003) siRNA function in RNAi: a chemical modification analysis. RNA 9:1034–1048

Ciapponi L, Cenci G, Ducau J, Flores C, Johnson-Schlitz D, Gorski MM, Engels WR, Gatti M (2004) The Drosophila Mre11/Rad50 complex is required to prevent both telomeric fusion and chromosome breakage. Curr Biol 14:1360–1366

Coller J, Parker R (2004) Eukaryotic mRNA decapping. Annu Rev Biochem 73:861–890

Cortes A, Huertas D, Fanti L, Pimpinelli S, Marsellach FX, Pina B, Azorin F (1999) DDP1, a single-stranded nucleic acid-binding protein of Drosophila, associates with pericentric heterochromatin and is functionally homologous to the yeast Scp160p, which is involved in the control of cell ploidy. EMBO J 18:3820–3833

Csink AK, Linsk R, Birchler JA (1994) The Lighten up (Lip) gene of Drosophila melanogaster, a modifier of retroelement expression, position effect variegation and white locus insertion alleles. Genetics 138:153–163

de Wit E, Greil F, van Steensel B (2005) Genome-wide HP1 binding in Drosophila: developmental plasticity and genomic targeting signals. Genome Res 15:1265–1273

DeCerbo J, Carmichael GG (2005) Retention and repression: fates of hyperedited RNAs in the nucleus. Curr Opin Cell Biol 17:302–308

Deng H, Zhang W, Bao X, Martin JN, Girton J, Johansen J, Johansen KM (2005) The JIL-1 kinase regulates the structure of Drosophila polytene chromosomes. Chromosoma 114:173–182

Deshpande G, Calhoun G, Schedl P (2005) Drosophila argonaute-2 is required early in embryogenesis for the assembly of centric/centromeric heterochromatin, nuclear division, nuclear migration, and germ-cell formation. Genes Dev 19:1680–1685

Doench JG, Petersen CP, Sharp PA (2003) siRNAs can function as miRNAs. Genes Dev 17:438–442

Elbashir SM, Lendeckel W, Tuschl T (2001a) RNA interference is mediated by 21- and 22-nucleotide RNAs. Genes Dev 15:188–200

Elbashir SM, Martinez J, Patkaniowska A, Lendeckel W, Tuschl T (2001b) Functional anatomy of siRNAs for mediating efficient RNAi in Drosophila melanogaster embryo lysate. EMBO J 20:6877–6888

Fire A, Xu S, Montgomery MK, Kostas SA, Driver SE, Mello CC (1998) Potent and specific genetic interference by double-stranded RNA in Caenorhabditis elegans. Nature 391:806–811

Forstemann K, Tomari Y, Du T, Vagin VV, Denli AM, Bratu DP, Klattenhoff C, Theurkauf WE, Zamore PD (2005) Normal microRNA maturation and germ-line stem cell maintenance requires Loquacious, a double-stranded RNA-binding domain protein. PLoS Biol 3:e236

Frolov MV, Birchler JA (1998) Mutation in P0, a dual function ribosomal protein/apurinic/apyrimidinic endonuclease, modifies gene expression and position effect variegation in Drosophila. Genetics 150:1487–1495

Galiana-Arnoux D, Dostert C, Schneemann A, Hoffman JA, Imler JL (2006) Essential function in vivo for Dicer-2 in host defense against RNA viruses in Drosophila. Nat Immunol 7:590–597

Gazzani S, Lawrenson T, Woodward C, Headon D, Sablowski R (2004) A link between mRNA turnover and RNA interference in Arabidopsis. Science 306:1046–1048

Girard A, Sachidanandam R, Hannon GJ, Carmell M (2006) A germline-specific class of small RNAs binds mammalian Piwi proteins. Nature 442:199–202

Green CM, Almouzni G (2003) Local action of the chromatin assembly factor CAF-1 at sites of nucleotide excision repair in vivo. EMBO J 22:5163–5174

Grimaud C, Bantignies F, Pal-Bhadra M, Bhadra U, Cavalli G (2006) RNAi components are required for nuclear clustering of Polycomb Group Response Elements. Cell 124:957–971

Gunawardane LS, Saito K, Nishida KM, Miyoshi K, Kawamura Y, Nagami T, Siomi H, Siomi MC (2007) A slicer-mediated mechanisms for repeat-associated siRNA 5′ end formation in Drosophila. Science 315:1587–1590

Guo S, Kemphues KJ (1994) par-1, a gene required for establishing polarity in C. elegans embryos, encodes a putative Ser/Thr kinase that is asymmetrically distributed. Cell 81:611–620

Haley B, Zamore PD (2004) Kinetic analysis of the RNAi enzyme complex. Nat Struct Mol Biol 11:599–606

Haley KJ, Stuart JR, Raymond JD, Niemi JB, Simmons MJ (2005) Impairment of cytotype regulation of P-element activity in Drosophila melanogaster by mutations in the Su(var)205 gene. Genetics 171:583–595

Hall IM, Noma K, Grewal SI (2003) RNA interference machinery regulates chromosome dynamics during mitosis and meiosis in fission yeast. Proc Natl Acad Sci USA 100:193–198

Hamilton A, Voinnet O, Chappell L, Baulcombe D (2002) Two classes of short interfering RNA in RNA silencing. EMBO J 21:4671–4679

Han J, Lee Y, Yeom KH, Kim YK, Jin H, Kim VN (2004) The Drosha-DGCR8 complex in primary microRNA processing. Genes Dev 18:3016–3027

Hannon GJ, Conklin DS (2004) RNA interference by short hairpin RNAs expressed in vertebrate cells. Methods Mol Biol 257:255–266

Haussecker D, Proudfoot NJ (2005) Dicer-dependent turnover of intergenic transcripts from the human beta-globin gene cluster. Mol Cell Biol 25:9724–9733

Haynes KA, Caudy AA, Collins L, Elgin SCR (2006) Element 1360 and RNAi components contribute to HP1-dependent silencing of a pericentric reporter. Curr Biol 16:2222–2227

Huertas D, Cortes A, Casanova J, Azorin F (2004) Drosophila DDP1, a multi-KH-domain protein, contributes to centromeric silencing and chromosome segregation. Curr Biol 14:1611–1620

Ishizuka A, Siomi MC, Siomi H (2002) A Drosophila fragile X protein interacts with components of RNAi and ribosomal proteins. Genes Dev 16:2497–2508

Jacque JM, Triques K, Stevenson M (2002) Modulation of HIV-1 replication by RNA interference. Nature 418:435–438

Jakymiw A, Lian S, Eystathioy T, Li S, Satoh M, Hamel JC, Fritzler MJ, Chan EK (2005) Disruption of GW bodies impairs mammalian RNA interference. Nat Cell Biol 7:1167–1174

Jensen S, Gassama MP, Heidmann T (1999a) Cosuppression of I transposon activity in Drosophila by I-containing sense and antisense transgenes. Genetics 153:1767–1774

Jensen S, Gassama MP, Heidmann T (1999b) Taming of transposable elements by homology-dependent gene silencing. Nat Genet 21:209–212

Jeong Br BR, Wu-Scharf D, Zhang C, Cerutti H (2002) Suppressors of transcriptional transgenic silencing in Chlamydomonas are sensitive to DNA-damaging agents and reactivate transposable elements. Proc Natl Acad Sci USA 99:1076–1081

Kalmykova AI, Klenov MS, Gvozdev VA (2005) Argonaute protein PIWI controls mobilization of retrotransposons in the Drosophila male germline. Nucleic Acids Res 33:2052–2059

Kaminker JS, Bergman CM, Kronmiller B, Carlson J, Svirskas R, Patel S, Frise E, Wheeler DA, Lewis SE, Rubin GM, Ashburner M, Celniker SE (2002) The transposable elements of the Drosophila melanogaster euchromatin: a genomics perspective. Genome Biol 3: RESEARCH0084

Kanellopoulou C, Muljo SA, Kung AL, Ganesan S, Drapkin R, Jenuwein T, Livingston DM, Rajewsky K (2005) Dicer-deficient mouse embryonic stem cells are defective in differentiation and centromeric silencing. Genes Dev 19:489–501

Karpen GH, Spradling AC (1992) Analysis of subtelomeric heterochromatin in the Drosophila minichromosome Dp1187 by single P element insertional mutagenesis. Genetics 132:737–753

Kassis JA, VanSickle EP, Sensabaugh SM (1991) A fragment of engrailed regulatory DNA can mediate transvection of the white gene in Drosophila. Genetics 128:751–761

Kato H, Goto DB, Martienssen RA, Urano T, Furukawa K, Murakami Y (2005) RNA polymerase II is required for RNAi-dependent heterochromatin assembly. Science 309:467–469

Kelley RL, Kuroda MI (2003) The Drosophila roX1 RNA gene can overcome silent chromatin by recruiting the male-specific lethal dosage compensation complex. Genetics 164:565–574

Kelley RL, Meller VH, Gordadze PR, Roman G, Davis RL, Kuroda MI (1999) Epigenetic spreading of the Drosophila dosage compensation complex from roX RNA genes into flanking chromatin. Cell 98:513–522

Kennerdell JR, Carthew RW (2000) Heritable gene silencing in Drosophila using double-stranded RNA. Nat Biotechnol 18:896–898

Kennerdell JR, Yamaguchi S, Carthew RW (2002) RNAi is activated during Drosophila oocyte maturation in a manner dependent on aubergine and spindle-E. Genes Dev 16:1884–1889

Klenov MS, Lavrov SA, Stolyarenko AD, Ryazansky SS, Aravin AA, Tuschl T, Gvozdev VA (2007) Repeat-associated short interfering RNAs are involved in chromatin silencing of retrotransposons in the Drosophila melanogaster germline. Nucleic Acids Res Aug 15 [Epub ahead of print]

Kraynack BA, Baker BF (2005) Small interfering RNAs containing full 2′-O-methylribonucle-otide-modified sense strands display Argonaute2/eIF2C2-dependent activity. RNA 12:163–176

Kruse C, Grunweller A, Willkomm DK, Pfeiffer T, Hartmann RK, Muller PK (1998) tRNA is entrapped in similar, but distinct, nuclear and cytoplasmic ribonucleoprotein complexes, both of which contain vigilin and elongation factor 1 alpha. Biochem J 329:615–621

Kruse C, Willkomm DK, Grunweller A, Vollbrandt T, Sommer S, Busch S, Pfeiffer T, Brinkmann J, Hartmann RK, Muller PK (2000) Export and transport of tRNA are coupled to a multi-protein complex. Biochem J 346:107–115

Lee YS, Nakahara K, Pham JW, Kim K, He Z, Sontheimer EJ, Carthew RW (2004) Distinct roles for Drosophila Dicer-1 and Dicer-2 in the siRNA/miRNA silencing pathways. Cell 117:69–81

Lei EP, Corces VG (2006) RNA interference machinery influences the nuclear organization of a chromatin insulator. Nat Genet 38:936–941

Lemaitre B, Ronsseray S, Coen D (1993) Maternal repression of the P element promoter in the germline of Drosophila melanogaster: a model for the P cytotype. Genetics 135:149–160

Li AM, Watson A, Fridovich-Keil JL (2003) Scp160p associates with specific mRNAs in yeast. Nucleic Acids Res 31:1830–1837

Li H, Li WX, Ding SW (2002) Induction and suppression of RNA silencing by an animal virus. Science 296:1319–1321

Lipardi C, Wei Q, Paterson BM (2001) RNAi as random degradative PCR: siRNA primers convert mRNA into dsRNAs that are degraded to generate new siRNAs. Cell 107:297–307

Liu J, Carmell MA, Rivas FV, Marsden CG, Thomson JM, Song JJ, Hammond SM, Joshua-Tor L, Hannon GJ (2004) Argonaute2 is the catalytic engine of mammalian RNAi. Science 305:1437–1441

Liu J, Rivas FV, Wohlschlegel J, Yates JR 3rd, Parker R, Hannon GJ (2005a) A role for the P-body component GW182 in microRNA function. Nat Cell Biol 7:1161–1166

Liu J, Valencia-Sanchez MA, Hannon GJ, Parker R (2005b) MicroRNA-dependent localization of targeted mRNAs to mammalian P-bodies. Nat Cell Biol 7:719–723

Liu LP, Ni JQ, Shi YD, Oakeley EJ, Sun FL (2005) Sex-specific role of Drosophila melanogaster HP1 in regulating chromatin structure and gene transcription. Nat Genet 37:1361–1366

Liu Q, Rand TA, Kalidas S, Du F, Kim HE, Smith DP, Wang X (2003) R2D2, a bridge between the initiation and effector steps of the Drosophila RNAi pathway. Science 301:1921–1925

Liu X, Jiang F, Kalidas S, Smith D, Liu Q (2006) Dicer-2 and R2D2 coordinately bind siRNA to promote assembly of the siRISC complexes. RNA 12:1514–1520

Llave C, Kasschau KD, Rector MA, Carrington JC (2002) Endogenous and silencing-associated small RNAs in plants. Plant Cell 14:1605–1619

Lozovskaya ER, Scheinker VS, Evgenev MB (1990) A hybrid dysgeneis syndrome in Drosophila virilis. Genetics 126:619–623

Ma JB, Yuan YR, Meister G, Pei Y, Tuschl T, Patel DJ (2005) Structural basis for 5′-end-specific recognition of guide RNA by the A. fulgidus Piwi protein. Nature 434:666–670

Malinsky S, Bucheton A, Busseau I (2000) New insights on homology-dependent silencing of I factor activity by transgenes containing ORF1 in Drosophila melanogaster. Genetics 156:1147–1155

Matranga C, Tomari Y, Shin C, Bartel DP, Zamore PD (2005) Passenger-strand cleavage facilitates assembly of siRNA into Ago2-containing RNAi enzyme complexes. Cell 123:607–620

Matzke MA, Primig M, Trnovsky J, Matzke AJM (1989) Reversible methylation and inactivation of marker genes in sequentially transformed tobacco plants. EMBO J 8:643–649

McLean C, Bucheton A, Finnegan DJ (1993) The 5′ untranslated region of the I factor, a long interspersed nuclear element-like retrotransposon of Drosophila melanogaster, contains an internal promoter and sequences that regulate expression. Mol Cell Biol 13:1042–1050

Meister G, Landthaler M, Patkaniowska A, Dorsett Y, Teng G, Tuschl T (2004) Human Argonaute2 mediates RNA cleavage targeted by miRNAs and siRNAs. Mol Cell 15:185–197

Mette MF, van der Winden J, Matzke M, Matzke AJ (2002) Short RNAs can identify new candidate transposable element families in Arabidopsis. Plant Physiol 130:6–9

Miyoshi K, Tsukumo H, Nagami T, Siomi H, Siomi MC (2005) Slicer function of Drosophila Argonautes and its involvement in RISC formation. Genes Dev 19:2837–2848

Napoli C, Lemieux C, Jorgenson R (1990) Introduction of a chimeric chalcone synthase gene in Petunia results in reversible co-suppression of homologous genes in trans. Plant Cell 2:279–289

O'Hare K, Driver A, McGrath S, Johnson-Schiltz DM (1992) Distribution and structure of cloned P elements from the Drosophila melanogaster P strain pi2. Genet Res 60:33–41

Oikemus SR, McGinnis N, Queiroz-Machado J, Tukachinsky H, Takada S, Sunkel CE, Brodsky MH (2004) Drosophila atm/telomere fusion is required for telomeric localization of HP1 and telomere position effect. Genes Dev 18:1850–1861

Okamura K, Ishizuka A, Siomi H, Siomi MC (2004) Distinct roles for Argonaute proteins in small RNA-directed RNA cleavage pathways. Genes Dev 18:1655–1666

Paddison PJ, Caudy AA, Hannon GJ (2002) Stable suppression of gene expression by RNAi in mammalian cells. Proc Natl Acad Sci USA 99:1443–1448

Pal-Bhadra M, Bhadra U, Birchler JA (1997) Cosuppression in Drosophila: gene silencing of Alcohol dehydrogenase by white-Adh transgenes is Polycomb dependent. Cell 90:479–490

Pal-Bhadra M, Bhadra U, Birchler JA (1999) Cosuppression of nonhomologous transgenes in Drosophila involves mutually related endogenous sequences. Cell 99:35–46

Pal-Bhadra M, Bhadra U, Birchler JA (2002) RNAi related mechanisms affect both transcriptional and post-transcriptional transgene silencing in Drosophila. Mol Cell 9:315–327

Pal-Bhadra M, Bhadra U, Birchler JA (2004a) Interrelationship of RNA interference and transcriptional gene silencing in Drosophila. Cold Spring Harb Symp Quant Biol 69:433–438

Pal-Bhadra M, Leibovitch BA, Gandhi SG, Rao M, Bhadra U, Birchler JA, Elgin SC (2004b) Heterochromatic silencing and HP1 localization in Drosophila are dependent on the RNAi machinery. Science 303:669–672

Pal-Bhadra M, Bhadra U, Kundu J, Birchler JA (2005) Gene expression analysis of the function of the MSL complex in Drosophila. Genetics 169:2061–2074

Pane A, Wehr K, Schupbach T (2007) Zucchini and squash encode two putative nucleases required for rasiRNA production in the Drosophila germline. Dev Cell 12:851–862

Parker JS, Roe SM, Barford D (2005) Structural insights into mRNA recognition from a PIWI domain-siRNA guide complex. Nature 434:663–666

Peng JC, Karpen GH (2007) H3K9 methylation and RNA interference regulate nucleolar organization and repeated DNA stability. Nat Cell Biol 9:25–35

Pham JW, Sontheimer EJ (2005) Molecular requirements for RNA-induced silencing complex assembly in the Drosophila RNA interference pathway. J Biol Chem 280:39278–39283

Pham JW, Pellino JL, Lee YS, Carthew RW, Sontheimer EJ (2004) A Dicer-2-dependent 80s complex cleaves targeted mRNAs during RNAi in Drosophila. Cell 117:83–94

Picard G (1976) Non-Mendelian female sterility in Drosophila melanogaster: hereditary transmission of I factor. Genetics 83:107–123

Quivy JP, Roche D, Kirschner D, Tagami H, Nakatani Y, Almouzni G (2004) A CAF-1 dependent pool of HP1 during heterochromatin duplication. EMBO J 23:3516–3526

Rabinow L, Nguyen-Huynh A, Birchler JA (1991) A trans-acting regulatory gene that inversely affects the expression of the white, brown and scarlet loci in Drosophila melanogaster. Genetics 129:463–480

Rabinow L, Chiang SL, Birchler JA (1993) Mutations at the Darkener of apricot locus modulate transcript levels of copia and copia-induced mutations in Drosophila melanogaster. Genetics 134:1175–1185

Reinhart BJ, Bartel DP (2002) Small RNAs correspond to centromere heterochromatic repeats. Science 297:1831

Reiss D, Josse T, Anxolabehere D, Ronsseray S (2004) Aubergine mutations in Drosophila mela-nogaster impair P cytotype determination by telomeric P elements inserted in heterochromatin. Mol Genet Genomics 272:336–343

Rio DC, Laski FA, Rubin GM (1986) Identification and immunochemical analysis of biologically active Drosophila P element transposase. Cell 44:21–32

Rivas FV, Tolia NH, Song JJ, Aragon JP, Liu J, Hannon GJ, Joshua-Tor L (2005) Purified Argonaute2 and an siRNA form recombinant human RISC. Nat Struct Mol Biol 12:340–349

Robin S, Chambeyron S, Bucheton A, Busseau I (2003) Gene silencing triggered by non-LTR retrotransposons in the female germline of Drosophila melanogaster. Genetics 164:521–531

Roche SE, Schiff M, Rio DC (1995) P-element repressor autoregulation involves germ-line tran-scriptional repression and reduction of third intron splicing. Genes Dev 9:1278–1288

Ronsseray S, Lehmann M, Anxolabehere D (1991) The maternally inherited regulation of P ele-ments in Drosophila melanogaster can be elicited by two P copies at cytological site 1A on the X chromosome. Genetics 129:501–512

Ronsseray S, Lehmann M, Nouaud D, Anxolabehere D (1996) The regulatory properties of autonomous subtelomeric P elements are sensitive to a suppressor of variegation in Drosophila melanogaster. Genetics 143:1663–1674

Ronsseray S, Marin L, Lehmann M, Anxolabehere D (1998) Repression of hybrid dysgenesis in Drosophila melanogaster by combinations of telomeric P-element reporters and naturally occurring P elements. Genetics 149:1857–1866

Ronsseray S, Josse T, Boivin A, Anxolabehere D (2003) Telomeric transgenes and trans-silencing in Drosophila. Genetica 117:327–335

Rubin GM, Kidwell MG, Bingham PM (1982) The molecular basis of P-M hybrid dysgenesis: the nature of induced mutations. Cell 29:987–994

Saito K, Nishida KM, Mori T, Kawamura Y, Miyoshi K, Nagami T, Siomi H, Siomi MC (2006) Specific association of Piwi with rasiRNAs derived from retrotransposon and heterochromatic regions in the Drosophila genome. Genes Dev 20:2214–2222

Savitsky M, Kwon D, Georgiev P, Kalmykova A, Gvozdev V (2006) Telomere elongation is under the control of the RNAi-based mechanism in the Drosophila germline. Genes Dev 20:345–354

Scadden AD (2005) The RISC subunit Tudor-SN binds to hyper-edited double-stranded RNA and promotes its cleavage. Nat Struct Mol Biol 12:489–496

Scadden AD, Smith CW (2001) RNAi is antagonized by A I hyper-editing. EMBO Rep 2:1107–1111

Schramke V, Sheedy DM, Denli AM, Bonila C, Ekwall K, Hannon GJ, Allshire RC (2005) RNA-interference-directed chromatin modification coupled to RNA polymerase II transcription. Nature 435:1275–1279

Schwarz DS, Hutvagner G, Haley B, Zamore PD (2002) Evidence that siRNAs function as guides, not primers, in the Drosophila and human RNAi pathways. Mol Cell 10:537–548

Schwarz DS, Tomari Y, Zamore PD (2004) The RNA-induced silencing complex is a Mg^{2+}-dependent endonuclease. Curr Biol 14:787–791

Sijen T, Plasterk RH (2003) Transposon silencing in the Caenorhabditis elegans germ line by natural RNAi. Nature 426:310–314

Simmons MJ, Raymond JD, Grimes CD, Belinco C, Haake BC, Jordan M, Lund C, Ojala TA, Papermaster D (1996) Repression of hybrid dysgenesis in Drosophila melanogaster by heat-shock-inducible sense and antisense P-element constructs. Genetics 144:1529–1544

Simmons MJ, Raymond JD, Niemi JB, Stuart JR, Merriman PJ (2004) The P cytotype in Drosophila melanogaster: a maternally transmitted regulatory state of the germ line associated with telomeric P elements. Genetics 166:243–254

Siomi MC, Tsukumo H, Ishizuka A, Nagami T, Siomi H (2005) A potential link between transgene silencing and poly(A) tails. RNA 11:1004–1011

Song K, Jung Y, Jung D, Lee I (2001) Human Ku70 interacts with heterochromatin protein 1alpha. J Biol Chem 276:8321–8327

Song YH, Mirey G, Betson M, Haber DA, Settleman J (2004) The Drosophila ATM ortholog, dATM, mediates the response to ionizing radiation and to spontaneous DNA damage during development. Curr Biol 14:1354–1359

Sontheimer EJ (2005) Assembly and function of RNA silencing complexes. Nat Rev Mol Cell Biol 6:127–138

Sontheimer EJ, Carthew RW (2004) Molecular biology. Argonaute journeys into the heart of RISC. Science 305:1409–1410

Spierer A, Seum C, Delattre M, Spierer P (2005) Loss of the modifiers of variegation Su(var)3-7 or HP1 impacts male X polytene chromosome morphology and dosage compensation. J Cell Sci 118:5047–5057

Stuart JR, Haley KJ, Swedzinski D, Lockner S, Kocian PE, Merriman PJ, Simmons MJ (2002) Telomeric P elements associated with cytotype regulation of the P transposon family in Drosophila melanogaster. Genetics 162:1641–1654

Sun FL, Haynes K, Simpson CL, Lee SD, Collins L, Wuller J, Eissenberg JC, Elgin SCR (2004) cis-Acting determinants of heterochromatin formation on Drosophila melanogaster chromosome four. Mol Cell Biol 24:8210–8220

Tahbaz N, Kolb FA, Zhang H, Jaronczyk K, Filipowicz W, Hobman TC (2004) Characterization of the interactions between mammalian PAZ PIWI domain proteins and Dicer. EMBO Rep 5:189–194

Takeda S, Tadele Z, Hofmann I, Probst AV, Angelis KJ, Kaya H, Araki T, Mengiste T, Mittelsten Scheid O, Shibahara K, Scheel D, Paszkowski J (2004) BRU1, a novel link between responses to DNA damage and epigenetic gene silencing in Arabidopsis. Genes Dev 18:782–793

Thacker J, Zdzienicka MZ (2004) The XRCC genes: expanding roles in DNA double-strand break repair. DNA Repair (Amst) 3:1081–1090

Tomari Y, Du T, Haley B, Schwarz DS, Bennett R, Cook HA, Koppetsch BS, Theurkauf WE, Zamore PD (2004a) RISC assembly defects in the Drosophila RNAi mutant armitage. Cell 116:831–841

Tomari Y, Matranga C, Haley B, Martinez N, Zamore PD (2004b) A protein sensor for siRNA asymmetry. Science 306:1377–1380

Tonkin LA, Bass BL (2003) Mutations in RNAi rescue aberrant chemotaxis of ADAR mutants. Science 302:1725

Tonkin LA, Saccomanno L, Morse DP, Brodigan T, Krause M, Bass BL (2002) RNA editing by ADARs is important for normal behavior in Caenorhabditis elegans. EMBO J 21:6025–6035

Tulin A, Stewart D, Spradling AC (2002) The Drosophila heterochromatic gene encoding poly(ADP-ribose) polymerase (PARP) is required to modulate chromatin structure during development. Genes Dev 16:2108–2119

Tulin AV, Kogan GL, Filipp D, Balakireva MD, Gvozdev VA (1997) Heterochromatic Stellate gene cluster in Drosophila melanogaster: structure and molecular evolution. Genetics 146:253–262

Usakin L, Abad J, Vagin VV, de Pablos B, Villasante A, Gvozdov VA (2007) Transcription of the 1.688 satellite DNA family is under the control of RNA interference machinery in Drosophila melanogaster ovaries. Genetics 176:1343–1349

Uziel T, Lerenthal Y, Moyal L, Andegeko Y, Mittelman L, Shiloh Y (2003) Requirement of the MRN complex for ATM activation by DNA damage. EMBO J 22:5612–5621

Vagin VV, Klenov MS, Kalmykova AI, Stolyarenko AD, Kotelnikov RN, Gvozdev VA (2004) The RNA interference proteins and vasa locus are involved in the silencing of retrotransposons in the female germline of Drosophila melanogaster. RNA Biol 1:54–58

Vagin VV, Sigova A, Li C, Seitz H, Gvozdev V, Zamore P (2006) A distinct small RNA pathway silences selfish genetic elements in the germline. Science 313:320–324

van der Krol AR, Mur LA, Beld M, Mol JNM, Stuitje AR (1990) Flavonoid genes in Petunia: addition of a limited number of gene copies may lead to a suppression of gene expression. Plant Cell 2:291–299

Verdel A, Jia S, Gerber S, Sugiyama T, Gygi S, Grewal SI, Moazed D (2004) RNAi-mediated targeting of heterochromatin by the RITS complex. Science 303:672–676

Vermeulen A, Behlen L, Reynolds A, Wolfson A, Marshall WS, Karpilow J, Khvorova A (2005) The contributions of dsRNA structure to Dicer specificity and efficiency. RNA 11:674–682

Volpe T, Schramke V, Hamilton GL, White SA, Teng G, Martienssen RA, Allshire RC (2003) RNA interference is required for normal centromere function in fission yeast. Chromosome Res 11:137–146

Volpe TA, Kidner C, Hall IM, Teng G, Grewal SI, Martienssen RA (2002) Regulation of heterochromatic silencing and histone H3 lysine-9 methylation by RNAi. Science 297:1833–1837

Wang Q, Zhang Z, Blackwell K, Carmichael GG (2005) Vigilins bind to promiscuously A-to-I-edited RNAs and are involved in the formation of heterochromatin. Curr Biol 15:384–391

Wang XH, Aliyari R, Li WX, Li HW, Kim K, Carthew R, Atkinson P, Ding SW (2006) RNA interference directs innate immunity against viruses in adult *Drosophila*. Science 312:452–454

Wang Y, Zhang W, Jin Y, Johansen J, Johansen KM (2001) The JIL-1 tandem kinase mediates histone H3 phosphorylation and is required for maintenance of chromatin structure in Drosophila. Cell 105:433–443

Williams RW, Rubin GM (2002) Argonaute1 is required for efficient RNA interference in Drosophila embryos. Proc Natl Acad Sci USA 99:6889–6894

Yang W, Wan, Q, Howell KL, Lee JT, Cho DS, Murray JM, Nishikurg K (2005) ADAR1 RNA deaminase limits short interfering RNA efficacy in mammalian cells. J Biol Chem 280:3946–3953

Zhang H, Kolb FA, Brondani V, Billy E, Filipowicz W (2002) Human Dicer preferentially cleaves dsRNAs at their termini without a requirement for ATP. EMBO J 21:5875–5885

Zhang H, Kolb FA, Jaskiewicz L, Westhof E, Filipowicz W (2004) Single processing center models for human Dicer and bacterial RNase III. Cell 118:57–68

Zhang W, Deng H, Bao X, Lerach S, Girton J, Johansen J, Johansen KM (2006) The JIL-1 histone H3S10 kinase regulates dimethyl H3K9 modifications and heterochromatic spreading in Drosophila. Development 133:229–235

Zhang Z, Carmichael GG (2001) The fate of dsRNA in the nucleus: a p54^{nrb}-containing complex mediates the nuclear retention of promiscuously A-to-I edited RNAs. Cell 106:465–475

Role of Dicer in Posttranscriptional RNA Silencing

Lukasz Jaskiewicz and Witold Filipowicz(✉)

Abstract Dicer, an RNase III type endonuclease, is the key enzyme involved in RNA interference (RNAi) and microRNA (miRNA) pathways. It is required for biogenesis of miRNAs and small interfering RNAs (siRNAs), and also plays an important role in an effector step of RNA silencing, the RNA-induced silencing complex (RISC) assembly. In this article we describe different functions of Dicer in posttranscriptional regulation. We review the current knowledge about Dicers in different organisms and the functions of individual domains of the enzyme. We also discuss information about Dicer-associated proteins and their role in the biogenesis of small RNAs and assembly of RISC.

1 Introduction

RNA interference (RNAi) and microRNA (miRNA)-mediated reactions have emerged as major pathways regulating gene expression in eukaryotic organisms. The specificity of these processes is dependent on 20- to 25-nt small interfering

Witold Filipowicz
Friedrich Miescher Institute for Biomedical Research, 4002 Basel, Switzerland
Witold.Filipowicz@fmi.ch

P.J. Paddison and P.K. Vogt (eds.), *RNA Interference.*
Current Topics in Microbiology and Immunology 320.
© Springer-Verlag Berlin Heidelberg 2008

RNAs (siRNAs) and miRNAs, acting as guides recognizing sequences of target RNAs. To perform their effector function, siRNAs and miRNAs are incorporated into ribonucleoprotein (RNP) complexes, referred to as si- or mi-RISCs (RNA-induced silencing complexes, acting posttranscriptionally) or RITS (RNA-induced transcriptional silencing complexes, acting at the chromatin level). The biogenesis of both miRNAs and siRNAs requires endonucleolytic enzymes, members of the RNase III family, which are able to process double-stranded RNA (dsRNA). MiRNAs are generated from the genome-encoded precursor hairpins by the sequential action of two RNase III-type nucleases, Drosha and Dicer. Dicer is also responsible for the excision of siRNAs from long dsRNA molecules, either experimentally expressed in cells or accumulating in cells as a result of antisense transcription or viral infection (reviewed by Kim 2005; Tomari and Zamore 2005).

Fire et al. (1998) were the first to demonstrate that sequence-specific gene silencing is induced in *Caenorhabditis elegans* by dsRNA. It soon became recognized that dsRNA is processed in cells into small double-stranded fragments, siRNAs, that act as effectors of RNA silencing (Hamilton and Baulcombe 1999; Zamore et al. 2000; Hammond et al. 2000). The enzyme responsible for processing of dsRNA to siRNAs was subsequently identified in *Drosophila* and named Dicer (Bernstein et al. 2001). Similar enzymes were then identified in other organisms, including mammals (Bernstein et al. 2001; Billy et al. 2001; Hutvagner et al. 2001), *C. elegans* (Grishok et al. 2001; Ketting et al. 2001), and plants (Reinhart et al. 2002), and their role in siRNA and miRNA biogenesis was documented.

In this article we review our current knowledge about Dicer and Dicer-associated proteins in RNA silencing in different organisms, and the role these proteins play in the biogenesis of small RNAs and assembly of RISC. Our review is focused on the function of Dicer in posttranscriptional regulation. The function of small RNAs in chromatin silencing has been reviewed elsewhere (Matzke and Birchler 2005; Grewal and Jia 2007; Zaratiegui et al. 2007). Dicer, and RNase III enzymes in general, are also discussed in some other recent articles (Nicholson 2003; Drider and Condon 2004; Murchison and Hannon 2004; Cerutti and Casas-Mollano 2006).

2   RNase III Family

The discovery that RNase III enzymes are involved in RNAi and miRNA pathways in different organisms has renewed interest in this class of proteins. DsRNA-specific RNase III was first identified in *Escherichia coli*. Among many functions of bacterial and fungal RNases III, the most prominent is their involvement in pre-ribosomal RNA (pre-rRNA) processing (reviewed by Nicholson 2003). A classification scheme proposed by Blaszczyk et al. (2001) divided RNase III orthologs into three classes: class I, which includes eubacterial enzymes and the yeast ortholog Rnt1p; class II, containing Drosha proteins; and class III, comprising Dicer homologs. Placement of Drosha and Dicer in separate classes was mainly based on differences in the domain organization of the proteins known at that time. With the identification of "primitive"

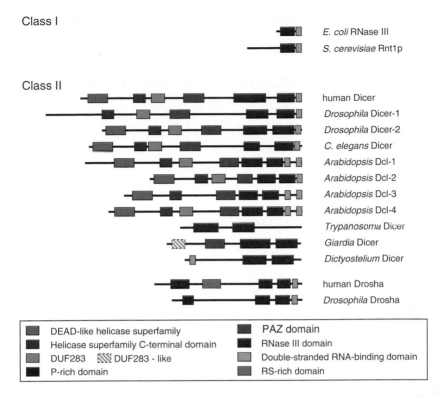

Fig. 1 A new classification for RNase III enzymes. Class I contains bacterial and fungal RNase III orthologs, class II contains Dicer and Drosha proteins. Drosha enzymes are found only in animals. Schematic domain organization of selected proteins of the RNase III family is shown

Dicers in unicellular eukaryotes such as *Giardia intestinalis* and *Trypanosoma brucei* (Macrae et al. 2006; Shi et al. 2006), the complexity of domain organization is no longer a distinguishing feature of Drosha and Dicer proteins. We therefore propose a new classification that divides RNase III orthologs into just two classes (Fig. 1): class I, comprising enzymes that contain a single RNase III domain and function as homodimers, and class II, which encompasses enzymes bearing two catalytic RNase III domains active as monomers. As in the old classification, class I embraces bacterial and fungal proteins that contain, in addition to a single RNase III domain, a C-terminal dsRNA-binding domain (dsRBD). The yeast Rnt1p also contains an N-terminal extension, shown to be important for enzyme dimerization (Lamontagne et al. 2000). Class II encompasses all Drosha and Dicer proteins. They invariably contain two RNase III domains, but the composition of additional domains varies considerably and can involve dsRBD, ATPase/helicase, PAZ (Piwi/Argonaute/Zwille), and DUF283 (domain of unknown function) domains (Fig. 1). Drosha enzymes generally contain a variable-length N-terminal region with proline-rich and/or arginine/serine-rich domains. For the human Drosha, the middle part, lacking a distinguishable motif, is responsible for interaction with a partner protein, DGCR8 (Han et al. 2004). For three enzymes of the Dicer/Drosha class, evidence is available that they indeed function as monomeric proteins, the two RNase III domains forming an intramolecular pseudo-dimer-type catalytic domain (Zhang et al. 2004; Han et al. 2004; Macrae et al. 2006). In the case of human Drosha, two such monomers may additionally dimerize to form a heterotetrameric complex with DGCR8 (Han et al. 2006). The finding that one of the *Arabidopsis* Dicers, Dcl-1, exerts the function of both Drosha and Dicer during pre-miRNA processing (Kurihara and Watanabe 2004) provides an additional argument for grouping the Drosha and Dicer enzymes together.

3   Dicer Proteins in Different Organisms

Dicers are large multidomain proteins found in most eukaryotes (e.g., animals, plants, and *Schizosaccharomyces pombe*, but not in *Saccharomyces cerevisiae*). Metazoan and plant Dicer proteins generally contain ATPase/helicase, DUF283, PAZ, two RNase III, and a dsRBD, but Dicers of lower eukaryotes frequently have a less complex domain organization (Fig. 1). The PAZ, dsRBD, and RNase III domains are involved in dsRNA binding and cleavage. The PAZ domain is also found in PPD (PAZ and Piwi domain) or Argonaute proteins that are also involved in RNAi and miRNA pathways. The presence of the helicase/ATPase domain could explain the observation that the generation of siRNAs by the *C. elegans* Dicer and one of the two *Drosophila* Dicers is stimulated by addition of ATP (Bernstein et al. 2001; Ketting et al. 2001; Liu et al. 2003; Nykanen et al. 2001). However, ATP has no significant effect on the activity of the mammalian enzyme even though it contains the ATPase/helicase domain (Zhang et al. 2002). Dicers of *G. intestinalis, Dictyostelium discoideum*, and *T. brucei* are devoid of the helicase/ATPase domain (Martens et al. 2002; Macrae et al. 2006; Shi et al. 2006). Interestingly, the *G. intestinalis* Dicer that lacks the helicase domain can complement the RNAi functions of the *S. pombe* strain deleted from the endogenous Dicer, even though the latter contains the helicase domain (Macrae et al. 2006). In *D. discoideum*, a domain with homology to the Dicer ATPase/helicase domain is present in the RNA-dependent-RNA polymerase(RdRP)-like protein (Martens et al. 2002).

Mammalian genomes encode only one Dicer protein. On the other hand, plants, such as *Arabidopsis thaliana*, poplar, and rice express four Dicer-like proteins (Dcl). Fungi, such as *Neurospora crassa*, and insects (e.g., *Drosophila* and mosquito) contain two Dicer genes. The four plant Dcls have distinct roles: Dcl-1 processes miRNA precursors, both the long primary miRNA transcripts (pri-miRNAs) and the precursor miRNA (pre-miRNAs); Dcl-2 generates siRNAs associated with antiviral defense; Dcl-3 produces siRNAs that are involved in chromatin modification and transcriptional silencing; and Dcl-4 generates *trans*-acting siRNAs (tasiRNAs) that originate from non-coding RNAs and regulate expression of their target mRNAs (Park et al. 2002; Kurihara and Watanabe 2004; Vazquez et al. 2004; Xie et al. 2004; Borsani et al. 2005; Gasciolli et al. 2005; Xie et al. 2005). Since small RNAs produced by individual Dcls are involved in diverse processes, there must be a mechanism for efficient discrimination between different RNA substrates and the subsequent incorporation of products into correct effector complexes. It has been suggested (Margis et al. 2006) that the dsRBDs of Dicer might be involved in mediating this process. Dcl-1, Dcl-3, and Dcl-4 each contain two dsRBDs, while Dcl-2 contains only one. Proteins associating with different Dcls may likewise contribute to the specificity (see below).

Distinct roles in RNA silencing have been established for the two *Drosophila* Dicer proteins. Dicer-1 is essential for pre-miRNA processing while Dicer-2 is necessary for siRNA production and the RNAi pathway. The functional separation of the *Drosophila* Dicers, however, is not absolute. Although Dicer-1 and Dicer-2 generate distinct types of small RNAs, both enzymes are required for siRNA-directed target mRNA cleavage and gene silencing (Lee et al. 2004b).

The subcellular localization of Dicer has been investigated in various systems. In plants, green fluorescent protein (GFP)-fusions of Dcl-1, Dcl-3, and Dcl-4 localized to the nucleus (Xie et al. 2004; Hiraguri et al. 2005), a finding that is consistent with the roles played by these proteins. On the other hand, in mammalian cells, endogenous Dicer and protein expressed either as a cyan fluorescent protein fusion or myc-tagged was found to localize to the cytoplasm (Billy et al. 2001; Provost et al. 2002). However, Dicer may also have a nuclear function in mammalian cells.

4   Proteins Interacting with Dicer

Although recombinant Dicer is active as a dsRNA-specific endonuclease in vitro, in cells it generally functions in association with other proteins as a component of multiprotein complexes (Table 1 and Fig. 2).

4.1   *dsRBD-Containing Cofactors of Dicer*

Cleavage of pre-miRNA and dsRNA substrates seems to be invariably catalyzed by Dicer in association with dsRBD-domain protein cofactors (Fig. 2). The first such dsRBD protein, Rde-4 (RNAi deficient-4), was identified in a genetic screen in *C. elegans* (Tabara et al. 1999). It is required for the initiation step of RNAi in worms, but its activity is not required for miRNA processing or worm development (Grishok et al. 2000). In *Drosophila*, Dicer-1 and Dicer-2 are associated with Loquacious (Loqs) and R2D2, respectively (Forstemann et al. 2005; Saito et al. 2005; Liu et al. 2003). The Dicer-2/R2D2 complex functions in directing the strand-specific incorporation of the siRNA into the RISC. A heterodimer of Dicer-2 and R2D2 senses the stability of the siRNA duplex ends and determines which strand will enter the RISC. Photocrosslinking to siRNAs containing 5-iodouracil

Table 1 Proteins interacting with Dicer

Name	Organism	References
1. dsRBD proteins		
RDE–4	*C. elegans*	Tabara et al. 1999
Loqs	*Drosophila*, Dicer–1	Forstemann et al. 2005; Saito et al. 2005
R2D2	*Drosophila*, Dicer–2	Liu et al. 2003
TRBP	Mammals	Chendrimada et al. 2005; Haase et al. 2005
PACT	Mammals	Lee et al. 2006
HYL1/DRB	Plants	Hiraguri et al. 2005
2. PPD proteins		
Ago–1	*Drosophila*, Dicer–1	Okamura et al. 2004
Ago–2	*Drosophila*, Dicer–2	Liu et al. 2003
Ago–2	Mammals	Tahbaz et al. 2004
Hiwi	Mammals	Tahbaz et al. 2004
3. Other proteins		
DRH–1	*C. elegans*	Tabara et al. 2002
FMRP	Mammals	Jin et al. 2004
dFXR	*Drosophila*	Caudy et al. 2002; Ishizuka et al. 2002
MVH	Mammals	Kotaja et al. 2006

4. Identified in C. elegans by Duchaine et al. (2006)	
Name	Structural description
a. Required for RNAi, known previously	
RDE–1	Piwi/PAZ
RDE–4	dsRBD
DRH–1	DEAH/D
DRH–2	DEAH/D
b. PIR–1 group, required for RNAi and development	
PIR–1	RNA phosphatase
DRH–3	DEAH/D
c. ERI proteins	
ERI–1	SAP domain, exonuclease
ERI–3	Also expressed as a fusion with TAF–6.1
ERI–5	Tudor domain
TAF–6.1	TATA box binding protein-associated factor, also expressed as a fusion with ERI–3
RRF–3	RdRP
d. Required for miRNA and development	
ALG–1	Piwi/PAZ
ALG–2	Piwi/PAZ
LIN–41	RBCC
e. Without determined function in small RNA-related silencing	
EFT–2	GTPase
SNR–3	SM domain
F38E11.5	WD repeats
B0001.2	DUF272
T06A10.3	
C32A3.2	

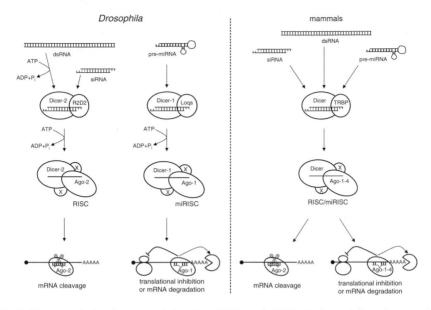

Fig. 2 Posttranscriptional gene regulation by miRNAs and siRNAs in *Drosophila* and mammals. Potential additional proteins are marked with X

residues at different positions revealed that Dicer binds to the thermodynamically less stable and R2D2 to the more stable siRNA end. The strand with the 5′ end at the less stable siRNA end is subsequently incorporated into the RISC complex (Tomari et al. 2004b; Fig. 2). Depletion of Loqs, which associates with Dicer-1, causes the accumulation of pre-miRNAs, demonstrating that Loqs is essential for efficient substrate processing by Dicer-1 (Forstemann et al. 2005; Saito et al. 2005). Loqs also increases the substrate specificity of Dicer-1, because the Dicer-1/Loqs complex apparently does not show the activity toward dsRNA exhibited by Dicer-1 alone (Saito et al. 2005).

In human cells, TRBP [human immunodeficiency virus (HIV-1) transactivating-response (TAR) RNA-binding protein] was found to be a dsRBD protein partner of Dicer (Chendrimada et al. 2005; Haase et al. 2005). TRBP is required for optimal RNA silencing mediated by siRNAs and endogenous miRNAs. However, evidence that TRBP is involved like R2D2 in the definition of siRNA asymmetry is still lacking. TRBP has previously been assigned several functions, including inhibition of the interferon-induced dsRNA-regulated protein kinase R (PKR) (Daher et al. 2001), modulation of HIV-1 gene expression through its association with the TAR hairpin (Dorin et al. 2003), and control of cell growth (Benkirane et al. 1997; Lee et al. 2004a). A mouse TRBP ortholog, Prbp, was shown to function as a translational regulator during spermatogenesis, and mice depleted of Prbp are male sterile and usually die at the time of weaning (Zhong et al. 1999). Another mammalian dsRBD protein, PKR activator (PACT), which is 42% identical to TRBP, has also been recently found to interact with Dicer. Its depletion strongly affected the accumulation of mature miRNAs in human cells (Lee et al. 2006). In contrast to TRBP, which inhibits PKR, PACT has a stimulatory effect on this kinase. The effects of TRBP and PACT on PKR activity are mediated by the C-terminal dsRBDs, which have no detectable dsRNA-binding activity (Gupta et al. 2003). In addition to effects on PKR, the C-terminal domains of PACT and TRBP can mediate homodimerization of both proteins (Daher et al. 2001). The C-terminal dsRBD of TRBP is also involved in association with Dicer (Haase et al. 2005), raising the possibility that RNAi and PKR pathways are interconnected and regulated by the aforementioned protein–protein interactions. TRBP may indeed be important for Dicer function in vivo since its titration by overexpression of TAR RNA in human cells leads to the inhibition of Dicer activity (Bennasser et al. 2006).

In plants, members of the HYL1/DRB family of proteins were identified as Dcl-interacting dsRBD partners and implicated in small RNA pathways in *Arabidopsis* (Hiraguri et al. 2005). Fusion proteins containing both dsRBD domains of Dcl-1, Dcl-3, and Dcl-4 can bind to members of the HYL1/DRB family. A model has been proposed in which the Dicer dsRBD domains along with PAZ and RNase III domains recognize and process specific RNA substrates and, by interacting with cognate HYL1/DRB members, direct the newly generated small RNAs to appropriate effector complexes (Margis et al. 2006).

4.2   Argonautes/PPD Proteins

Another group of well-characterized Dicer partners is represented by PPD or Argonaute proteins. Members of the PPD protein family contain two signature domains: a PAZ domain in the center and a PIWI domain at the carboxyl terminus (Carmell et al. 2002; Tolia and Joshua-Tor 2007). Genetic and biochemical studies have indicated that PPD proteins are involved in control of stem cell differentiation, tissue development (Carmell et al. 2002), and chromatin modification (Verdel et al. 2004; Irvine et al. 2006). PPD proteins can be divided into two subgroups: those that are homologous to the *Arabidopsis* Argonaute-1 and are ubiquitously expressed, and those that are most similar to the *Drosophila* Piwi, expressed in germline stem cells (Carmell et al. 2002; Tolia and Joshua-Tor 2007). These subgroups are referred to as Argonaute (Ago) and Piwi proteins. Different Ago proteins have been identified as components of the RISC in different organisms (Tabara et al. 1999; Hammond et al. 2001; Caudy and Hannon 2004; Pham et al. 2004; Tomari et al. 2004a), and mammalian Ago-2 was demonstrated to catalyze the mRNA cleavage (Liu et al. 2004; Meister et al. 2004; Rivas et al. 2005). The interaction between human Dicer and two PPD proteins, Ago-2 and Hiwi, has been investigated in detail (Tahbaz et al. 2004), revealing that a subregion of the PIWI domain, the PIWI-box, binds directly to the Dicer RNase III domain. Ago-2, Hiwi, and Dicer are present in soluble and membrane-associated fractions, indicating that interactions between these two types of protein may occur in multiple cellular compartments. A stable association between PPD proteins and Dicer is dependent on the activity of the Hsp90 protein, as the association can be inhibited by geldanamycin, a specific Hsp90 inhibitor (Tahbaz et al. 2004).

PPD-related proteins are also expressed in some prokaryotes, though their function in these organisms remains unclear. Recent crystallization efforts resulted in the determination of the structure of PfAgo from *Pyrococcus furiosus* (Song et al. 2004), AfPiwi from *Archaeoglobus fulgidus* (Parker et al. 2004; Parker et al. 2005; Ma et al. 2005) and of an Argonaute from *Aquifex aeolicus* (Yuan et al. 2005; Yuan et al. 2006), either as proteins alone or in a complex with siRNA mimics. PIWI domains of all these proteins bear striking similarity to RNase H, an enzyme that cleaves the RNA strand in DNA–RNA hybrids. This suggested that the PIWI domain of Ago proteins is responsible for the "Slicer" activity, catalyzing the siRNA-directed endonucleolytic cleavage of mRNA in the RISC. RNase H contains a triad of conserved acidic amino acids, DDE, essential for catalysis. A related set of residues, DDH, is conserved in PfAgo and some eukaryotic Ago proteins, for example Ago-2 (Tolia and Joshua-Tor 2007). Mutagenesis of human Ago-2 demonstrated that all three DDH triad amino acids are involved in the mRNA cleavage by the RISC (Liu et al. 2004; Rivas et al. 2005). The demonstration that human Ago-2, expressed and purified from *E. coli*, is able to cleave mRNA targeted by a complementary single-stranded siRNA provided the ultimate proof that Ago-2 acts as a Slicer in the RISC (Rivas et al. 2005).

4.3   Other Proteins Interacting with Dicer

Several other proteins have been found to interact with Dicer. In *C. elegans*, the RNA-helicase-related protein DRH-1, which is required for RNAi, was found to interact with Rde-4 and Dicer (Tabara et al. 2002). FMRP, an mRNA-binding protein involved in the pathogenesis of fragile X syndrome, has been shown to interact with Dicer and Ago-1 in mammalian cells (Jin et al. 2004), and *Drosophila* dFXR, a fly ortholog of FMRP, interacts with Dicer-1 and Ago-2 (Caudy et al. 2002; Ishizuka et al. 2002). In mammalian male germ cells, Dicer was shown to interact with mouse vasa homolog (MVH), with both proteins localizing to the P body-related structure known as a chromatoid body (Kotaja et al. 2006).

A major proteomic effort was undertaken to characterize proteins interacting with Dicer in *C. elegans* (Duchaine et al. 2006). A total of 108 candidate proteins were identified. The authors focused on the top 20 proteins most reproducibly co-purifying with Dicer. They were divided into five groups: (1) previously known to be required for RNAi (like Rde-1 and Rde-4); (2) the PIR-1 group, required for RNAi and development; (3) enhancers of RNAi (ERI) proteins; (4) proteins required for miRNA function and development; and (5) proteins without a well-defined function in small RNA silencing (Table 1). PIR-1, a homolog of an RNA-phosphatase, conserved in animals, is required for processing the RdRP-amplified Dicer substrate and accumulation of the resulting secondary siRNAs. Its putative role is dephosphorylation of the 5′-triphosphate-bearing secondary siRNAs synthesized by RdRP (reviewed by Ketting 2006). Another PIR-1 group protein is the helicase DRH-3. DRH-3 is related to the mammalian helicase RIG-I (Yoneyama et al. 2004) and is required for RNAi in the germline. Worms with mutations in proteins from the ERI-1 group exhibit enhanced RNAi phenotypes in response to exogenous dsRNA and accumulate higher levels of dsRNA-derived siRNAs. Identification of so many Dicer-interacting proteins indicates that in *C. elegans*, and most likely in other organisms also, Dicer participates in many cellular processes.

5   Mechanism of dsRNA and Pre-miRNA Processing by Dicer

The mechanism of dsRNA and pre-miRNA processing has been most extensively studied with the human Dicer. The protein was overexpressed in insect cells and purified. The ribonuclease activity of Dicer requires the presence of Mg^{2+} ions but Mn^{2+} and Co^{2+} can partially replace Mg^{2+}. Dicer can cleave with similar efficiency dsRNAs ranging from 30 to 130 bp, yielding siRNAs of approx. 20 bp (Zhang et al. 2002; Provost et al. 2002). Dicer preferentially processes dsRNA from the ends of the substrate, as demonstrated by accumulation of processing intermediates diagnostic of the gradual removal of siRNA units from substrate ends (Zhang et al. 2002). However, blocking the ends of dsRNA with RNA tetraloops or DNA–RNA duplexes revealed that free ends are not absolutely required: the terminally blocked dsRNA was cleaved internally, with reduced kinetics. After the initial internal cleavage, normal kinetics were restored as 2-nt 3′-overhang-containing ends became available (Zhang et al. 2002). Interestingly, preincubation of recombinant Dicer with proteinase K causes a significant increase in enzyme activity. Such a stimulatory effect is also seen with an endogenous Dicer immunoprecipitated from mammalian cell extracts (Zhang et al. 2002). It is possible that limited proteolysis removes a Dicer region that partially occludes the active site.

Processing of miRNA precursors by recombinant Dicer was investigated in detail using pre-let-7 miRNA as a model substrate. Native gel electrophoresis showed that pre-let-7 RNA is effectively processed by Dicer in vitro to yield the double-stranded siRNA-like product (Zhang et al. 2004). Processing of both dsRNA and pre-let-7 RNA by the recombinant human Dicer occurs with a very low turnover rate, most probably because the product of the reaction remains associated with the enzyme (Zhang et al. 2002, 2004). Cleavage of the substrate by either recombinant or endogenous human Dicer is ATP independent (Billy et al. 2001; Zhang et al. 2002; Provost et al. 2002). Addition of other nucleotide triphosphates or nonhydrolyzable ATP analogs has no appreciable effect on Dicer activity. In addition, mutation of the conserved lysine residue in the nucleotide-binding site (P-loop motif) has no impact on Dicer activity (Zhang et al. 2002). So far, ATPase activity could not be demonstrated in preparations of recombinant human Dicer, suggesting that activity of the ATPase/helicase domain is regulated by additional factors.

Mutagenesis studies indicated that residues Asp1320 and Glu1652 from RNase IIIa, and Asp1709 and Glu1813 from RNase IIIb that are involved in Mg^{2+} coordination are essential for cleavage activity of Dicer. Equivalent mutations in the *E. coli* RNase III also rendered this class I enzyme inactive, demonstrating that a similar cleavage mechanism is used by all members of the RNase III family. Analysis of cleavage products generated by individual RNase IIIa or IIIb domain mutants demonstrated that Dicer accesses its substrates in a polar fashion, with the RNase IIIa domain always processing the protruding 3'-OH-bearing RNA strand, and RNase IIIb cutting the opposite 5'-phosphate-containing strand (Zhang et al. 2004). To understand the role of the PAZ domain, residues F960, YY971/972, and E1036, all implicated in RNA binding, were substituted by alanines. The PAZ mutants exhibited reduced dsRNA-processing activity (Zhang et al. 2004). The PAZ domain was demonstrated to recognize the 3'-protruding nucleotides at the siRNA end (Lingel et al. 2003; Song et al. 2003; Yan et al. 2003; Ma et al. 2004). Consistent with these findings, Dicer cleaves dsRNA and pre-miRNA substrates containing 3'-overhang nucleotides more efficiently that those containing blunt ends (Zhang et al. 2004).

In a model based on the mutagenic studies, Dicer functions as an intramolecular pseudo-dimer with RNase IIIa and IIIb domains forming a single processing center containing two independent catalytic "half sites," each capable of cutting one RNA strand of the duplex to generate products with 2-nt 3'-overhangs (Zhang et al. 2004). The 3'-overhang-containing end of the substrate is recognized by the PAZ domain. In the model, the dsRNA substrate is placed in the positively charged valley on the surface of the catalytic domains. This model has been nicely validated by the determination of the crystal structure of the full-length Dicer from the protozoan *G. intestinalis* (Macrae et al. 2006).

The *G. intestinalis* Dicer is smaller than its orthologs in higher organisms. It lacks the N-terminal ATPase/helicase domain and the C-terminal dsRBD (Fig. 3). Structural studies revealed that it forms an elongated molecule that may act as a molecular ruler measuring the distance between the dsRNA end and the site of enzymatic cleavage (Macrae et al. 2006). The RNase III domains form the catalytic center and the PAZ domain is connected to RNase III domains by a long α-helix dubbed the "connector" helix, which is implicated in determining the product length. The PAZ domain of the *Giardia* Dicer shares similarity with PAZ domains of *Drosophila* Ago-1 and Ago-2 and resembles the oligonucleotide-binding (OB) fold, consistent with the RNA-binding activity of the domain (Lingel et al. 2003; Song et al. 2003; Yan et al. 2003). Structural study of the *Giardia* Dicer shed some light on a possible role of the conserved "domain of unknown function 283" (DUF283). Low but significant sequence homology exists between the N-terminal domain of *Giardia* Dicer and DUF283 of metazoan Dicers (Fig. 1). The DUF283-like domain of *Giardia* Dicer forms a platform-like structure providing support for the connector helix (Macrae et al. 2006).

A

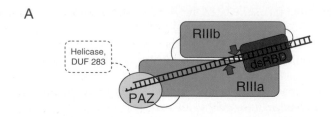

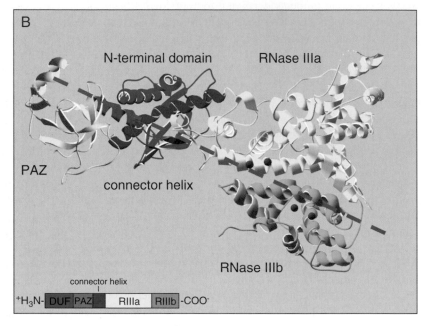

Fig. 3 **A** A model of dsRNA processing by human Dicer (Zhang et al. 2004). Individual domains of Dicer are shown in different colors. The enzyme contains a single dsRNA cleavage center with two independent catalytic sites. The center is formed by intramolecular dimerization of the RNase IIIa and RNase IIIb domains. The placement of the RIIIa domain illustrates the fact that this domain cleaves the 3′-OH-bearing and protruding RNA strand. DsRBD positioning is arbitrary. **B** Crystal structure of *Giardia intestinalis* Dicer (Macrae et al. 2006). This ribbon representation of Dicer shows the N-terminal platform domain (*blue*), the PAZ domain (*orange*), the connector helix (*red*), the RNase IIIa domain (*yellow*), and the RNase IIIb domain (*green*). Predicted location of dsRNA is indicated by a *dashed line*. PDB_id 2ffl was rendered using DeepView (Guex and Peitsch 1997) and POV-Ray 3.6 (www.povray.org)

6 Function of Dicer in the Assembly of Effector Complexes

The roles of Dicer are not confined to miRNA and siRNA biogenesis. The enzyme also appears to be essential for the effector step of RNA silencing (Fig. 2). The involvement of Dicer in RISC formation has been studied in most detail in *Drosophila* (Pham et al. 2004; Tomari et al. 2004a). Three distinct siRNA-containing complexes, R1, R2, and R3, have been identified as intermediates in RISC formation by Pham et al. (2004). The R1 complex corresponds to the 360-kDa RISC described previously (Nykanen et al. 2001). It consists of Dicer-2, R2D2, and possibly one or more unidentified proteins. The function of R1 may be to process long dsRNA and possibly determine the guide/passenger strand asymmetry of siRNA, as described below. R1 serves as a precursor to R2 and R3 (Pham et al. 2004). R2 is formed at a high rate, suggesting that it may be derived from the binding of R1 to another as-yet-unidentified preassembled complex. The R2 complex is thought to function in siRNA duplex unwinding. The unwinding of the siRNA may be initiated by the Dicer-2–R2D2 complex, but can proceed only in the presence of Ago-2 (Tomari et al. 2004b). A DEA(H/D)-box ATPase/helicase Armitage has been implicated in the unwinding process (Tomari et al. 2004a; Cook et al. 2004). The approx. 80S R3 or a "holo-RISC" complex whose formation requires ATP contains siRNAs, Dicer-1, Dicer-2, R2D2, Ago-2, and a few other proteins identified previously as associated with the RISC (VIG, Tudor-SN, dFXR). The R3 complex co-fractionates with rRNA of small and large ribosomal subunits, suggesting that it is ribosome associated. R3, the RNAi effector complex, may contain regulatory factors that are not absolutely necessary for the mRNA cleavage in vitro (Pham et al. 2004). Complexes similar to those described above were also characterized by Tomari et al. (2004a). According to these authors, the assembly of RISC begins with the formation of "complex B" that contains dsRNA and other unidentified proteins. Complex B is a precursor to the RISC loading complex (RLC) that, like R1 and R2, contains Dicer-2 and R2D2.

The dynamics of RISC assembly in mammals is not as well understood as in *Drosophila*. Chendrimada et al. (2005) reported that human cells contain a preassembled complex of Dicer, TRBP, and Ago-2 capable of binding siRNA duplexes. This complex was subsequently found to be able to determine the asymmetry of the siRNA-like miRNA duplex and to incorporate correctly the guide miRNA strand for mRNA cleavage (Gregory et al. 2005). Interestingly, assembly of RISC initiated with pre-miRNA was more efficient than that with pre-cut miRNA duplex, consistent with the cleavage and effector steps of RNAi being tightly coupled. Maniataki and Mourelatos (2005) identified a similar complex containing Dicer, Ago-2, and TRBP. The complex was active in processing of pre-miRNAs and incorporated a proper miRNA strand able to guide the cleavage of a complementary RNA mimicking the mRNA. However, the complex could not assemble when a perfect siRNA duplex was used in place of pre-miRNA. Another possible intermediate of the mammalian RISC, named complex D, has also been described from human cell extracts incubated with the exogenous siRNA duplex. Complex D contains Dicer associated with siRNA; based on the estimated size of 250–300 kDa, it might be an equivalent of the *Drosophila* R1 complex (Pellino et al. 2005). Some other data indicate that Dicer may not be essential for RISC formation in mammals. HeLa cell extracts immunodepleted of Dicer retain siRNA-mediated RISC activity (Martinez et al. 2002), and mouse Dicer-null embryonic stem cells are capable of mounting RNAi in response to transfected siRNA (Kanellopoulou et al. 2005). It is possible that Dicer plays a merely stimulatory role in the assembly and function of the mammalian RISC. The observation that approx. 30-bp dsRNAs, which Dicer processes to induce RNAi, are more efficient than siRNAs at triggering the RNAi response in human cells (Kim et al. 2005; Rose et al. 2005; Siolas et al. 2005) is consistent with such a possibility.

For the siRNA to act as a guide for mRNA cleavage, the siRNA duplex must be unwound into individual strands during RISC assembly. The strand that is incorporated into the RISC is referred to as a guide strand, while the discarded strand is called a passenger. A strand selection mechanism exists to ensure effective siRNA loading to the RISC. Thermodynamic differences in the base-pairing stabilities of the 5′ ends of the two siRNA strands determine which strand is assembled into the RISC (Khvorova et al. 2003; Schwarz et al. 2003). In *Drosophila*, strand selection is achieved by an appropriate orientation of the siRNA duplex in the Dicer-2/R2D2 heterodimer. The siRNA end with stronger thermodynamic stability interacts with R2D2, while the less stable end is bound by Dicer. The strand with its 5′ terminus at the less stable end is then selected as a guide and becomes part of an active RISC (Tomari et al. 2004b; Preall et al. 2006; Fig. 2). Thermodynamic stability rules have to be considered when designing siRNAs in order to ensure that the guide strand is indeed preferentially incorporated into the RISC, and to minimize the potential off-targeting effects resulting from the inclusion of the passenger strand into the RISC.

The strand selection mechanism described above is easy to follow when the reaction is initiated with preformed siRNAs. It is, however, less clear how the siRNA asymmetry is recognized when siRNAs are excised from long dsRNA. Clearly, Dicer or the Dicer/R2D2 complex is unable to sense the thermodynamic asymmetry of siRNA segments that are embedded in a sequence of long dsRNA. Since Dicer generally liberates siRNAs from dsRNA ends (Elbashir et al. 2001; Zhang et al. 2002), on average only a half of the generated siRNAs will be "optimally aligned" on the surface of the Dicer/R2D2 complex to comply with the thermodynamic rules required for siRNA strand selection. Importantly, Preall et al. (2006) have demonstrated that siRNA strand selection is independent of the dsRNA processing polarity during *Drosophila* RISC assembly in vitro. These data indicate that the guide strand selection is not defined at the Dicer processing step even though Dicer processes dsRNA in a strictly defined mode, with the strand containing the 3′ protruding end always being cleaved by the RNase IIIa domain (see the previous section). Hence, *Drosophila* Dicer-2 does not directly hand over newly generated siRNAs into the RISC but probably releases the siRNAs into solution to rebind them again in a proper orientation. The mechanism underlying such an "siRNA flipping" process is unknown.

Pre-miRNA processing by Dicer in vitro (Zhang et al. 2004), and very likely also in vivo, yields double-stranded siRNA-like products and a similar thermodynamic, stability-based strand selection mechanism also functions during miRISC formation. This is consistent with the observation that mature miRNAs can originate from either ascending or descending strands of the pre-miRNA hairpin. Like siRNAs, miRNAs in their double-stranded form show the thermodynamic polarity of ends that defines the strand of the pre-miRNA hairpin to be selected as a mature and active miRNA (Khvorova et al. 2003; Krol et al. 2004).

7   Role of Dicer *In Vivo*

Knockout experiments indicated that Dicer is essential for vertebrate development. Disruption of the Dicer gene in mice arrests embryogenesis at day 8.5 (Bernstein et al. 2003), while mice with a strong hypomorphic mutation, resulting from the deletion of the first two Dicer exons, die between 12.5 and 14.5 days of gestation and display defects in angiogenesis (Yang et al. 2005). Effects of different tissue-specific Dicer knockouts have also been analyzed. Mouse oocytes lacking Dicer fail to accumulate mature miRNAs and are unable to progress through first meiotic division, displaying disorganized spindles and chromosome congression defects (Murchison et al. 2007; Tang et al. 2007). These observations suggest that miRNAs play an essential role during the earliest stages of embryonic development, when maternally encoded transcripts have to undergo specific downregulation (Giraldez et al. 2006). In addition, Dicer may be involved in the protection of germ cells from the movement of transposable elements, since in oocytes lacking Dicer transcripts levels of some transposons are elevated (Murchison et al. 2007). In mice with the epidermal-specific Dicer knockout, proper morphogenesis and maintenance of hair follicles is affected (Andl et al. 2006). Dicer function was also found to be essential for lung epithelium morphogenesis (Harris et al. 2006) and limb development (Harfe et al. 2005).

Dicer-deficient mouse embryonic stem (ES) cells display proliferation and differentiation defects and, as expected, are defective in dsRNA-induced RNAi and generation of miRNAs (Kanellopoulou et al. 2005; Murchison et al. 2005). Epigenetic silencing of centromeric repeats is also reduced in these cells (Kanellopoulou et al. 2005). Likewise, in the chicken-human hybrid DT40 cell line, loss of Dicer leads to premature sister chromatid separation due to abnormalities in heterochromatin formation (Fukagawa et al. 2004). Dicer function was also found to be essential for zebrafish development and many processes in *C. elegans*. In *Drosophila*, Dicer-1, which is involved in miRNA biogenesis, is likewise an essential gene (reviewed by Wienholds and Plasterk 2005; Giraldez et al. 2006). Most of the phenotypes associated with Dicer knockouts are probably mainly caused by the depletion of miRNAs. However, other mechanisms controlled by Dicer, related to RNAi, such as the formation of heterochromatic structures and centromeric silencing, may also contribute to developmental or cellular defects discussed above (reviewed by Grewal and Jia 2007; Zaratiegui et al. 2007).

References

Andl T, Murchison EP, Liu F, Zhang Y, Yunta-Gonzalez M, Tobias JW, Andl CD, Seykora JT, Hannon GJ, Millar SE (2006) The miRNA-processing enzyme dicer is essential for the morphogenesis and maintenance of hair follicles. Curr Biol 16:1041–1049

Benkirane M, Neuveut C, Chun RF, Smith SM, Samuel CE, Gatignol A, Jeang KT (1997) Oncogenic potential of TAR RNA binding protein TRBP and its regulatory interaction with RNA-dependent protein kinase PKR. EMBO J 16:611–624

Bennasser Y, Yeung ML, Jeang KT (2006) HIV-1 TAR RNA subverts RNA interference in trans-
    fected cells through sequestration of TAR RNA-binding protein, TRBP. J Biol Chem
    281:27674–27678
Bernstein E, Caudy AA, Hammond SM, Hannon GJ (2001) Role for a bidentate ribonuclease in
    the initiation step of RNA interference. Nature 409:363–366
Bernstein E, Kim SY, Carmell MA, Murchison EP, Alcorn H, Li MZ, Mills AA, Elledge SJ,
    Anderson KV, Hannon GJ (2003) Dicer is essential for mouse development. Nat Genet
    35:215–217
Billy E, Brondani V, Zhang H, Muller U, Filipowicz W (2001) Specific interference with gene
    expression induced by long, double-stranded RNA in mouse embryonal teratocarcinoma cell
    lines. Proc Natl Acad Sci USA 98:14428–14433
Blaszczyk J, Tropea JE, Bubunenko M, Routzahn KM, Waugh DS, Court DL, Ji X (2001)
    Crystallographic and modeling studies of RNase III suggest a mechanism for double-stranded
    RNA cleavage. Structure 9:1225–1236
Borsani O, Zhu J, Verslues PE, Sunkar R, Zhu JK (2005) Endogenous siRNAs derived from a pair
    of natural cis-antisense transcripts regulate salt tolerance in Arabidopsis. Cell
    123:1279–1291
Carmell MA, Xuan Z, Zhang MQ, Hannon GJ (2002) The Argonaute family: tentacles that reach
    into RNAi, developmental control, stem cell maintenance, and tumorigenesis. Genes Dev
    16:2733–2742
Caudy AA, Hannon GJ (2004) Induction and biochemical purification of RNA-induced silencing
    complex from Drosophila S2 cells. Methods Mol Biol 265:59–72
Caudy AA, Myers M, Hannon GJ, Hammond SM (2002) Fragile X-related protein and VIG asso-
    ciate with the RNA interference machinery. Genes Dev 16:2491–2496
Cerutti H, Casas-Mollano JA (2006) On the origin and functions of RNA-mediated silencing:
    from protists to man. Curr Genet 50:81–99
Chendrimada TP, Gregory RI, Kumaraswamy E, Norman J, Cooch N, Nishikura K, Shiekhattar R
    (2005) TRBP recruits the Dicer complex to Ago2 for microRNA processing and gene silenc-
    ing. Nature 436:740–744
Cook HA, Koppetsch BS, Wu J, Theurkauf WE (2004) The Drosophila SDE3 homolog armit-
    age is required for oskar mRNA silencing and embryonic axis specification. Cell 116:
    817–829
Daher A, Longuet M, Dorin D, Bois F, Segeral E, Bannwarth S, Battisti PL, Purcell DF, Benarous R,
    Vaquero C, Meurs EF, Gatignol A (2001) Two dimerization domains in the trans-activation
    response RNA-binding protein (TRBP) individually reverse the protein kinase R inhibition of
    HIV-1 long terminal repeat expression. J Biol Chem 276:33899–33905
Dorin D, Bonnet MC, Bannwarth S, Gatignol A, Meurs EF, Vaquero C (2003) The TAR RNA-
    binding protein, TRBP, stimulates the expression of TAR-containing RNAs in vitro and in vivo
    independently of its ability to inhibit the dsRNA-dependent kinase PKR. J Biol Chem
    278:4440–4448
Drider D, Condon C (2004) The continuing story of endoribonuclease III. J Mol Microbiol
    Biotechnol 8:195–200
Duchaine TF, Wohlschlegel JA, Kennedy S, Bei Y, Conte D Jr, Pang K, Brownell DR, Harding S,
    Mitani S, Ruvkun G, Yates JR, 3rd Mello CC (2006) Functional proteomics reveals the bio-
    chemical niche of C. elegans DCR-1 in multiple small-RNA-mediated pathways. Cell
    124:343–354
Elbashir SM, Lendeckel W, Tuschl T (2001) RNA interference is mediated by 21- and 22-nucle-
    otide RNAs. Genes Dev 15:188–200
Fire A, Xu S, Montgomery MK, Kostas SA, Driver SE, Mello CC (1998) Potent and specific
    genetic interference by double-stranded RNA in Caenorhabditis elegans. Nature
    391:806–811
Forstemann K, Tomari Y, Du T, Vagin VV, Denli AM, Bratu DP, Klattenhoff C, Theurkauf WE,
    Zamore PD (2005) Normal microRNA maturation and germ-line stem cell maintenance
    requires loquacious, a double-stranded RNA-binding domain protein. PLoS Biol 3:e236

Fukagawa T, Nogami M, Yoshikawa M, Ikeno M, Okazaki T, Takami Y, Nakayama T, Oshimura M (2004) Dicer is essential for formation of the heterochromatin structure in vertebrate cells. Nat Cell Biol 6:784–791

Gasciolli V, Mallory AC, Bartel DP, Vaucheret H (2005) Partially redundant functions of Arabidopsis DICER-like enzymes and a role for DCL4 in producing trans-acting siRNAs. Curr Biol 15:1494–1500

Giraldez AJ, Mishima Y, Rihel J, Grocock RJ, Van Dongen S, Inoue K, Enright AJ, Schier AF (2006) Zebrafish MiR-430 promotes deadenylation and clearance of maternal mRNAs. Science 312:75–79

Gregory RI, Chendrimada TP, Cooch N, Shiekhattar R (2005) Human RISC couples microRNA biogenesis and posttranscriptional gene silencing. Cell 123:631–640

Grewal SI, Jia S (2007) Heterochromatin revisited. Nat Rev Genet 8:35–46

Grishok A, Tabara H, Mello CC (2000) Genetic requirements for inheritance of RNAi in C. elegans. Science 287:2494–2497

Grishok A, Pasquinelli AE, Conte D, Li N, Parrish S, Ha I, Baillie DL, Fire A, Ruvkun G, Mello CC (2001) Genes and mechanisms related to RNA interference regulate expression of the small temporal RNAs that control C. elegans developmental timing. Cell 106:23–34

Guex N, Peitsch MC (1997) SWISS-MODEL and the Swiss-PdbViewer: an environment for comparative protein modeling. Electrophoresis 18:2714–2723

Gupta V, Huang X, Patel RC (2003) The carboxy-terminal, M3 motifs of PACT and TRBP have opposite effects on PKR activity. Virology 315:283–291

Haase AD, Jaskiewicz L, Zhang H, Laine S, Sack R, Gatignol A, Filipowicz W (2005) TRBP, a regulator of cellular PKR and HIV-1 virus expression, interacts with Dicer and functions in RNA silencing. EMBO Rep 6:961–967

Hamilton AJ, Baulcombe DC (1999) A species of small antisense RNA in posttranscriptional gene silencing in plants. Science 286:950–952

Hammond SM, Bernstein E, Beach D, Hannon GJ (2000) An RNA-directed nuclease mediates post-transcriptional gene silencing in Drosophila cells. Nature 404:293–296

Hammond SM, Boettcher S, Caudy AA, Kobayashi R, Hannon GJ (2001) Argonaute2, a link between genetic and biochemical analyses of RNAi. Science 293:1146–1150

Han J, Lee Y, Yeom KH, Kim YK, Jin H, Kim VN (2004) The Drosha-DGCR8 complex in primary microRNA processing. Genes Dev 18:3016–3027

Han J, Lee Y, Yeom KH, Nam JW, Heo I, Rhee JK, Sohn SY, Cho Y, Zhang BT, Kim VN (2006) Molecular basis for the recognition of primary microRNAs by the Drosha-DGCR8 complex. Cell 125:887–901

Harfe BD, McManus MT, Mansfield JH, Hornstein E, Tabin CJ (2005) The RNaseIII enzyme Dicer is required for morphogenesis but not patterning of the vertebrate limb. Proc Natl Acad Sci USA 102:10898–10903

Harris KS, Zhang Z, McManus MT, Harfe BD, Sun X (2006) Dicer function is essential for lung epithelium morphogenesis. Proc Natl Acad Sci USA 103:2208–2213

Hiraguri A, Itoh R, Kondo N, Nomura Y, Aizawa D, Murai Y, Koiwa H, Seki M, Shinozaki K, Fukuhara T (2005) Specific interactions between Dicer-like proteins and HYL1/DRB-family dsRNA-binding proteins in Arabidopsis thaliana. Plant Mol Biol 57:173–188

Hutvagner G, McLachlan J, Pasquinelli AE, Balint E, Tuschl T, Zamore PD (2001) A cellular function for the RNA-interference enzyme Dicer in the maturation of the let-7 small temporal RNA. Science 293:834–838

Irvine DV, Zaratiegui M, Tolia NH, Goto DB, Chitwood DH, Vaughn MW, Joshua-Tor L, Martienssen RA (2006) Argonaute slicing is required for heterochromatic silencing and spreading. Science 313:1134–1137

Ishizuka A, Siomi MC, Siomi H (2002) A Drosophila fragile X protein interacts with components of RNAi and ribosomal proteins. Genes Dev 16:2497–2508

Jin P, Zarnescu DC, Ceman S, Nakamoto M, Mowrey J, Jongens TA, Nelson DL, Moses K, Warren ST (2004) Biochemical and genetic interaction between the fragile X mental retardation protein and the microRNA pathway. Nat Neurosci 7:113–117

Kanellopoulou C, Muljo SA, Kung AL, Ganesan S, Drapkin R, Jenuwein T, Livingston DM, Rajewsky K (2005) Dicer-deficient mouse embryonic stem cells are defective in differentiation and centromeric silencing. Genes Dev 19:489–501

Ketting RF (2006) Partners in dicing. Genome Biol 7:210

Ketting RF, Fischer SE, Bernstein E, Sijen T, Hannon GJ, Plasterk RH (2001) Dicer functions in RNA interference and in synthesis of small RNA involved in developmental timing in C. elegans. Genes Dev 15:2654–2659

Khvorova A, Reynolds A, Jayasena SD (2003) Functional siRNAs and miRNAs exhibit strand bias. Cell 115:209–216

Kim DH, Behlke MA, Rose SD, Chang MS, Choi S, Rossi JJ (2005) Synthetic dsRNA Dicer substrates enhance RNAi potency and efficacy. Nat Biotechnol 23:222–226

Kim VN (2005) MicroRNA biogenesis: coordinated cropping and dicing. Nat Rev Mol Cell Biol 6:376–385

Kotaja N, Bhattacharyya SN, Jaskiewicz L, Kimmins S, Parvinen M, Filipowicz W, Sassone-Corsi P (2006) The chromatoid body of male germ cells: similarity with processing bodies and presence of Dicer and microRNA pathway components. Proc Natl Acad Sci USA 103: 2647–2652

Krol J, Sobczak K, Wilczynska U, Drath M, Jasinska A, Kaczynska D, Krzyzosiak WJ (2004) Structural features of microRNA (miRNA) precursors and their relevance to miRNA biogenesis and small interfering RNA/short hairpin RNA design. J Biol Chem 279: 42230–42239

Kurihara Y, Watanabe Y (2004) Arabidopsis micro-RNA biogenesis through Dicer-like 1 protein functions. Proc Natl Acad Sci USA 101:12753–12758

Lamontagne B, Tremblay A, Abou Elela S (2000) The N-terminal domain that distinguishes yeast from bacterial RNase III contains a dimerization signal required for efficient double-stranded RNA cleavage. Mol Cell Biol 20:1104–1115

Lee JY, Kim H, Ryu CH, Kim JY, Choi BH, Lim Y, Huh PW, Kim YH, Lee KH, Jun TY, Rha HK, Kang JK, Choi CR (2004a) Merlin, a tumor suppressor, interacts with transactivation-responsive RNA-binding protein and inhibits its oncogenic activity. J Biol Chem 279: 30265–30273

Lee Y, Hur I, Park SY, Kim YK, Suh MR, Kim VN (2006) The role of PACT in the RNA silencing pathway. EMBO J 25:522–532

Lee YS, Nakahara K, Pham JW, Kim K, He Z, Sontheimer EJ, Carthew RW (2004b) Distinct roles for Drosophila Dicer-1 and Dicer-2 in the siRNA/miRNA silencing pathways. Cell 117:69–81

Lingel A, Simon B, Izaurralde E, Sattler M (2003) Structure and nucleic-acid binding of the Drosophila Argonaute 2 PAZ domain. Nature 426:465–469

Liu J, Carmell MA, Rivas FV, Marsden CG, Thomson JM, Song JJ, Hammond SM, Joshua-Tor L, Hannon GJ (2004) Argonaute2 is the catalytic engine of mammalian RNAi. Science 305: 1437–1441

Liu Q, Rand TA, Kalidas S, Du F, Kim HE, Smith DP, Wang X (2003) R2D2, a bridge between the initiation and effector steps of the Drosophila RNAi pathway. Science 301:1921–1925

Ma JB, Ye K, Patel DJ (2004) Structural basis for overhang-specific small interfering RNA recognition by the PAZ domain. Nature 429:318–322

Ma JB, Yuan YR, Meister G, Pei Y, Tuschl T, Patel DJ (2005) Structural basis for 5′-end-specific recognition of guide RNA by the A. fulgidus Piwi protein. Nature 434:666–670

Macrae IJ, Zhou K, Li F, Repic A, Brooks AN, Cande WZ, Adams PD, Doudna JA (2006) Structural basis for double-stranded RNA processing by Dicer. Science 311:195–198

Maniataki E, Mourelatos Z (2005) A human, ATP-independent, RISC assembly machine fueled by pre-miRNA. Genes Dev 19:2979–2990

Margis R, Fusaro AF, Smith NA, Curtin SJ, Watson JM, Finnegan EJ, Waterhouse PM (2006) The evolution and diversification of Dicers in plants. FEBS Lett 580:2442–2450

Martens H, Novotny J, Oberstrass J, Steck TL, Postlethwait P, Nellen W (2002) RNAi in Dictyostelium: the role of RNA-directed RNA polymerases and double-stranded RNase. Mol Cell Biol 13:445–453

Martinez J, Patkaniowska A, Urlaub H, Luhrmann R, Tuschl T (2002) Single-stranded antisense siRNAs guide target RNA cleavage in RNAi. Cell 110:563–574

Matzke MA, Birchler JA (2005) RNAi-mediated pathways in the nucleus. Nat Rev Genet 6:24–35

Meister G, Landthaler M, Patkaniowska A, Dorsett Y, Teng G, Tuschl T (2004) Human Argonaute2 mediates RNA cleavage targeted by miRNAs and siRNAs. Mol Cell 15:185–197

Murchison EP, Hannon GJ (2004) miRNAs on the move: miRNA biogenesis and the RNAi machinery. Curr Opin Cell Biol 16:223–229

Murchison EP, Partridge JF, Tam OH, Cheloufi S, Hannon GJ (2005) Characterization of Dicer-deficient murine embryonic stem cells. Proc Natl Acad Sci USA 102:12135–12140

Murchison EP, Stein P, Xuan Z, Pan H, Zhang MQ, Schultz RM, Hannon GJ (2007) Critical roles for Dicer in the female germline. Genes Dev 21:682–693

Nicholson AW (2003) The ribonuclease III superfamily: forms and functions in RNA maturation, decay, and gene silencing. In: Hannon GJ (ed) RNAi—a guide to gene silencing. Cold Spring Harbor Laboratory Press, New York, pp 149–174

Nykanen A, Haley B, Zamore PD (2001) ATP requirements and small interfering RNA structure in the RNA interference pathway. Cell 107:309–321

Okamura K, Ishizuka A, Siomi H, Siomi MC (2004) Distinct roles for Argonaute proteins in small RNA-directed RNA cleavage pathways. Genes Dev 18:1655–1666

Park W, Li J, Song R, Messing J, Chen X (2002) CARPEL FACTORY, a Dicer homolog, and HEN1, a novel protein, act in microRNA metabolism in Arabidopsis thaliana. Curr Biol 12:1484–1495

Parker JS, Roe SM, Barford D (2004) Crystal structure of a PIWI protein suggests mechanisms for siRNA recognition and slicer activity. EMBO J 23:4727–4737

Parker JS, Roe SM, Barford D (2005) Structural insights into mRNA recognition from a PIWI domain-siRNA guide complex. Nature 434:663–666

Pellino JL, Jaskiewicz L, Filipowicz W, Sontheimer EJ (2005) ATP modulates siRNA interactions with an endogenous human Dicer complex. RNA 11:1719–1724

Pham JW, Pellino JL, Lee YS, Carthew RW, Sontheimer EJ (2004) A Dicer-2-dependent 80 s complex cleaves targeted mRNAs during RNAi in Drosophila. Cell 117:83–94

Preall JB, He Z, Gorra JM, Sontheimer EJ (2006) Short interfering RNA strand selection is independent of dsRNA processing polarity during RNAi in Drosophila. Curr Biol 16:530–535

Provost P, Dishart D, Doucet J, Frendewey D, Samuelsson B, Radmark O (2002) Ribonuclease activity and RNA binding of recombinant human Dicer. EMBO J 21:5864–5874

Reinhart BJ, Weinstein EG, Rhoades MW, Bartel B, Bartel DP (2002) MicroRNAs in plants. Genes Dev 16:1616–1626

Rivas FV, Tolia NH, Song JJ, Aragon JP, Liu J, Hannon GJ, Joshua-Tor L (2005) Purified Argonaute2 and an siRNA form recombinant human RISC. Nat Struct Mol Biol 12:340–349

Rose SD, Kim DH, Amarzguioui M, Heidel JD, Collingwood MA, Davis ME, Rossi JJ, Behlke MA (2005) Functional polarity is introduced by Dicer processing of short substrate RNAs. Nucleic Acids Res 33:4140–4156

Saito K, Ishizuka A, Siomi H, Siomi MC (2005) Processing of pre-microRNAs by the Dicer-1-loquacious complex in Drosophila cells. PLoS Biol 3:e235

Schwarz DS, Hutvagner G, Du T, Xu Z, Aronin N, Zamore PD (2003) Asymmetry in the assembly of the RNAi enzyme complex. Cell 115:199–208

Shi H, Tschudi C, Ullu E (2006) An unusual Dicer-like1 protein fuels the RNA interference pathway in Trypanosoma brucei. RNA 12:2063–2072

Siolas D, Lerner C, Burchard J, Ge W, Linsley PS, Paddison PJ, Hannon GJ, Cleary MA (2005) Synthetic shRNAs as potent RNAi triggers. Nat Biotechnol 23:227–231

Song JJ, Liu J, Tolia NH, Schneiderman J, Smith SK, Martienssen RA, Hannon GJ, Joshua-Tor L (2003) The crystal structure of the Argonaute2 PAZ domain reveals an RNA binding motif in RNAi effector complexes. Nat Struct Biol 10:1026–1032

Song JJ, Smith SK, Hannon GJ, Joshua-Tor L (2004) Crystal structure of Argonaute and its implications for RISC slicer activity. Science 305:1434–1437

Tabara H, Sarkissian M, Kelly WG, Fleenor J, Grishok A, Timmons L, Fire A, Mello CC (1999) The rde-1 gene, RNA interference, and transposon silencing in C. elegans. Cell 99: 123–132

Tabara H, Yigit E, Siomi H, Mello CC (2002) The dsRNA binding protein RDE-4 interacts with RDE-1, DCR-1, and a DExH-box helicase to direct RNAi in C. elegans. Cell 109:861–871

Tahbaz N, Kolb FA, Zhang H, Jaronczyk K, Filipowicz W, Hobman TC (2004) Characterization of the interactions between mammalian PAZ PIWI domain proteins and Dicer. EMBO Rep 5:189–194

Tang F, Kaneda M, O'Carroll D, Hajkova P, Barton SC, Sun YA, Lee C, Tarakhovsky A, Lao K, Surani MA (2007) Maternal microRNAs are essential for mouse zygotic development. Genes Dev 21:644–648

Tolia NH, Joshua-Tor L (2007) Slicer and the argonautes. Nat Chem Biol 3:36–43

Tomari Y, Zamore PD (2005) Perspective: machines for RNAi. Genes Dev 19:517–529

Tomari Y, Du T, Haley B, Schwarz DS, Bennett R, Cook HA, Koppetsch BS, Theurkauf WE, Zamore PD (2004a) RISC assembly defects in the Drosophila RNAi mutant armitage. Cell 116:831–841

Tomari Y, Matranga C, Haley B, Martinez N, Zamore PD (2004b) A protein sensor for siRNA asymmetry. Science 306:1377–1380

Vazquez F, Vaucheret H, Rajagopalan R, Lepers C, Gasciolli V, Mallory AC, Hilbert JL, Bartel DP, Crete P (2004) Endogenous trans-acting siRNAs regulate the accumulation of Arabidopsis mRNAs. Mol Cell 16:69–79

Verdel A, Jia S, Gerber S, Sugiyama T, Gygi S, Grewal SI, Moazed D (2004) RNAi-mediated targeting of heterochromatin by the RITS complex. Science 303:672–676

Wienholds E, Plasterk RH (2005) MicroRNA function in animal development. FEBS Lett 579:5911–5922

Xie Z, Johansen LK, Gustafson AM, Kasschau KD, Lellis AD, Zilberman D, Jacobsen SE, Carrington JC (2004) Genetic and functional diversification of small RNA pathways in plants. PLoS Biol 2:E104

Xie Z, Allen E, Wilken A, Carrington JC (2005) DICER-LIKE 4 functions in trans-acting small interfering RNA biogenesis and vegetative phase change in Arabidopsis thaliana. Proc Natl Acad Sci USA 102:12984–12989

Yan KS, Yan S, Farooq A, Han A, Zeng L, Zhou MM (2003) Structure and conserved RNA binding of the PAZ domain. Nature 426:468–474

Yang WJ, Yang DD, Na S, Sandusky GE, Zhang Q, Zhao G (2005) Dicer is required for embryonic angiogenesis during mouse development. J Biol Chem 280:9330–9335

Yoneyama M, Kikuchi M, Natsukawa T, Shinobu N, Imaizumi T, Miyagishi M, Taira K, Akira S, Fujita T (2004) The RNA helicase RIG-I has an essential function in double-stranded RNA-induced innate antiviral responses. Nat Immunol 5:730–737

Yuan YR, Pei Y, Ma JB, Kuryavyi V, Zhadina M, Meister G, Chen HY, Dauter Z, Tuschl T, Patel DJ (2005) Crystal structure of A. aeolicus argonaute, a site-specific DNA-guided endoribonuclease, provides insights into RISC-mediated mRNA cleavage. Mol Cell 19: 405–419

Yuan YR, Pei Y, Chen HY, Tuschl T, Patel DJ (2006) A potential protein-RNA recognition event along the RISC-loading pathway from the structure of A. aeolicus Argonaute with externally bound siRNA. Structure 14:1557–1565

Zamore PD, Tuschl T, Sharp PA, Bartel DP (2000) RNAi: double-stranded RNA directs the ATP-dependent cleavage of mRNA at 21 to 23 nucleotide intervals. Cell 101:25–33

Zaratiegui M, Irvine DV, Martienssen RA (2007) Noncoding RNAs and gene silencing. Cell 128:763–776

Zhang H, Kolb FA, Brondani V, Billy E, Filipowicz W (2002) Human Dicer preferentially cleaves dsRNAs at their termini without a requirement for ATP. EMBO J 21:5875–5885

Zhang H, Kolb FA, Jaskiewicz L, Westhof E, Filipowicz W (2004) Single processing center models for human Dicer and bacterial RNase III. Cell 118:57–68

Zhong J, Peters AH, Lee K, Braun RE (1999) A double-stranded RNA binding protein required for activation of repressed messages in mammalian germ cells. Nat Genet 22:171–174

The Mechanism of RNase III Action:
How Dicer Dices

Xinhua Ji

Abstract Members of the Ribonuclease III (RNase III) family are double-stranded (ds) RNA-specific endoribonucleases, characterized by a signature motif in their active centers and a 2-nucleotide (nt) 3′ overhang in their products. Dicer functions as a dsRNA-processing enzyme, producing small interfering RNA (siRNA) of approx. 24 nt in length (approx. 20-basepair RNA duplex with a 2-nt 3′ overhang on each end). Bacterial RNase III functions not only as a processing enzyme, but also as a binding protein that binds dsRNA without cleaving it. As a processing enzyme it produces siRNA-like RNA of approx. 13 nt in length (approx. 9-basepair duplex with a 2-nt 3′ overhang on each end) as well as various types of mature RNA. Dicer is structurally most complicated member of the family; bacterial RNase III is comparatively much simpler. One structure is known for Dicer in its RNA-free form (MacRae, Zhou, Li, Repic, Brooks, Cande, Adams, and Doudna, *Science* 311:195–198); many structures are available for bacterial RNase III, including the

Xinhua Ji

Macromolecular Crystallography laboratory, National Cancer Institute, National Institutes of Health, Frederick, MD 21702-1201, USA

jix@ncifcrf.gov

P.J. Paddison and P.K. Vogt (eds.), *RNA Interference.*
Current Topics in Microbiology and Immunology 320.
© Springer-Verlag Berlin Heidelberg 2008

first catalytic complex of the entire family (Gan, Tropea, Austin, Court, Waugh, and Ji, *Cell* 124:355–366). In light of the structural and biochemical information on the RNase III proteins and the structure of a non-Dicer PAZ (Piwi Argonaute Zwille) domain in complex with a 7-basepair RNA duplex with a 2-nt 3′ overhang on each end (Ma, Ye, and Patel, *Nature* 429:318–322), the structure and function of Dicer is being elucidated.

Abbreviations Aa-RNase III: *Aquifex aeolicus* RNase III; Ago: Argonaute; ds: Double-stranded; dsRBD: dsRNA-binding domain; endoND: Endonuclease domain; Ec-RNase III: *Escherichia coli* RNase III; Gi-Dicer: *Giardia intestinalis* Dicer; Hs-Ago1; *Homo sapiens* Ago1; Hs-Dicer: *Homo sapiens* Dicer; nt: Nucleotide; PAZ: Piwi Argonaute Zwille; PDB: Protein Data Bank; siRNA: Small interfering RNA; ss: Single-stranded; RISC: RNA-induced silencing complex; RMSD: Root-mean-square deviation; RNAi: RNA interference; RNase III: Ribonuclease III; Sp-Dicer: *Schizosaccharomyces pombe* Dicer

1 Introduction

In the mechanism of RNA interference (RNAi), three consecutive events have been demonstrated. First, Dicer processes a double-stranded (ds) RNA into small interfering RNA (siRNA) molecules (Bernstein et al. 2001; Carthew 2001). Second, a dsRNA-binding protein (Chendrimada et al. 2005) recruits a Dicer–siRNA complex to Argonaute2 (Ago2), and the Ago2 cleaves the anti-guide strand of the siRNA duplex (Rand et al. 2005). Third, the passenger-strand cleavage facilitates assembly of the remaining single-stranded (ss) antisense siRNA along with the Ago2 into an RNA-induced silencing complex (RISC) (Matranga et al. 2005), where the ss antisense siRNA guides the cleavage of target RNA by Ago2 (Martinez et al. 2002). Hence, Dicer (and homologs) and Ago2 (and homologs) are responsible for the cleavage of dsRNA and ssRNA, respectively, in the RNAi pathway.

Dicer belongs to the ribonuclease III (RNase III) family, a highly conserved family of dsRNA-specific endoribonucleases (Robertson et al. 1968; Court 1993; Nicholson 1996; Krainer 1997; Nicholson 1999; Filippov et al. 2000), playing important roles in RNA processing (Robertson et al. 1968), posttranscriptional gene expression control (Court 1993; Krainer 1997; Wu et al. 2000), and defense against virus infection (Saleh et al. 2004; van Rij and Andino 2006). In plants and fungi, the substrates of Dicer are genome-encoded precursors folded as dsRNA-like hairpins; whereas in animals, the dsRNA substrates are formed in cells by DNA- or RNA-dependent synthesis (Caplen et al. 2001; Elbashir et al. 2001; Filipowicz 2005). The production of siRNA by Dicer requires the occurrence of two cleavage events, one cut on each RNA strand, creating a 2-nt 3′ overhang at each end of the siRNA, which is essential for downstream gene silencing (Ohmichi et al. 2002). Therefore, how each cleavage is carried out, how the 2-nt 3′ overhang is created, and how the length of siRNA is determined are three fundamental questions for the catalytic mechanism of Dicer.

The RNase III family, ranging in length from approx. 200 to approx. 2,000 amino acid residues, can be divided into four classes with increasing molecular weight and complexity of the polypeptide chain, exemplified by bacterial RNase III, *Saccharomyces cerevisiae* Rnt1p, *Drosophila melanogaster* Drosha, and *Homo sapiens* Dicer (Hs-Dicer), respectively (Blaszczyk et al. 2004). The bacterial RNase III proteins are composed of an endonuclease domain (endoND) followed by a dsRNA-binding domain (dsRBD). In addition to an endoND and a dsRBD, Rnt1p has an N-terminal domain of approx. 200 amino acid residues (Lamontagne et al. 2001). Drosha has a large N-terminal extension of approx. 900 amino acid residues followed by two endoNDs and one dsRBD (Filippov et al. 2000). Finally, Dicer has two endoNDs, one dsRBD, and an even larger N-terminal extension of approx. 1,500 amino acid residues that includes an RNA helicase domain and a Piwi Argonaute Zwille (PAZ) domain (Bernstein et al. 2001). Figure 1A depicts the domain structures of four RNase III proteins, including Hs-Dicer, *Schizosaccharomyces pombe* Dicer (Sp-Dicer), *Giardia intestinalis* Dicer (Gi-Dicer), and *Aquifex aeolicus* RNase III (Aa-RNase III). The sequence of each endoND is characterized by a stretch of eight conserved residues, which is known as the RNase III signature

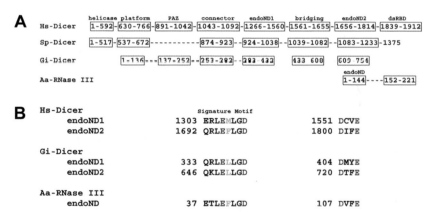

Fig. 1 A, B RNase III proteins and catalytic residues. **A** Domain structure of RNase III proteins: Hs-Dicer (SWISS-PROT Q9UPY3), Sp-Dicer (SWISS-PROT Q09884), Gi-Dicer (SWISS-PROT Q7R2M2), and Aa-RNase III (SWISS-PROT O67082). The domain boundaries (indicated with *boxed ranges* of amino acid sequence) for Gi-Dicer and Aa-RNase III are derived from crystal structures (PDB entries 2FFL and 2EZ6, Table 1) while those for Hs- and Sp-Dicer are on the basis of sequence analysis. The size of gaps between domains is not proportional to the length of amino acid sequences. **B** RNase III signature motif in the endoND and the catalytic residues (in *red*) of Hs-Dicer, Gi-Dicer, and Aa-RNase III. Indicated in *green* is the ball residue of the ball-and-socket junction

motif (Fig. 1B). Bacterial RNase III (and Rnt1p) contains one endoND and functions as a homodimer (Robertson et al. 1968; Gan et al. 2006), whereas Dicer (and Drosha) contains two endoNDs and functions as a monomer (Zhang et al. 2004; MacRae et al. 2006).

2 Domain Structure and Function of RNase III Proteins

To date, 16 three-dimensional structures of RNase III in various liganded forms have been reported (Table 1). Although the *Escherichia coli* enzyme is the most extensively studied member of the RNase III family, structural information for RNase III has thus far been restricted to enzymes from other organisms, especially *A. aeolicus*. Accordingly, in the following sections, the amino acid residue numbers of Aa-RNase III will be used unless otherwise stated. The structures that are most

Table 1 Three-dimensional structures of RNase III proteins

Source	Protein	Mutation	Ligands	$\mathring{A}^a$	PDB[b] accession code
G. intestinalis	Dicer		Mn^{2+}	3.30	2FFL (MacRae et al. 2006)
S. cerevisiae	dsRBD		RNA hairpin[c]	NMR	1T4L (Wu et al. 2004)
	dsRBD			NMR	1T4N (Leulliot et al. 2004)
	dsRBD			2.50	1T4O (Leulliot et al. 2004)
E. coli	dsRBD			NMR	N/A[d] (Kharrat et al. 1995)
T. maritima	RNase III			2.00	1O0W[e]
M. tuberculosis	endoND		Ca^{2+}	2.10	2A11 (Akey and Berger 2005)
A. aeolicus	endoND			2.15	1I4S (Blaszczyk et al. 2001)
	endoND		Mn^{2+}	2.15	1JFZ (Blaszczyk et al. 2001)
	endoND		Mg^{2+}	2.30	1RC5 (Blaszczyk et al. 2004)
	RNase III	E110K	dsRNA[f]	2.15	1RC7 (Blaszczyk et al. 2004)
	RNase III		dsRNA[g]	2.50	1YYK (Gan et al. 2005)
	RNase III	E110K	dsRNA[g]	2.90	1YYO (Gan et al. 2005)
	RNase III		dsRNA[h]	2.80	1YYW (Gan et al. 2005)
	RNase III	E110Q	dsRNA[i]	2.10	1YY9 (Gan et al. 2005)
	RNase III	D44N	Mg^{2+}, dsRNA[j]	2.05	2EZ6 (Gan et al. 2006)

[a]For crystal structures only
[b]Protein Data Bank (Berman et al. 2000)
[c]The 5' terminal RNA hairpin of Snr47 precursor
[d]Coordinates are not available
[e]Primary reference is not available
[f]dsRNA formed by self-complimentary sequence 5'-GGCGCGCGCC–3'
[g]dsRNA formed by self-complementary sequence 5'-CGCGAAUUCGCG–3'
[h]dsRNA formed by self-complementary sequence 5'-AAAUAUAUAUUU–3'
[i]dsRNA formed by self-complementary sequence 5'-CGAACUUCGCG–3'
[j]A dsRNA-like hairpin, product of a dsRNA cleavage reaction, of the sequence
5'-AAAGGUCAUUCGCAAGAGUGGCCUUUAU–3'

informative within the scope of this study include the 3.3-Å structure of Gi-Dicer in complex with Mn^{2+} (PDB entry 2FFL, Table 1) and the 2.05-Å structure of Aa-RNase III in complex with dsRNA and Mg^{2+} (PDB entry 2EZ6, Table 1). In addition, the 2.6-Å structure of the PAZ domain of human Ago1 (Hs-Ago1) in complex with a siRNA-like duplex (PDB entry 1SI3) suggests possible interactions between the PAZ domain and RNA in Dicer (Ma et al. 2004). The three structures, Gi-Dicer • Mn^{2+} (2FFL), Aa-RNase III • dsRNA • Mg^{2+} (2EZ6), and Hs-Ago1-PAZ • dsRNA (1SI3), are depicted in Fig. 2.

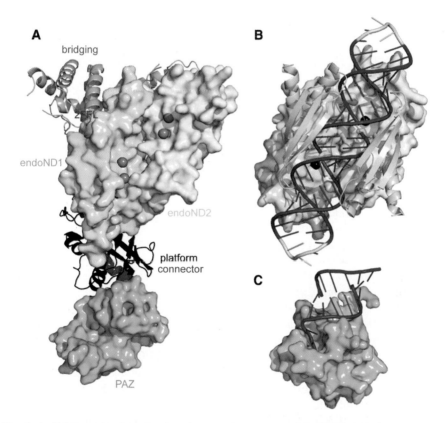

Fig. 2 A–C Schematic view showing the crystal structures of **A** Gi-Dicer • Mn^{2+} (PDB entry 2FFL, Table 1), **B** Aa-RNase III • dsRNA • Mg^{2+} (2EZ6, Table 1), and **C** Hs-Ago1-PAZ • dsRNA (1SI3). Proteins are illustrated as surface representations and ribbon diagrams (helices as *spirals*, β-strands as *arrows*, and loops as *pipes*), RNA as *rod* (backbone) and *sticks* (bases), and metal ions as *spheres*. The proteins are color-coded on the basis of their domain structures (Fig. 1A): platform in *black*, PAZ in *green*, connector in *red*, endoND in *cyan* or *yellow*, spacer in *pink*, and dsRBD in *gray*. The Mn^{2+} ions are *gray* and Mg^{2+} are *black*. The dsRNA strands are in *red* and *blue*, and the stem-loop in *gray*. The orientations of the three structures are consistent on the basis of Cα-trace alignment between corresponding domains

2.1   The Helicase Domain: Unclear Function

RNA helicases dissociate RNA duplexes in an ATP-dependent manner (Cordin et al. 2006). However, the in vitro dsRNA processing activity is not ATP-dependent for Hs-Dicer (Provost et al. 2002; Zhang et al. 2002), whereas it is ATP-dependent for *Drosophila melanogaster* Dicer-2 (Nykanen et al. 2001; Liu et al. 2003; Lee et al. 2004). The reason for this discrepancy on the ATP dependence of Dicer function is not clear (Meister and Tuschl 2004). Gi-Dicer does not have an N-terminal helicase domain (Fig. 1A) but is fully functional both in vitro and in vivo (MacRae et al. 2006), indicating that the helicase domain is dispensable for the function of Dicer.

2.2   The PAZ Domain: Indispensable for Dicer Function

The PAZ domain is highly conserved exclusively in Dicer and Ago proteins (Cerutti et al. 2000; Carmell et al. 2002). The three-dimensional structure of Ago-PAZ has been elucidated as a stand-alone domain structure (Lingel et al. 2003; Yan et al. 2003; Lingel et al. 2004; Ma et al. 2004), as a maltose-binding protein fusion (Song et al. 2003), and embedded in Ago2 (Song et al. 2004; Rivas et al. 2005; Yuan et al. 2005). Among these structures, the crystal structure of Hs-Ago1-PAZ•dsRNA, in which the 9-nt RNA forms an siRNA mimic with a 7-basepair A-form duplex and a 2-nt 3′ overhang at each end, suggests that the PAZ serves as an siRNA-end-binding module for siRNA transfer in the RNAi pathway and as an anchoring site for the 3′ end of guide RNA within the RISC (PDB entry 1SI3; Ma et al. 2004).

The superposition of Hs-Ago1-PAZ•dsRNA (1SI3) and the PAZ domain in Gi-Dicer•Mn^{2+} (PDB entry 2FFL, Table 1) indicates that the anchoring site for the 2-nt 3′ overhang of the PAZ in Gi-Dicer is located on the same side of the molecule with the RNase III catalytic valley (Fig. 2), suggesting that the Dicer-PAZ is also responsible for recognizing the 2-nt 3′ overhang of substrate and that the size of the siRNA product is linked to this recognition (Cook and Conti 2006; MacRae et al. 2006). Being involved in substrate recognition and functioning as a determinant for product size, the PAZ domain appears to be indispensable for Dicer function. Indeed, the purified C-terminal fragment of Hs-Dicer, encompassing the endoND1, endoND2, and dsRBD, did not show cleavage activity (Zhang et al. 2004). However, a PAZ domain has not been recognized in the sequence of Sp-Dicer (Fig. 1A). It remains to be seen whether the PAZ function in Sp-Dicer is fulfilled by a different structural motif or a PAZ-like domain is formed from a different amino acid sequence.

A seven-turn helix connects the PAZ domain and the endoND dimer. This helical connector is supported and perhaps also stabilized by the surrounding secondary structural elements formed by the platform domain (Fig. 1A and 2A). In addition to its structural role, this neck-like structure may also provide some flexibility to the Dicer molecule (Fig. 2). On the basis of sequence homology, it has been predicted that the structure formed by the helical connector and the platform domain should also exist in other Dicer proteins (MacRae et al. 2006).

2.3 The EndoND Dimer: Essential for RNase III Function

The endoND is strictly conserved in all RNase III proteins. All reported structures show that two endoNDs form a tight dimer. Aa-RNase III contains one endoND (Fig. 1A); the endoNDs from two molecules form a tight dimer (PDB entries 1I4S to 2EZ6, Table 1). It is also the case for the RNase III proteins from *Thermotoga maritime* and *Mycobacterium tuberculosis* (PDB entries 1O0 W and 2A11, Table 1). Gi-Dicer has two endoNDs (Fig. 1A); the two endoNDs dimerize intramolecularly (PDB entry 2FFL, Table 1). The endoND dimer of Aa-RNase III and that of Gi-Dicer superimpose well with a root-mean-square deviation (RMSD) of 2.2 Å for 234 pairs of Cα positions (Fig. 3A). Among the superimposed secondary structural elements, two α-helices display the smallest RMSDs, leading to virtually identical positioning of functionally important residues 40, 41, 44, 107, and 110 (Fig. 3A).

A bridging sequence in Gi-Dicer (Fig. 1A) forms a domain structure, which is packed against the endoND dimer (Fig. 2A). In the bridging domain among Dicer sequences, a stretch of conserved amino acid sequence (approx. 20 residues) has been identified and speculated as part of the Ago-binding site of Dicer (MacRae et al. 2006).

2.3.1 Subunit Interface

The subunit interface in the endoND dimer is a hydrophobic surface. A "ball-and-socket" junction is formed between the two subunits at each end of the interface. The ball from one endoND is the side-chain of residue 41. In the middle of the signature motif, it is a Phe in Aa-RNase III, but a Leu in Gi-Dicer (Fig. 1B). The socket is a cavity on the partner endoND (Fig. 3B and 3C). To assess the importance of the ball-and-socket junction, the ball residue in *E. coli* RNase III (Ec-RNase III) was mutated and tested for RNase III activity (Blaszczyk et al. 2001). The Gly, Asp, and Arg substitutions gave rise to a defective enzyme, whereas the Met and Trp mutants were functional (Table 2). It appears that the hydrophobic side-chains of the latter mutants can still function as the ball of the junction, but this interaction is precluded by the charged side-chains (Asp and Arg) or in the absence of any side-chain in this position (Gly). Interestingly, in the first signature motif of Hs-Dicer, a Met is located in the position of the ball residue (Fig. 1B).

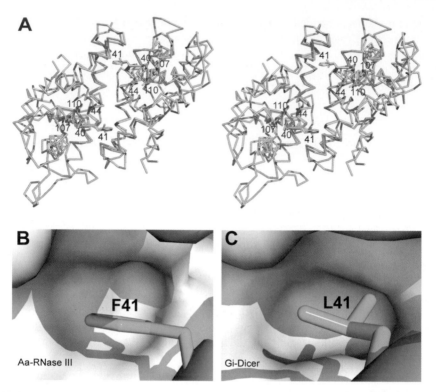

Fig. 3 A–C The endoND dimer of RNase III proteins. **A** Stereoview showing the Cα-trace super-position of the endoND dimer in Aa-RNase III(D44N)•dsRNA•Mg²⁺ (in *orange*, PDB entry 2EZ6, Table 1) and that in Gi-Dicer•Mn²⁺ (in *cyan*, 2FFL, Table 1). The side-chains of residues 40, 41, 44, 107, and 110 in each endoND are shown as *stick models*, in *orange* for Aa-RNase III and in atomic color scheme for Gi-Dicer (carbon in *cyan*, nitrogen in *blue*, and oxygen in *red*). **B** The ball-and-socket junction in the endoND dimer of Aa-RNase III (2EZ6). **C** The ball-and-socket junction in the endoND dimer of Gi-Dicer (2FFL). The stick model in *green* represents the side-chain of the ball residue from one subunit while the surface in *gray* illustrates the socket on the partner subunit

2.3.2 Catalytic Valley

The dimerization of endoND creates a large valley, 50 Å long and 20 Å wide, which accommodates a dsRNA substrate and is therefore referred to as the "catalytic valley" (Fig. 2A and B). The two ball-and-socket junctions appear to be responsible for accurately positioning the two signature motifs in the catalytic valley and the protein fold locates residues E107 and E110, which are distant in the polypeptide chain, in proximity to the signature motif, giving rise to two catalytic sites in the catalytic valley (Fig. 3A).

Table 2 Catalytic site mutations of *E. coli* RNase III and Hs-Dicer and their activities

Residue[a]	Protein	Mutation	In vitro dsRNA Binding	In vitro dsRNA Processing	In vivo activity	Reference(s)
E40	Ec-RNase III	A		-/+[b]		Sun et al. 2004
F41	Ec-RNase III	G			-	Blaszczyk et al. 2001
		D			-	Blaszczyk et al. 2001
		R			-	Blaszczyk et al. 2001
		M			+	Blaszczyk et al. 2001
		W			+	Blaszczyk et al. 2001
D44	Ec-RNase III	A			-	Blaszczyk et al. 2001
		A		-		Zhang et al. 2004
		A	+	-[c,d]		Sun et al. 2004
		E	+	[c,d]		Sun et al. 2004
		N	+	-[c,d]		Sun et al. 2004
	Hs-Dicer	A		-		Zhang et al. 2004
D107	Ec-RNase III	A		-/+[b]		Sun et al. 2004
E110	Ec-RNase III	K	+		-	Inada et al. 1989; Li and Nicholson 1996; Dasgupta et al. 1998
		Q	+		-	Sun and Nicholson 2001
		D	+	-[c,d]		Sun and Nicholson 2001
		A	+		-	Li and Nicholson 1996
		A		-		Zhang et al. 2004
	Hs-Dicer	A		-		Zhang et al. 2004

[a]The amino acid numbering system of Aa-RNase III is used
[b][Mg^{2+}]-dependent, exhibiting 108% and 52% (D107A), 36% and 5% (E40A) wildtype level cleavage activities in 10 and 1 mM Mg^{2+}, respectively
[c]Low level of cleavage activity is observed at extended reaction times and high enzyme concentrations
[d]Partial cleavage activity (~5,000-fold lower for the D44 mutants; ~2,700-fold lower for E110D) can be rescued by Mn^{2+}

2.3.3 Catalytic Site

The RNase III-catalyzed dsRNA cleavage is Mg^{2+}-dependent and probably proceeds in a single step via an S_N2 (bimolecular nucleophilic substitution)-type mechanism (Robertson et al. 1968; Dunn 1982; Li and Nicholson 1996; Sun and Nicholson 2001;

Campbell et al. 2002). Near each end of the catalytic valley is located a metal ion-coordinated cluster of four acidic side-chains, E40, D44, D107, and E110 (Fig. 3A). The four side-chains are conserved, among which E40 and D44 is also part of the signature motif (Fig. 1B). The recent structure of Aa-RNase III in complex with product of dsRNA cleavage (PDB entry 2EZ6, Table 1) reveals that this metal-coordinated cluster of acidic side-chains is the center of catalytic site (Gan et al. 2006).

Each catalytic site is composed of amino acid residues E40, D44, D107, and E110, nucleotide residues R−1, R 0, and R+1, and Mg^{2+} ion and water molecules (Fig. 4). Among the four acidic side-chains, the significance of E40 and D107 in catalysis is Mg^{2+}-concentration dependent, and therefore, redundant roles in metal binding have been proposed for these two side-chains (Table 2). In contrast, side-chains D44 and E110 are essential for catalysis because there is a stringent functional requirement for both the charge and size of these two side-chains (Table 2), which, together with their relationship with other components of the catalytic site, suggests the involvement of a second metal ion in the mechanism of RNase III. The crystal

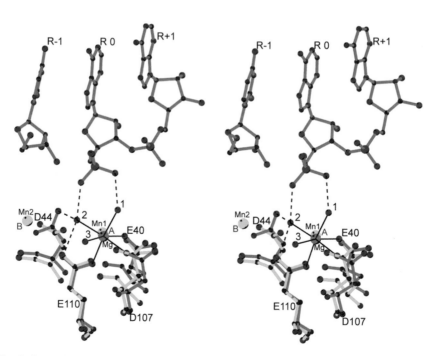

Fig. 4 Stereoview showing the catalytic site observed in Aa-RNase III • dsRNA • Mg^{2+} (in *orange*, PDB entry 2EZ6, Table 1) superimposed with that in Gi-Dicer • Mn^{2+} (in cyan, 2FFL, Table 1). Residues are shown as ball-and-stick models in atomic color scheme (carbon in *black*, nitrogen in *blue*, oxygen in *red*, phosphorous in *purple*, magnesium in *orange*, and manganese in *cyan*). Metal coordination bonds are indicated with *solid lines*, while hydrogen bonds with *dashed lines*. Metal sites A and B are indicated with *capital letters* in *red*

structure of Gi-Dicer•Mn^{2+} (PDB entry 2FFL, Table 1) suggests a position for a second metal ion (Fig. 4).

2.3.4   Metal Ions

RNase III enzymes belong to a superfamily of polynucleotidyl transferases that include RNases (MacRae et al. 2006), DNases, and transposases. Two-metal-ion catalysis was established for both Tn5 transposase (Davies et al. 2000; Steiniger-White et al. 2004) and RNase H (Nowotny et al. 2005; Nowotny and Yang 2006), and was predicted for RNase III on the basis of biochemical data (Sun et al. 2005) and related structural information (Gan et al. 2006; Yang et al. 2006).

To date, five crystal structures of RNase III proteins in complex with metal ions have been reported, including Aa-endoND•Mn^{2+} (PDB entry 1JFZ), Aa-endoND•Mg^{2+} (1RC5), Aa-RNase III(D44N)•dsRNA•Mg^{2+} (2EZ6), Gi-Dicer•Mn^{2+} (2FFL), and Mt-endoND•Ca^{2+} (2A11, Table 1). In all three structures of *A. aeolicus* protein (1JFZ, 1RC5, 2EZ6), only one metal ion (either Mn^{2+} or Mg^{2+}) was observed per endoND in the same position (named as metal site A, Fig. 4). In the Gi-Dicer•Mn^{2+} structure (2FFL), two Mn^{2+} ions were found close to the catalytic site in each endoND. One Mn^{2+} occupies metal site A, but the second Mn^{2+} occupies different positions in the two endoNDs. In one endoND, the second Mn^{2+} is located between the side-chains of D44 and E110 and near the scissile bond (named as metal site B, Fig. 4); whereas in the other, the second Mn^{2+} is located between the side-chains of E40 and D107 and the phosphate bridge between R 0 and R+1 (named metal site C, not shown). In the Mt-endoND•Ca^{2+} structure (2A11), two Ca^{2+} ions were identified per endoND; one occupies metal site A and the other occupies metal site C (not shown).

Metal A is a catalytic cation. In the Aa-RNase III(D44N)•dsRNA•Mg^{2+} structure (2EZ6), it coordinates with three acidic side-chains (E40, D107, and E110) and three water molecules (1, 2, and 3), assuming the geometry of an octahedron; also, it interacts with the side-chain of D44 via a water molecule (Fig. 4). In addition to interacting with the metal ion, E110 is also hydrogen bonded to water 2 that, together with water 1, interacts with the 5′ phosphate of RNA. Metal B is most likely the second catalytic cation as suggested by its location in proximity to the scissile bond and the D44 and E110 side-chains (Fig. 4).

The catalytic valley of RNase III is highly negatively charged (Blaszczyk et al. 2001); additional metal ions, including metal C, may be involved in the binding of dsRNA.

2.3.5   Hallmarks of RNase III Reaction Products

The crystal structure of the RNase III-product complex (PDB entry 2EZ6, Table 1) indicates that a single cleavage event occurs on each strand of the RNA within each catalytic site, which creates terminal phosphate group at the 5′ end of each strand

(Fig. 4), and the two RNA cleavage events together create the 2-nt 3′ overhang (Fig. 2B). The 3′-hydroxyl and 5′-phosphate groups and the 2-nt 3′ overhang are hallmarks of RNase III reaction products. It has been suggested that the 5′ phosphate groups of each strand are essential for the incorporation of siRNAs into the RNAi pathway (Schwarz et al. 2002). It has also been shown that short RNA duplexes without the 2-nt 3′ overhang do not initiate RNAi (Ohmichi et al. 2002).

The detailed mechanism for the hydrolysis of each scissile bond remains to be seen when the structure of an RNase III-substrate complex becomes available. Most likely, it resembles that of RNase H (Nowotny et al. 2005; Nowotny and Yang 2006). Although RNase H is specific for a RNA/DNA hybrid while RNase III is specific for dsRNA, the basic catalytic events by the two enzymes are the same, i.e., metal-dependent and sequence-nonspecific hydrolysis of an RNA phosphodiester bond. A comparison between the catalytic sites in the two enzymes can be found in Gan et al. (2006).

2.4   The dsRBD: Dynamic yet Dispensable

Comparative analysis of seven crystal structures of bacterial RNase III with or without bound dsRNA (PDB entries 1OOW, 1RC7, 1YYK, 1YYO, 1YYW, 1YY9, and 2EZ6, Table 1) demonstrates that the relative orientation between the endoND and the dsRBD varies dramatically. Both the endoND and the dsRBD are relatively rigid. Thus, the flexibility of a seven-residue linker between the two domains (Fig. 1A) is responsible for major conformational changes within the molecule (Gan et al. 2005, 2006). It was also shown that the length of the linker may vary; extension of the linker from 9 to 20 amino acids in Ec-RNase III does not affect the accuracy of scissile bond selection (Conrad et al. 2001).

In Hs-Dicer, the sequence between the endoND2 and dsRBD contains 24 amino acid residues (Fig. 1A). Therefore, the flexibility of the linker appears to be guaranteed. In the catalytic complex of Hs-Dicer, the dsRBD may interact with endoND2 and RNA in a similar manner as observed for the Aa-RNase III complex (Fig. 2B).

Gi-Dicer does not have a dsRBD (Fig. 1A), but it is fully functional both in vitro and in vivo (MacRae et al. 2006). A truncated form of Ec-RNase III without dsRBD was shown to accurately cleave certain processing substrates in vitro (Sun et al. 2001). The RNase III proteins in bacteria *Mycoplasma genitalium* and *Mycoplasma pneumoniae* do not have dsRBD (Tian et al. 2004). Therefore, the dsRBD is dispensable for the dsRNA-processing activity of RNase III proteins.

3   Minimal Functional Core of RNase III Proteins

Both the helicase domain and the dsRBD are dispensable for the enzymatic function of RNase III proteins. Thus, the minimal functional core of bacterial RNase III is the endoND dimer and that of Dicer is the platform-to-endoND2 fragment (Fig. 1).

3.1 The EndoND Dimer of Bacterial RNase III

Figure 5A depicts the minimal functional core of bacterial RNase III in complex with a cleaved RNA and four Mg^{2+} ions. The entire structure is taken from Aa-RNase III•dsRNA•Mg^{2+} (PDB entry 2EZ6, Table 1), except that the two Mg^{2+} ions in gray are modeled on the basis of the Gi-Dicer•Mn^{2+} structure (PDB entry 2FFL).

In the crystal structure of Aa-RNase III•dsRNA•Mg^{2+} (PDB entry 2EZ6), four RNA-binding motifs (RBMs 1 4) are identified, among which RBMs 1 and 2 are located in the dsRBD and RBMs 3 and 4 in the endoND (Gan et al. 2006). The four RBMs collectively recognize and bind a dsRNA substrate by forming seven hydrogen bonds with O2′ hydroxyls and projecting two loops (RBMs 2 and 4) into the minor groove. RBMs 1 and 2 play dominant roles in the initial recognition and binding of dsRNA, whereas RBM 3 and 4 are dominant in substrate specificity and scissile bond selection. Note that RBMs 1 and 2 do not discriminate against nonsubstrate dsRNA. It is RBMs 3 and 4 that discriminate against nonsubstrate dsRNA (Gan et al. 2006).

Without dsRBD, RBMs 1 and 2 are missing, which certainly reduces the affinity of the protein for dsRNA, but does not abolish its catalytic activity. Each RBM 3 interacts with one RNA strand and helps to define a scissile bond, while RBM 4 recognizes the minor groove of the RNA substrate (Fig. 5A). A typical product of bacterial RNase III is a 9-basepair dsRNA molecule with a 2-nt 3′ overhang on each end of the duplex, which fits perfectly the distance between the catalytic sites (as indicated by the metal ions) and RBM 4 (Fig. 5A).

3.2 The Platform-to-EndoND2 Fragment of Dicer

Figure 5B illustrates the minimal functional core of Dicer in complex with a cleaved RNA and four Mg^{2+} ions. The platform-to-endoND2 fragment is from the Gi-Dicer•Mn^{2+} structure (PDB entry 2FFL, Table 1), the RNA and the two Mg^{2+} ions in black are from the Aa-RNase III•dsRNA•Mg^{2+} structure (2EZ6) with an extension of the RNA to include an siRNA molecule, and the two Mg^{2+} ions in gray are modeled on the basis of the Gi-Dicer•Mn^{2+} structure (2FFL).

This structure-based model of Dicer•dsRNA•Mg^{2+} may represent a snapshot before product release in the catalytic cycle of stem-loop dsRNA processing (Fig. 5B). It is shown that a siRNA, containing a 20-bp A-form duplex with a 2-nt 3′ overhang on each end, fits the distance between the catalytic sites (as indicated with the metal ions) and the 2-nt 3′ overhang-anchoring site of the PAZ domain. Flexibility of the protein, RNA, or both is required for substrate binding. The neck-like structure of Dicer formed by the platform domain and the helical connector may provide certain amount of flexibility (Fig. 5B).

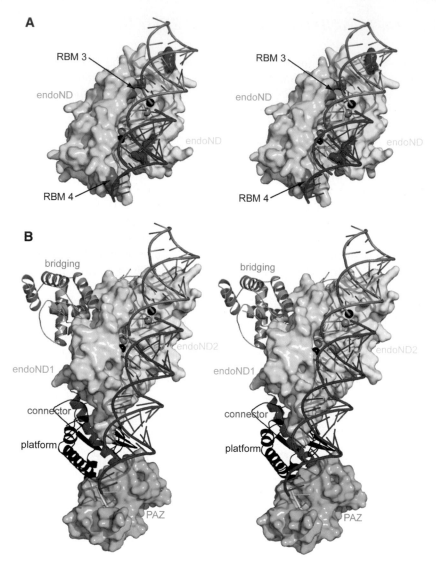

Fig. 5 A, B Stereoviews illustrating the minimal functional core of RNase III proteins. **A** The endoND dimer of bacterial RNase III is shown with dsRNA and four Mg^{2+} ions. The protein, RNA, and two Mg^{2+} ions are part of the Aa-RNase III·dsRNA·Mg^{2+} structure (PDB entry 2EZ6, Table 1). The two endoNDs are shown as molecular surfaces and colored in *cyan* and *yellow*, respectively. RNA-binding motifs (RBMs) 3 and 4 are highlighted in *blue* in one endoND and in *purple* in the other and are labeled for one set only. The RNA is shown as *rod* (backbone) and *sticks* (bases) with the product molecule highlighted as *red and blue strands*. The two Mg^{2+} ions from the Aa-RNase III·dsRNA·Mg^{2+} structure (2EZ6) are shown as a *black sphere*, while the other two, modeled according to the Gi-Dicer·Mn^{2+} structure (2FFL), are shown in *gray*. **B** The platform-to-endoND2 fragment of Dicer is shown with dsRNA and four Mg^{2+} ions. The protein is the Gi-Dicer·Mn^{2+} structure (2FFL). The RNA is part of the Aa-RNase III·dsRNA·Mg^{2+} structure (2EZ6) with an extension to include a typical siRNA that contains a 20-bp A-form dsRNA with a 2-nt 3' overhang on each end of the duplex. The PAZ domain and the two endoNDs are shown as

4   Conclusions

The dimerization of endoNDs, either intermolecularly (bacterial RNase III and Rnt1p) or intramolecularly (Drosha and Dicer), is essential for dsRNA-processing activity of RNase III proteins. A catalytic valley formed upon dimerization accommodates a dsRNA substrate. Two catalytic sites are located in the catalytic valley. The accurate arrangement of the two catalytic sites is achieved with the help of a ball-and-socket junction at each end of the dimer interface. The center of each catalytic site is the cluster of metal-coordinated side-chains E40, D44, D107, and E110. The hydrolysis of each RNA strand involves both endoNDs. Residues from one endoND (RBM 3 residues) are involved in the binding of the strand and the selection of the scissile bond, while those from the partner endoND (D44 and E110) are involved in the cleavage chemistry. The cleavage of both strands of a dsRNA substrate creates the characteristic 2-nt $3'$ overhang with $3'$-OH and $5'$-phosphate ends. The available structural and biochemical data suggest the requirement of a second divalent cation in the hydrolysis of each RNA strand.

Both the helicase domain and the dsRBD are dispensable for the dsRNA-processing activity of RNase III proteins. Therefore, the minimal functional core of bacterial RNase III is the endoND dimer, whereas that of Dicer is the platform-to-endoND2 fragment. The function of helicase domain is not clear. When the dsRBD is present, however, induced fit occurs during protein–RNA recognition and substrate binding, which is facilitated by a flexible linker connecting the dsRBD to the upstream endoND. In Dicer, a second event of induced fit may be facilitated by a neck-like structure formed by the platform domain and the connector between the PAZ domain and the endoND dimer. The PAZ domain may be involved in the recognition of the 2-nt $3'$ overhang of dsRNA substrate and serve as a determinant for the length of the products of dsRNA processing by Dicer.

Acknowledgements   I would like to thank all my co-workers who contributed to the work cited from this laboratory. I am particularly indebted to Drs. Jianhua Gan, Joseph Tropea, and Jaroslaw Blaszczyk for their invaluable contributions. This research was supported by the Intramural Research Program of the NIH, National Cancer Institute, Center for Cancer Research.

Fig. 5 (continued) molecular surfaces (in *green*, *cyan*, and *yellow*, respectively); the platform domain, the connector, and the bridging domain are shown as ribbon diagrams (in *black*, *red*, and *pink*, respectively). The 2-nt RNA segment in *gray* on the PAZ domain indicates the anchoring site for the 2-nt $3'$ overhang as suggested by the best achievable alignment between the Cα-traces of the two PAZ domains (1SI3 and 2FFL). The Mg^{2+} ions, modeled according to the Aa-RNase III·dsRNA·Mg^{2+} (2EZ6) and Gi-Dicer (2FFL) structure, are shown in *black* and *gray*, respectively

References

Akey DL, Berger JM (2005) Structure of the nuclease domain of ribonuclease III from M. tuberculosis at 2.1 Å. Protein Sci 14:2744–2750

Berman HM, Westbrook J, Feng Z, Gilliland G, Bhat TN, Weissig H, Shindyalov IN, Bourne PE (2000) The Protein Data Bank. Nucleic Acids Res 28:235–242

Bernstein E, Caudy AA, Hammond SM, Hannon GJ (2001) Role for a bidentate ribonuclease in the initiation step of RNA interference. Nature 409:363–366

Blaszczyk J, Tropea JE, Bubunenko M, Routzahn KM, Waugh DS, Court DL, Ji X (2001) Crystallographic and modeling studies of RNase III suggest a mechanism for double-stranded RNA cleavage. Structure 9:1225–1236

Blaszczyk J, Gan J, Tropea JE, Court DL, Waugh DS, Ji X (2004) Noncatalytic assembly of ribonuclease III with double-stranded RNA. Structure (Camb) 12:457–466

Campbell FE Jr, Cassano AG, Anderson VE, Harris ME (2002) Pre-steady-state and stopped-flow fluorescence analysis of Escherichia coli ribonuclease III: insights into mechanism and conformational changes associated with binding and catalysis. J Mol Biol 317:21–40

Caplen NJ, Parrish S, Imani F, Fire A, Morgan RA (2001) Specific inhibition of gene expression by small double-stranded RNAs in invertebrate and vertebrate systems. Proc Natl Acad Sci USA 98:9742–9747

Carmell MA, Xuan Z, Zhang MQ, Hannon GJ (2002) The Argonaute family: tentacles that reach into RNAi, developmental control, stem cell maintenance, and tumorigenesis. Genes Dev 16:2733–2742

Carthew RW (2001) Gene silencing by double-stranded RNA. Curr Opin Cell Biol 13:244–248

Cerutti L, Mian N, Bateman A (2000) Domains in gene silencing and cell differentiation proteins: the novel PAZ domain and redefinition of the Piwi domain. Trends Biochem Sci 25:481–482

Chendrimada TP, Gregory RI, Kumaraswamy E, Norman J, Cooch N, Nishikura K, Shiekhattar R (2005) TRBP recruits the Dicer complex to Ago2 for microRNA processing and gene silencing. Nature 436:740–744

Conrad C, Evguenieva-Hackenberg E, Klug G (2001) Both N-terminal catalytic and C-terminal RNA binding domain contribute to substrate specificity and cleavage site selection of RNase III. FEBS Lett 509:53–58

Cook A, Conti E (2006) Dicer measures up. Nat Struct Mol Biol 13:190–192

Cordin O, Banroques J, Tanner NK, Linder P (2006) The DEAD-box protein family of RNA helicases. Gene 367:17–37

Court D (1993) RNA processing and degradation by RNase III. In: Belasco JG, Braverman G (eds) Control of Messenger RNA Stability. Academic Press, New York, pp 71–116

Dasgupta S, Fernandez L, Kameyama L, Inada T, Nakamura Y, Pappas A, Court DL (1998) Genetic uncoupling of the dsRNA-binding and RNA cleavage activities of the Escherichia coli endoribonuclease RNase III—the effect of dsRNA binding on gene expression. Mol Microbiol 28:629–640

Davies DR, Goryshin IY, Reznikoff WS, Rayment I (2000) Three-dimensional structure of the Tn5 synaptic complex transposition intermediate. Science 289:77–85

Dunn JJ (1982) Ribonuclease III. In: Boyer P (ed) The enzymes. Academic Press, New York, pp 485–499

Elbashir SM, Harborth J, Lendeckel W, Yalcin A, Weber K, Tuschl T (2001) Duplexes of 21-nucleotide RNAs mediate RNA interference in cultured mammalian cells. Nature 411:494–498

Filipowicz W (2005) RNAi: the nuts and bolts of the RISC machine. Cell 122:17–20

Filippov V, Solovyev V, Filippova M, Gill SS (2000) A novel type of RNase III family proteins in eukaryotes. Gene 245:213–221

Gan J, Tropea JE, Austin BP, Court DL, Waugh DS, Ji X (2005) Intermediate states of ribonuclease III in complex with double-stranded RNA. Structure (Camb) 13:1435–1442

Gan J, Tropea JE, Austin BP, Court DL, Waugh DS, Ji X (2006) Structural insight into the mechanism of double-stranded RNA processing by ribonuclease III. Cell 124:355–366

Inada T, Kawakami K, Chen SM, Takiff HE, Court DL, Nakamura Y (1989) Temperature-sensitive lethal mutant of ERA, a G protein in Escherichia coli. J Bacteriol 171:5017–5024

Kharrat A, Macias MJ, Gibson TJ, Nilges M, Pastore A (1995) Structure of the dsRNA binding
domain of E. coli RNase III. EMBO J 14:3572–3584

Krainer A (1997) Eukaryotic mRNA processing. IRL Press, New York

Lamontagne B, Larose S, Boulanger J, Elela SA (2001) The RNase III family: a conserved structure and expanding functions in eukaryotic dsRNA metabolism. Curr Issues Mol Biol
3:71–78

Lee YS, Nakahara K, Pham JW, Kim K, He Z, Sontheimer EJ, Carthew RW (2004) Distinct roles
for Drosophila Dicer-1 and Dicer-2 in the siRNA/miRNA silencing pathways. Cell
117:69–81

Leulliot N, Quevillon-Cheruel S, Graille M, van Tilbeurgh H, Leeper TC, Godin KS, Edwards TE,
Sigurdsson ST, Rozenkrants N, Nagel RJ, Ares M, Varani G (2004) A new alpha-helical extension promotes RNA binding by the dsRBD of Rnt1p RNAse III. EMBO J 23:2468–2477

Li H, Nicholson AW (1996) Defining the enzyme binding domain of a ribonuclease III processing
signal. Ethylation interference and hydroxyl radical footprinting using catalytically inactive
RNase III mutants. EMBO J 15:1421–1433

Lingel A, Simon B, Izaurralde E, Sattler M (2003) Structure and nucleic-acid binding of the
Drosophila Argonaute 2 PAZ domain. Nature 426:465–469

Lingel A, Simon B, Izaurralde E, Sattler M (2004) Nucleic acid 3′-end recognition by the
Argonaute2 PAZ domain. Nat Struct Mol Biol 11:576–577

Liu Q, Rand TA, Kalidas S, Du F, Kim HE, Smith DP, Wang X (2003) R2D2, a bridge between
the initiation and effector steps of the Drosophila RNAi pathway. Science 301:1921–1925

Ma JB, Ye K, Patel DJ (2004) Structural basis for overhang-specific small interfering RNA recognition by the PAZ domain. Nature 429:318–322

MacRae IJ, Zhou K, Li F, Repic A, Brooks AN, Cande WZ, Adams PD, Doudna JA (2006)
Structural basis for double-stranded RNA processing by Dicer. Science 311:195–198

Martinez J, Patkaniowska A, Urlaub H, Luhrmann R, Tuschl T (2002) Single-stranded antisense
siRNAs guide target RNA cleavage in RNAi. Cell 110:563–574

Matranga C, Tomari Y, Shin C, Bartel DP, Zamore PD (2005) Passenger-strand cleavage facilitates
assembly of siRNA into Ago2-containing RNAi enzyme complexes. Cell 123:607–620

Meister G, Tuschl T (2004) Mechanisms of gene silencing by double-stranded RNA. Nature
431:343–349

Nicholson AW (1996) Structure, reactivity, and biology of double-stranded RNA. Prog Nucleic
Acid Res Mol Biol 52:1–65

Nicholson AW (1999) Function, mechanism and regulation of bacterial ribonucleases. FEMS
Microbiol Rev 23:371–390

Nowotny M, Yang W (2006) Stepwise analyses of metal ions in RNase H catalysis from substrate
destabilization to product release. EMBO J 25:1924–1933

Nowotny M, Gaidamakov SA, Crouch RJ, Yang W (2005) Crystal structures of RNase H bound
to an RNA/DNA hybrid: substrate specificity and metal-dependent catalysis. Cell
121:1005–1016

Nykanen A, Haley B, Zamore PD (2001) ATP requirements and small interfering RNA structure
in the RNA interference pathway. Cell 107:309–321

Ohmichi T, Karimata H, Sugimoto N (2002) Effect of secondary structure of short double-
stranded RNA on RNAi efficiency. Nucleic Acids Res Suppl 63–64

Provost P, Dishart D, Doucet J, Frendewey D, Samuelsson B, Radmark O (2002) Ribonuclease
activity and RNA binding of recombinant human Dicer. EMBO J 21:5864–5874

Rand TA, Petersen S, Du F, Wang X (2005) Argonaute2 cleaves the anti-guide strand of siRNA
during RISC activation. Cell 123:621–629

Rivas FV, Tolia NH, Song JJ, Aragon JP, Liu J, Hannon GJ, Joshua-Tor L (2005) Purified
Argonaute2 and an siRNA form recombinant human RISC. Nat Struct Mol Biol 12:340–349

Robertson HD, Webster RE, Zinder ND (1968) Purification and properties of ribonuclease III from Escherichia coli. J Biol Chem 243:82–91

Saleh MC, Van Rij RP, Andino R (2004) RNA silencing in viral infections: insights from poliovirus. Virus Res 102:11–17

Schwarz DS, Hutvagner G, Haley B, Zamore PD (2002) Evidence that siRNAs function as guides, not primers, in the Drosophila and human RNAi pathways. Mol Cell 10:537–548

Song JJ, Liu J, Tolia NH, Schneiderman J, Smith SK, Martienssen RA, Hannon GJ, Joshua-Tor L (2003) The crystal structure of the Argonaute2 PAZ domain reveals an RNA binding motif in RNAi effector complexes. Nat Struct Biol 10:1026–1032

Song JJ, Smith SK, Hannon GJ, Joshua-Tor L (2004) Crystal structure of Argonaute and its implications for RISC slicer activity. Science 305:1434–1437

Steiniger-White M, Rayment I, Reznikoff WS (2004) Structure/function insights into Tn5 transposition. Curr Opin Struct Biol 14:50–57

Sun W, Nicholson AW (2001) Mechanism of action of Escherichia coli ribonuclease III. Stringent chemical requirement for the glutamic acid 117 side-chain and Mn(2+) rescue of the Glu117Asp mutant. Biochemistry 40:5102–5110

Sun W, Jun E, Nicholson AW (2001) Intrinsic double-stranded-RNA processing activity of Escherichia coli ribonuclease III lacking the dsRNA-binding domain. Biochemistry 40:14976–14984

Sun W, Li G, Nicholson AW (2004) Mutational analysis of the nuclease domain of Escherichia coli ribonuclease III. Identification of conserved acidic residues that are important for catalytic function in vitro. Biochemistry 43:13054–13062

Sun W, Pertzev A, Nicholson AW (2005) Catalytic mechanism of Escherichia coli ribonuclease III: kinetic and inhibitor evidence for the involvement of two magnesium ions in RNA phosphodiester hydrolysis. Nucleic Acids Res 33:807–815

Tian B, Bevilacqua PC, Diegelman-Parente A, Mathews MB (2004) The double-stranded-RNA-binding motif: interference and much more. Nat Rev Mol Cell Biol 5:1013–1023

van Rij RP, Andino R (2006) The silent treatment: RNAi as a defense against virus infection in mammals. Trends Biotechnol 24:186–193

Wu H, Xu H, Miraglia LJ, Crooke ST (2000) Human RNase III is a 160-kDa protein involved in preribosomal RNA processing. J Biol Chem 275:36957–36965

Wu H, Henras A, Chanfreau G, Feigon J (2004) Structural basis for recognition of the AGNN tetraloop RNA fold by the double-stranded RNA-binding domain of Rnt1p RNase III. Proc Natl Acad Sci USA 101:8307–8312

Yan KS, Yan S, Farooq A, Han A, Zeng L, Zhou MM (2003) Structure and conserved RNA binding of the PAZ domain. Nature 426:468–474

Yang W, Lee JY, Nowotny M (2006) Making and breaking nucleic acids: two-Mg2+-ion catalysis and substrate specificity. Mol Cell 22:5–13

Yuan YR, Pei Y, Ma JB, Kuryavyi V, Zhadina M, Meister G, Chen HY, Dauter Z, Tuschl T, Patel DJ (2005) Crystal structure of A. aeolicus argonaute, a site-specific DNA-guided endoribonuclease, provides insights into RISC-mediated mRNA cleavage. Mol Cell 19:405–419

Zhang H, Kolb FA, Brondani V, Billy E, Filipowicz W (2002) Human Dicer preferentially cleaves dsRNAs at their termini without a requirement for ATP. EMBO J 21:5875–5885

Zhang H, Kolb FA, Jaskiewicz L, Westhof E, Filipowicz W (2004) Single processing center models for human Dicer and bacterial RNase III. Cell 118:57–68

MicroRNA Metabolism in Plants

Xuemei Chen

Abstract MicroRNAs (miRNAs) are 21- to 24-nucleotide (nt) RNAs that are the final products of nonprotein-coding genes. miRNAs are processed from single-stranded precursors that form hairpin structures, with the miRNAs residing in one arm of the stems. miRNAs were first isolated and recognized as regulators of protein-coding genes through forward genetic screens in *Caenorhabditis elegans*, but were not recognized as universal regulators of gene expression in animals until three landmark studies in year 2001 demonstrated the widespread

Xuemei Chen
Department of Botany and Plant Sciences, University of California, Riverside, Riverside, CA 92521, USA
xuemei.chen@ucr.edu

P.J. Paddison and P.K. Vogt (eds.), *RNA Interference.*
Current Topics in Microbiology and Immunology 320.
© Springer-Verlag Berlin Heidelberg 2008

existence of miRNAs in animals. Soon after, studies from a few groups identified a number of miRNAs from *Arabidopsis*, providing the first evidence for the existence of these regulatory molecules in plants. Since then, numerous miRNAs from a number of land plants ranging from mosses to flowering plants were identified, and functional studies in *Arabidopsis* established a framework of understanding of miRNA biogenesis and function. This chapter summarizes the current knowledge as well as gaps in our understanding of plant miRNA biogenesis and function.

1   MicroRNA Discovery in Plants

The discovery of microRNAs (miRNAs) in plants is still an ongoing process. Although much effort has been directed toward miRNA identification in *Arabidopsis* and rice, many economically or evolutionarily important species have yet to be examined, and more miRNAs likely remain to be discovered even in the species that have been extensively studied. One limiting factor in the miRNA discovery process is the availability of a sequenced genome, without which a comprehensive analysis of the potential precursor structures of cloned small RNAs is not possible. During the initial cloning of small RNAs from *Arabidopsis* and rice, it became clear that plants are extremely rich in endogenous small RNAs and that only a small portion of cloned small RNAs corresponds to miRNAs (Llave et al. 2002a; Mette et al. 2002). The majority of endogenous small RNA species represents small interfering RNAs (siRNAs). The only difference between miRNAs and siRNAs lies in their biogenesis. While an miRNA and its miRNA* are the main, if not only, sequences resulting from the processing of a single-stranded precursor that forms hairpin structures, siRNAs are generated from long double-stranded RNAs (dsRNAs) or single-stranded RNAs that form hairpin structures. In the cases where siRNAs are derived from a single-stranded hairpin precursor, usually multiple species from the same precursor are produced. Therefore, it is crucial that sequences that flank a cloned small RNA be available to allow the analysis of the potential precursor structure. It is also important that enough small RNAs have been found from a particular locus to distinguish an miRNA-generating locus from an siRNA-generating locus.

In *Arabidopsis*, three major methods have been used for miRNA discovery: forward genetics, direct cloning and sequencing, and bioinformatic prediction. Although forward genetic studies have only resulted in the identification of a few miRNAs, this method provides hints to the functions of these miRNAs in addition to their isolation. For example, an early flowering mutant was isolated and the early flowering phenotype was caused by the overexpression of miR172 (Aukerman and Sakai 2003). Leaf wrinkling in a mutant was caused by the overexpression of miR-Jaw (Palatnik et al. 2003). In a genetic screen for floral patterning mutants, a mutant that produces extra petals in early flowers was isolated and the mutation was in one of the three members of the miR164 family (Baker et al. 2005). This loss-of-function mutant in one member of a small miRNA gene family demonstrates that the members of the gene family are not completely functionally redundant. A mutant that had extremely large and disorganized meristems was found to be due to the overexpression of miR166g (Williams et al. 2005). While a loss-of-function mutation in a *MIR* gene clearly indicates the function of this miRNA in the developmental process, the gain-of-function mutants resulting from overexpression of the miRNAs do not necessarily suggest a function of these miRNAs in the developmental processes but do indicate that proper control of the miRNA levels is important for the developmental processes.

A second approach to miRNA discovery was bioinformatic prediction. While a number of published studies employed several different algorithms to predict miRNAs, the features that the algorithms search for in the genomic sequences are based on our current knowledge of plant miRNAs and are largely similar among the studies (Bonnet et al. 2004; Jones-Rhoades and Bartel 2004; Wang et al. 2004; Adai et al. 2005). These features include the intergenic location of the *MIR* genes, the high degree of sequence complementarity of miRNAs to their mRNA targets, the hairpin structures of the precursors, and the conservation of some miRNAs between two species (*Arabidopsis* and rice). Most algorithms begin by extracting intergenic sequences, and then apply other filters such as conservation between rice and *Arabidopsis*, or complementarity to target mRNAs to further refine the prediction. Others start by extracting all sequence segments that have the potential to form hairpin RNAs, and then apply other filters such as conservation between rice and *Arabidopsis* or complementarity to mRNAs to further refine the search. One obvious drawback of the bioinformatic approach is that either the initial prediction phase or the subsequent refinement phase relies on sequence conservation, which makes it difficult to predict species-specific miRNAs.

A third, and perhaps the most effective, method for miRNA discovery was direct cloning and sequencing. In particular, deep sequencing of cloned small RNA libraries using massively parallel signature sequencing (MPSS) or pyrosequencing allowed the identification of numerous small RNAs from *Arabidopsis* and provided a picture of the genomic landscape of small RNAs (Lu et al. 2005, 2006; Axtell et al. 2006; Henderson et al. 2006; Rajagopalan et al. 2006; Fahlgren et al. 2007; Kasschau et al. 2007; Zhang et al. 2007). One added advantage of this approach is that most small RNA species from a particular genomic loci are exhibited, which helps discern whether the locus gives rise to an miRNA or multiple siRNAs. If multiple small RNAs mapping to both strands of a locus are present, these small RNAs are most likely siRNAs. Another advantage of deep sequencing is that the antisense strands to the small RNAs (also known as miRNA* or siRNA*) that are also released from the precursor during small RNA biogenesis are often detected, although at much lower frequency compared to the sense strands. This also helps identify the miRNAs from the small RNA populations since, by definition, the miRNA and the miRNA* should map to the same strand and should be separated by tens to hundreds of nucleotides.

2 MicroRNA Genes in Plants: Organization, Conservation, and Origin

As of June 2007, the miRBase (http://microrna.sanger.ac.uk/sequences/index.shtml) version 9.2 contains a total of 959 *MIR* genes from 10 plant species including moss, dicots, and monocots. Several features of plant *MIR* genes can be readily discerned from the current sets of miRNAs. First, plant *MIR* genes often have paralogs such that the 184 *Arabidopsis* miRNAs in miRBase version 9.2 represent approximately 100 families of related miRNAs. *MIR* gene families arose from the process of gene duplication and diversification that also drives the evolution of protein-coding gene families (Maher et al. 2006). Second, each species has an evolutionarily fluid set of miRNAs. Some miRNA families, such as miR156, miR160, miR319, and miR390, appear to be of ancient origin such that they are conserved from mosses to flowering plants (Arazi et al. 2005; Axtell and Bartel 2005). Since the complete genome of a nonflowering land plant is not currently available, it is not possible to determine how many miRNA families are conserved among land plants through homology searches. Some miRNA families evolved after mosses and flowering plants diverged but before the divergence of monocots and dicots. Intriguingly, a large set of miRNA families is not shared among two of the three sequenced angiosperm genomes (*Arabidopsis*, poplar, and rice), suggesting that these miRNAs are evolutionarily "young" miRNAs. Among the known families of miRNAs in *Arabidopsis*, 4 are conserved down to mosses, 20 are shared between *Arabidopsis* and rice, while 22 are conserved between *Arabidopsis* and poplar. The remaining families are so far unique to *Arabidopsis*, but as the genomes of species closely related to *Arabidopsis* become available, some of these families may be found to be common to these related species. Consistent with the notion that the nonconserved miRNAs represent evolutionarily "young" miRNAs, these miRNAs are predominantly found at single loci in the genome. Third, the great majority of plant miRNA genes are located in intergenic regions, which is in contrast to animal miRNA genes that tend to be localized in introns or exons of protein-coding genes (reviewed in Kim 2005). Finally, unlike animal miRNA genes that are often found in clusters and that are transcribed into a polycistronic RNA (reviewed in Kim 2005), plant miRNA genes are usually not arranged in tandem in the genome or co-expressed. In the current set of *Arabidopsis* miRNAs, only three pairs of *MIR* genes (*MIR169i* and *MIR169j*; *MIR169k* and *MIR169l*; *MIR169m* and *MIR169n*) are arranged such that the two miRNAs are in the same orientation and are within 500 bp of each other. It is possible that each gene pair is co-transcribed.

The fact that *Arabidopsis* has many *MIR* gene families that are not found in poplar or rice suggests that *MIR* genes continue to be generated during the evolution of land plants. Some of these "young" *Arabidopsis* miRNAs (such as miR161, miR163, miR826, miR841, miR842, and miR846) revealed one potential mechanism by which miRNA genes originate in evolution (Allen et al. 2004; Rajagopalan et al. 2006; Fahlgren et al. 2007). The precursors to these miRNAs show extensive sequence similarity to their target genes, which led to the model that de novo generation of miRNA genes results from an inverted duplication event of the target genes. Transcription through the inverted repeats, which are likely to diverge in sequence after the initial duplication event, would result in an RNA with an imperfect hairpin structure reminiscent of miRNA precursors.

Plants and animals were thought to have evolved miRNAs independently since they do not share common miRNAs. However, a recent study identified an *Arabidopsis* miRNA, miR854, that has potential homologs in four examined animal (including human) genomes, and these homologs only differ from miR854 by one nucleotide (Arteaga-Vazquez et al. 2006). Human and mice miR854 were detectable by RNA filter hybridization. *Arabidopsis* miR854 has multiple binding sites in the 3′ untranslated region (UTR) of the *UBP1* gene that encodes an hnRNP protein and causes translation inhibition of *UBP1* expression. The animal miR854 is also complementary to a site in the 3′ UTR of the *UBP1* homologs. If the animal miR854 is to be confirmed as a regulator of its predicted target in animals in the future, miR854 and its target gene will be the first example of a conserved miRNA/ target pair between plant and animal kingdoms.

3   MicroRNA Biogenesis in *Arabidopsis*

3.1   *Transcription*

All *Arabidopsis* miRNAs analyzed so far have their own transcriptional units such that each *MIR* gene is transcribed into a primary precursor known as pri-miRNA. This was first suggested by the intergenic location of *MIR* genes and later confirmed by the presence of expressed sequence tags (ESTs) corresponding to miRNA precursor transcripts. The first indications that plant *MIR* genes are transcribed by RNA polymerase II were that pri-miRNAs can be found to correspond to ESTs representing polyadenylated transcripts and that some pri-miRNAs that have been characterized contain introns. The most conclusive study showed that 5′ capped transcripts were detected for 52 of the 99 tested *MIR* genes (Xie et al. 2005a). The great majority of the pri-miRNAs begin with an adenosine, which is located within 40 nt downstream of a conserved TATA box-like sequence. A bioinformatic analysis of 800-nt regions upstream of the mapped transcription start sites in these genes identified binding motifs for a number of known transcription factors (Megraw et al. 2006).

3.2   *Dicer Processing*

Plant miRNAs, like their animal counterparts, are released from pri-miRNAs through at least two sequential processing steps by RNase III enzymes. In animals, pri-miRNAs are first processed by an RNase III enzyme Drosha to the hairpin RNAs, known as pre-miRNAs, the immediate precursors to miRNAs (reviewed in

Kim 2005). This processing step occurs in the nucleus and is assisted by the dsRNA-binding protein DGCR8. The pre-miRNAs are then exported to the cytoplasm by exportin 5 and the pre-miRNAs are further processed by another RNase III enzyme, Dicer, to a duplex of the miRNAs and the antisense strands (miRNA*s). Plants do not have Drosha homologs, and the two sequential processing steps are both carried out by Dicer-like 1 (DCL1), a Dicer homolog.

The requirement for DCL1 in miRNA processing was revealed by the fact that partial loss-of-function mutants in *DCL1* have greatly reduced accumulation of miRNAs and consequently exhibit pleiotropic developmental defects (Ray et al. 1996; Jacobsen et al. 1999; Park et al. 2002; Reinhardt et al. 2002). Null mutations in *DCL1* lead to embryonic lethality (Schwartz et al. 1994; McElver et al. 2001). Immunoprecipitated DCL1 from *Arabidopsis* was shown to be able to produce 21-nt small RNAs from long dsRNAs (Qi et al. 2005). This study, however, did not test whether DCL1 can release miRNAs from a pri- or pre-miRNA. That DCL1 converts pri-miRNAs to pre-miRNAs is inferred from the fact that pre-miRNAs are reduced in abundance while pri-miRNAs accumulate to higher levels in *dcl1* mutants (Kurihara and Watanabe 2004; Kurihara et al. 2006). The processing of pri-miRNAs to pre-miRNAs by DCL1 also requires two other proteins, HYPONASTIC LEAVES1 (HYL1) and SERRATE (SE). HYL1 belongs to a family of dsRNA-binding proteins in *Arabidopsis* (Lu and Fedoroff 2000; Hiraguri et al. 2005). Loss-of-function mutations in *HYL1* result in reduced accumulation of many miRNAs and elevated expression of miRNA target genes (Han et al. 2004; Vazquez et al. 2004a). The increased accumulation of pri-miRNAs and decreased levels of pre-miRNAs in *hyl1* mutants suggests that HYL1 is required for the processing of pri-miRNAs to pre-miRNAs (Kurihara et al. 2006). In fact, HYL1 has been found to interact with DCL1 in vitro and in a transient expression assay in *Nicotiana benthamiana* (Hiraguri et al. 2005; Kurihara et al. 2006). SE encodes a C2H2 zinc finger protein that was initially found to specify leaf polarity through promoting the accumulation of miR165/166 (Grigg et al. 2005). Later, it was demonstrated that SE plays a general role in the biogenesis of many miRNAs (Lobbes et al. 2006; Yang et al. 2006a). Since *se* mutants lead to increased accumulation of pri-miRNAs, SE likely acts in the processing of pri-miRNAs to pre-miRNAs (Lobbes et al. 2006; Yang et al. 2006a). This is consistent with the finding that SE interacts with HYL1 (Lobbes et al. 2006; Yang et al. 2006a). Although there is so far no direct genetic or biochemical evidence that DCL1 also processes pre-miRNAs, the fact that mutations in other *Arabidopsis* Dicer homologs (*DCL2*, *DCL3*, and *DCL4*) do not affect the accumulation of the great majority of miRNAs (Xie et al. 2004; Gasciolli et al. 2005; Xie et al. 2005b; Yoshikawa et al. 2005) suggests that this is most likely the case. Recently, a study showed that HYL1 immunoprecipitate from Arabidopsis was able to process pre-miRNAs in vitro (Wu et al. 2007). RNAi-mediated knockdown of *DCL1* in rice led to reduced accumulation of miRNAs and pleiotropic developmental phenotypes, suggesting that the function of DCL1 in miRNA biogenesis is conserved between monocots and dicots (Liu et al. 2005).

While DCL2, DCL3, and DCL4 are mainly responsible for processing long dsRNAs into siRNAs, a recent study showed that DCL4 also plays a minor role in the biogenesis of a small number of miRNAs in *Arabidopsis*. In particular, two "young" miRNAs, miR822 and miR839, still accumulate in *dcl1* mutants but fail to accumulate in *dcl4* mutants (Rajagopalan et al. 2006). Interestingly, the precursors of these two miRNAs are hairpins of relatively long double-stranded regions. The extensive double-strandedness of the precursors perhaps reflects a short evolutionary course after the initial duplication events that gave rise to the miRNA genes. miR822 was previously annotated as an siRNA due to its independence on DCL1 for biogenesis (Allen et al. 2004). However, deep sequencing revealed that this miRNA comes from a single-stranded hairpin RNA rather than a long dsRNA. In addition, the accumulation of this miRNA does not depend on RDR2 or RDR6, which are responsible for generating long dsRNAs in the biogenesis of siRNAs (Boutet et al. 2003; Vazquez et al. 2004b; Xie et al. 2004; Borsani et al. 2005; Yoshikawa et al. 2005; Katiyar-Agarwal et al. 2006). We may hypothesize that during the evolution of *MIR* genes, the inverted duplication of a locus initially gives rise to a hairpin RNA with perfect or near perfect double-strandedness and this hairpin is initially recognized by DCL4 (or may be DCL3 or DCL2). As the inverted repeat sequences diverge and the hairpin accumulates more and more bulges and mismatches, DCL4 fails to recognize the RNA and DCL1 gains access to the RNA.

It should also be noted that DCL1 is not limited to the production of miRNAs. DCL1 is required for the biogenesis of one class of siRNAs known as nat-siRNAs (Borsani et al. 2005; Katiyar-Agarwal et al. 2006), although the biochemical mechanism of DCL1 in this process is unknown.

3.3 Methylation

3.3.1 HEN1 Is a MicroRNA Methyltransferase

The biogenesis of plant miRNAs differs from that of animal miRNAs in that methylation of miRNAs occurs after Dicer processing. We discovered this additional step in plant miRNA biogenesis from our studies on a gene named *HEN1*, which was first isolated as a gene important in flower development (Chen et al. 2002). The fact that *hen1* mutants share similar developmental defects with partial loss-of-function *dcl1* mutants prompted us to test whether HEN1 is a general miRNA biogenesis factor. Indeed, we found that most miRNAs are reduced in abundance in *hen1* mutants, which confirmed a general role of HEN1 in miRNA biogenesis (Park et al. 2002). The clue that HEN1 may be a methyltransferase came from position-iterated basic local alignment search tool (PSI-BLAST) searches that showed that the C-terminal domain (~200 amino acid) of HEN1 resembles methyltransferases. In particular, a highly conserved *S*-adenosyl methionine (SAM)-binding site is found in this region of HEN1. The known *hen1* mutant alleles that carry point mutations, such as *hen1-1*, *hen1-2*, and *hen1-4*, all contain mutations in the methyltransferase region (Chen et al. 2002; Bonnet et al. 2004). Knowing that HEN1 serves as a general factor in miRNA biogenesis and that HEN1 has a potential methyltransferase domain, we postulated that HEN1 is an miRNA methyltransferase.

We tested our hypothesis by purifying glutathione S-transferase (GST)-HEN1 protein from *E. coli* and carrying out methyltransferase assays using various molecules in miRNA biogenesis as substrates. The substrates tested included pre-miRNAs, miRNAs, miRNA*s, and miRNA/miRNA* duplexes. The assay was set up such that the substrates were each incubated with GST-HEN1 or GST alone, C^{14}-SAM as the methyl donor, and buffer. After the reactions, the RNAs were extracted and analyzed by gel electrophoresis followed by autoradiography. We found that among the various intermediates in miRNA biogenesis tested as substrates, only miRNA/miRNA* duplexes were methylated by GST-HEN1 (Yu et al. 2005). A number of different miRNA/miRNA* duplexes were substrates of HEN1, indicating that HEN1 is a general, sequence-independent miRNA methyltransferase.

3.3.2 HEN1 Deposits a Methyl Group on the 2′ OH of the 3′ Terminal Nucleotide

We determined the features that HEN1 recognizes in its substrates. We found that HEN1 has a strict requirement for the 2 nt 3′ overhang in the miRNA/miRNA* duplex, a characteristic of Dicer products. Although blunt ends can be methylated at greatly reduced efficiency, miRNA/miRNA* duplexes with 1 nt, 3 nt, 4 nt, or 5 nt overhangs fail to be methylated (Yang et al. 2006b). We tested whether other features of Dicer products, such as 5′ P and 3′ OH, are recognized by HEN1. We found that the 3′ OH but not the 5′ P is a necessary feature of the HEN1 substrates (Yu et al. 2005). The 2′ OH of the 3′ terminal nucleotide is also necessary for HEN1-mediated methylation (Yu et al. 2005). Another feature of Dicer products is the specific size; *Arabidopsis* DCL proteins generate 21–24 nt small RNAs (Gasciolli et al. 2005; Xie et al. 2005b). We found that HEN1 is able to "measure" the size of the miRNA/miRNA* duplexes. While duplexes ranging from 19 nt to 27 nt in size can be methylated in vitro by HEN1, 21- to 24-nt duplexes are methylated with the best efficiency (Yang et al. 2006b). The strict requirement for the 2-nt overhang and the 3′ OH, and the preference for 21- to 24-nt duplexes, probably ensure that only Dicer products are methylated in vivo. miRNA/miRNA* duplexes often contain mismatches or bulges whereas siRNA/siRNA* duplexes do not. We found that HEN1 can methylate both miRNA/miRNA* and siRNA/siRNA* duplexes in vitro.

We determined where the methyl group(s) is deposited onto the miRNA after the in vitro reaction. The requirement for both the 2′ and 3′ OH on the ribose of the 3′ terminal nucleotide for methylation prompted us to test whether the methyl group(s) is deposited on one of the OH groups on the 3′ terminal nucleotide. We first tested whether the OH groups are blocked after the HEN1-mediated reaction. The status of the OH groups can be assayed with chemical reactions (periodate treatment followed by β elimination) that require the presence of both OH groups on the ribose of the 3′ terminal nucleotide. These chemical reactions lead to the elimination of the 3′ terminal nucleotide to result in an RNA that is shorter (by 1 nt) and contains a 3′ P (Alefelder et al. 1998). The resulting RNA can be distinguished from the original RNA by high-resolution gel electrophoresis. We assayed the miRNAs after the HEN-mediated in vitro reaction and found that the miRNAs are resistant to periodate/β elimination reactions, indicating that the methyl group(s) is on one of the OH groups on the 3′ terminal nucleotide (Yu et al. 2005). To determine whether methylation occurs on the 2′ OH, 3′ OH, or both, we established conditions that allowed us to separate 2′-O-methyl cytidine and 3′-O-methyl cytidine by HPLC. Analysis of the nucleosides from miRNAs methylated by HEN1 in vitro demonstrated that HEN1 deposits a methyl group exclusively onto the 2′ OH of the 3′ terminal nucleotide (Yang et al. 2006b).

3.3.3 Plant MicroRNAs and siRNAs Carry a Methyl Group

The fact that miRNAs are reduced in abundance in *hen1* mutants and that HEN1 possesses miRNA methyltransferase activity in vitro suggests that plant miRNAs carry a methyl group in vivo. This is indeed true. We first demonstrated that plant miRNAs from the wildtype but not the *hen1-1* genotype are resistant to periodate/β elimination reactions, suggesting that at least one of the OH groups on the 3′ terminal nucleotides of plant miRNAs is blocked through a process requiring HEN1 (Yu et al. 2005). Next we isolated miR173 from *Arabidopsis* through affinity purification and measured the mass of this miRNA. The molecular mass of this miRNA from *Arabidopsis* is 14 Da larger than that of an in vitro synthesized unmodified miR173, consistent with the presence of a methyl group in miR173 from plants (Yu et al. 2005).

We also examined all types of currently known siRNAs except nat-siRNAs with the periodate/β elimination assay. siRNAs from sense transgenes and inverted-repeat transgenes, *trans*-acting siRNAs, and heterochromatic siRNAs were all resistant to the chemical reactions in a HEN1-dependent manner, suggesting that all siRNAs are methylated in vivo by HEN1 (Li et al. 2005). An independent study also demonstrated the methylation of siRNAs (Ebhardt et al. 2005). Interestingly, not all siRNAs require HEN1 for accumulation despite the fact that they are all methylated by HEN1 (Boutet et al. 2003; Xie et al. 2004).

3.3.4 Lack of Methylation Results in Uridylation and Degradation of MicroRNAs

We uncovered a novel uridylation activity that targets unmethylated miRNAs. We found that miRNAs become heterogeneous in size in *hen1* mutants such that a ladder of bands with 1-nt increments (mostly larger than the miRNA in wildtype plants) is present in *hen1* for any particular miRNA when examined by RNA filter hybridization. Primer extension showed that the heterogeneous species have the same 5′ end and that the total abundance of the heterogeneous species is reduced as compared to wildtype (Li et al. 2005). This suggests that the heterogeneous species differ in their 3′ ends and that miRNAs in *hen1* contain additional nucleotides at their 3′ ends. Indeed, sequence analysis of miR173 and miR167 from wildtype and *hen1-1* plants confirmed the presence of 3′ additional nucleotides in *hen1-1*. These nucleotides do not correspond to those 3′ to the miRNAs in the pre-miRNAs, indicating that these nucleotides are added after the processing of the miRNAs from the precursors. These nucleotides are predominantly, but not exclusively, U residues. This led us to conclude that a novel polymerase activity, which we refer to as the uridylation activity, adds the additional nucleotides to miRNAs in the *hen1* mutant (Li et al. 2005).

The sequence analysis of miR167 and miR173 also revealed that unmethylated miRNAs are more susceptible to a 3′-to-5′ exonuclease activity. 3′ truncated miRNAs containing U tails were frequently found in *hen1-1* but were also present at a low frequency in wildtype (Li et al. 2005). We suspect that uridylation attracts an exonuclease to degrade the miRNA from the 3′ end and that the exonuclease is not highly processive so that it only truncates a few nucleotides at a time. The truncated miRNAs are again uridylated. However, it is also possible that uridylation and exonucleolytic degradation of miRNAs are two independent events.

3.4   RISC Assembly

A methylated miRNA/miRNA* duplex next undergoes RNA-induced silencing complex (RISC) assembly, a process in which the miRNA strand is incorporated into a protein complex whose major protein component is an Argonaute (AGO) protein. AGO proteins contain PAZ domains that bind RNA and piwi domains that assume a folded structure that resembles RNase H (Ma et al. 2004, 2005; Parker et al. 2004, 2005; Song et al. 2004). Some AGO proteins possess key catalytic residues in the piwi domain and cleave the target mRNA in the middle of the complementary region between the mRNA and the siRNA or miRNA (Liu et al. 2004; Meister et al. 2004; Miyoshi et al. 2005). Other AGO proteins lack the key catalytic residues and cannot cause mRNA cleavage. For human and *Drosophila* AGO2, which possesses the endonucleolytic, or slicer, activity, it has been shown that the slicer activity is crucial for RISC loading (Matranga et al. 2005; Miyoshi et al. 2005). The passenger strand (miRNA*) is cleaved by AGO2 and the cleaved fragments are released to result in the formation of RISC with one miRNA strand. The determination of which strand of the duplex ends up in RISC is largely based on the thermodynamic properties of the two ends of the duplex. The strand in which the 5′ end is less thermodynamically stable in the duplex becomes preferentially incorporated into RISC (Khvorova et al. 2003; Schwarz et al. 2003).

Plant miRNAs and siRNAs appear to follow this asymmetry rule in RISC loading. In fact, most plant miRNAs begin with a U residue such that the 5′ end of the miRNAs tend be engaged in A–U, rather than G–C, hydrogen bonding (Reinhart et al. 2002; Rajagopalan et al. 2006). There are 10 AGO proteins in *Arabidopsis* and most of these contain the key catalytic residues critical for slicer activity (reviewed in Herr 2005). *Arabidopsis* AGO1 has been demonstrated to be associated with most miRNAs and contains the slicer activity that cleaves miRNA targets (Baumberger and Baulcombe 2005; Qi et al. 2005; Qi et al. 2006). AGO1 is also associated with some siRNAs such as transgene siRNAs, *trans*-acting siRNAs, and viral siRNAs (Baumberger and Baulcombe 2005; Zhang et al. 2006). *ago1* mutants have severe developmental defects (Bohmert et al. 1998), suggesting that AGO1 probably mediates the functions of many miRNAs. AGO4 is required for heterochromatin formation and for the accumulation of repeat associated siRNAs (Zilberman et al. 2003). AGO4 also has the slicer activity and this activity is required for heterochromatin formation at some but not all loci (Qi et al. 2006). Intriguingly, while AGO4 binds 24-nt endogenous siRNAs, it is also found to bind some 21-nt miRNAs (Qi et al. 2006). Immunopurified AGO4 from *Arabidopsis* can lead to the cleavage of some miRNA targets.

3.5 Export

The production of miRNA/miRNA* duplexes occurs in the nucleus since DCL1 is a nuclear protein (Papp et al. 2003). Two processes that act on miRNA/miRNA* duplexes are methylation and incorporation of the miRNA strand into a protein complex named RISC. Since miRISCs are known to cause mRNA cleavage, miRISCs should be present in the cytoplasm where mRNAs are located. One plant miRNA has also been shown to trigger DNA methylation at the target genomic locus (Bao et al. 2004); therefore, some miRNAs should also be present in the nucleus. The nuclear generation of miRNAs and the functionality of miRNAs in the cytoplasm require an export step in miRNA biogenesis.

HASTY, the *Arabidopsis* homolog of exportin 5, plays a role in miRNA nuclear export (Bollman et al. 2003; Park et al. 2005). *hasty* mutants have pleiotropic developmental defects and reduced accumulation of most miRNAs. However, it is not known whether the cargo of HASTY is miRNA/miRNA* duplexes or miRISCs. *hasty* mutants show reduced levels of miRNAs in both nuclear and cytoplasmic fractions. In addition, in both cellular compartments, miRNA abundance is higher than that of the miRNA*, suggesting that detectable miRNAs are present in miRISCs in both compartments. Either RISC loading occurs in the nucleus followed by export of miRISC into the cytoplasm or RISC loading occurs in the cytoplasm following the export of miRNA/miRNA* duplexes. Perhaps some miRISCs can then be imported back into the nucleus. A recent study showed that a sequence motif in an animal miRNA specifies nuclear import of the miRNA (Hwang et al. 2007). If RISC loading occurs in the nucleus, then the methylation of the miRNA/miRNA* duplex should also occur in the nucleus because the singled-stranded miRNA in RISC cannot be methylated by HEN1. In the scenario whereby RISC loading occurs in the cytoplasm, methylation can theoretically occur in either the nucleus or the cytoplasm. The subcellular location of miRNA methylation is currently unknown.

4   Regulation of MicroRNA Biogenesis

4.1   Feedback Regulation

miRNA biogenesis is under feedback regulation such that two key players in miRNA biogenesis and function are themselves regulated by miRNAs. The *DCL1* gene may be regulated by the status of miRNA biogenesis by two different mechanisms. First, *DCL1* mRNA has a binding site for miR162, which leads to the cleavage of *DCL1* mRNA (Xie et al. 2003). Consistent with this, *DCL1* mRNA levels are elevated in the *hen1-1* mutant, in which the abundance of miR162 is reduced. Second, the 14th intron of the *DCL1* gene appears to harbor the precursor to miR838. Although not proved, it is possible that the precursor is not transcribed independently but is released from the 14th intron of *DCL1* pre-mRNA through DCL1-mediated processing. If this is the case, it is possible that miRNA biogenesis competes with the splicing of *DCL1* pre-mRNA. In fact, truncated forms of *DCL1* mRNAs were found (Xie et al. 2003), some of which may correspond to the fragments generated through the process that releases the pre-miR838 from the 14th intron (Rajagopalan et al. 2006).

The *AGO1* gene encoding the main miRISC component is also under the regulation by an miRNA. miR168 has a binding site in *AGO1* mRNA and leads to AGO1-mediated cleavage of *AGO1* mRNA (Vaucheret et al. 2004). Therefore, the amount of functional miR168 bound by AGO1 determines the levels of *AGO1* mRNA. In addition, *MIR168* and *AGO1* genes are transcribed in a similar pattern, which probably ensures that *AGO1* is under the regulation of miR168 at all times and in all the cells that express *AGO1*. Among all miRNAs tested so far, miR168 appears to be preferentially stabilized by AGO1 such that miR168 levels are the least sensitive to reduced DCL1 activity but are sensitive to changes in the levels of AGO1 protein. This probably ensures that *AGO1* mRNA levels are under tight control by the levels of functional AGO1 protein.

4.2   Viral RNA Silencing Suppressors Affect MicroRNA Metabolism

A number of virally encoded proteins that suppress RNA silencing also negatively affect miRNA metabolism (reviewed in Voinnet 2005). The viral proteins can affect miRNA metabolism or function at a number of steps in the miRNA pathway. Some of these proteins, such as P1/HcPro from *Turnip mosaic virus*, p19 from the *Tomato bushy stunt virus*, and p21 from the *Beet yellows virus*, when expressed in plants from transgenes, cause the plants to show developmental phenotypes reminiscent of those exhibited by weak *dcl1* mutants. HcPro, p19, and p21 bind to miRNA/miRNA* (Chapman et al. 2004; Dunoyer et al. 2004; Lakatos et al. 2006), which are products of DCL1, and prevent subsequent steps in miRNA biogenesis. For example, methylation by HEN1 is reduced in transgenic plants expressing these viral proteins (Yu et al. 2006). RISC assembly is presumably also affected because the relative ratio of miRNA*s to miRNAs is much higher in plants expressing these viral proteins (Chapman et al. 2004; Dunoyer et al. 2004). Despite the accumulation of miRNAs in the transgenic plants expressing the viral proteins, sometimes to higher levels than in wildtype, miRNA targets overaccumulate, suggesting that miRNAs are not RISC bound or are not functional. Another viral protein, Cucumber mosaic virus 2b, has been recently shown to interact with AGO1 and inhibit its slicer activity (Zhang et al. 2006).

5 Mode of Action of Plant MicroRNAs

Plant miRNAs have a high degree of sequence complementarity to their target mRNAs and direct the slicing of the target mRNAs in the middle of the complementary regions (Llave et al. 2002b; Tang et al. 2003). This has been demonstrated by the detection of 3' cleavage products that have 5' ends that start at the middle of the complementary regions. While this is probably mediated by AGO1 (Baumberger and Baulcombe 2005; Qi et al. 2005), other AGO proteins may also play a role in this process. For example, immunopurified AGO4 is able to cleave some miRNA targets in vitro (Qi et al. 2006).

The mRNA cleavage products are then further degraded by other mechanisms. The 3' cleavage products of some miRNA targets are degraded by the 5' to 3' exonuclease XRN4 such that they accumulate in *xrn4* mutants (Souret et al. 2004). The 3' cleavage products of other miRNA targets must be degraded by an XRN4-independent mechanism because they do not accumulate in *xrn4* mutants. The 5' cleavage products are usually undetectable by RNA filter hybridization but can be detected by sensitive, PCR-based methods. It was found that the 5' cleavage products tend to acquire an oligo U tail, and the presence of the U tail correlates with shortening of the RNA from the 5' ends, which leads to the conclusion that the oligo U tail causes 5' to 3' exonucleolytic degradation of the 5' cleavage products (Shen and Goodman 2004). Intriguingly, this mechanism is conserved in the unicellular alga *Chlamydomonas reinhardtii*. The 5' products of RISC-cleaved transcripts in *Chlamydomonas* tend to acquire an oligo A tail, which also correlates with the degradation of the 5' cleavage products (Ibrahim et al. 2006). The enzyme that adds the oligo A tail, MUT68, belongs to the broad polyA polymerase family. Other members of the family also have small RNA-related functions. For example, *C. elegans* rde-3 is necessary for RNAi and the Cid12 protein from *Schizosaccharomyces pombe* is required for the accumulation of heterochromatic siRNAs and heterochromatin formation (Motamedi et al. 2004; Chen et al. 2005).

Translation inhibition is also a mechanism of regulation by plant miRNAs. Overexpression of miR172 does not lead to decreased accumulation of the target *AP2* mRNA but does lead to the reduction of AP2 protein levels as well as phenotypes that imply compromised *AP2* function (Aukerman and Sakai 2003; Chen

2004). This suggests that miR172 inhibits the translation of its target mRNAs. It was also found that miR172 can lead to the cleavage of their target mRNAs including *AP2* mRNA (Aukerman and Sakai 2003; Schwab et al. 2005). The fact that miR172-mediated cleavage of *AP2* mRNA does not result in reduced *AP2* mRNA accumulation was likely due to feedback regulation such that *AP2* transcription is increased to compensate for the loss of *AP2* mRNA. Alternatively, the cleavage that was detected by the sensitive rapid amplification of cDNA ends (RACE)-PCR approach is not sufficient to result in a gross reduction in target mRNA levels. Regardless of the molecular mechanisms underlying the stable levels of *AP2* mRNA, it is clear that miR172 has to exert its effect on *AP2* mRNA at a level other than mRNA cleavage; otherwise, the reduction in AP2 protein levels by miR172 is hard to explain. Recently, it was also observed that miR156/157 and miR854 lead to reduced protein but not mRNA levels of their target genes (Arteaga-Vazquez et al. 2006; Gandikota et al. 2007).

6   Outstanding Questions

Despite the rapid progress in the field of miRNA research in plants, many outstanding questions remain to be addressed.

6.1   *The Dynamics of MicroRNA Evolution*

The fact that over half of the known miRNA families in *Arabidopsis* are not conserved in poplar or rice suggests that miRNA genes evolve rapidly in plants. It also suggests that homology-based miRNA gene discovery will result in gross underestimation of miRNA gene numbers. Deep sequencing of small RNAs under normal and various stress conditions will be necessary to uncover the full complement of miRNA genes in any plant species. To understand the evolutionary history of miRNAs in any species, it will also be necessary to obtain the full complements of miRNA genes in a number of species closely related to the species in question. Finally, uncovering miRNAs from key representative species spanning the entire evolutionary distance from unicellular plants to angiosperms will be necessary to provide a comprehensive picture of miRNA evolution in plants. It is worth noting that miRNAs have recently been identified from the unicellular green alga *C. reinhardtii* (Molnar et al. 2007; Zhao et al. 2007).

6.2   *Regulation of MicroRNA Biogenesis*

Other than negative feedback regulation of miRNA biogenesis, little is known about how miRNA biogenesis is regulated in plants. Viruses have evolved proteins that can repress miRNA biogenesis or function at multiple steps of the pathway. It is also possible that endogenous proteins regulate various steps in miRNA biogenesis or function in a negative manner. However, no such proteins have been identified so far. One of the challenges in the future would be to continue to identify the components of the miRNA pathway, especially genes that act negatively to regulate miRNA biogenesis.

Another obvious gap in our knowledge is that nothing is known about how miRNAs are turned over. Presumably miRNAs are subject to degradation by nucleases that, together with positive factors in miRNA biogenesis, determine the steady-state abundance of miRNAs. The identity of these nucleases needs to be revealed.

6.3   Mode of Action of Plant MicroRNAs

Based on the fact that most plant miRNAs lead to characteristic RISC-mediated cleavage of target mRNAs, it has been widely assumed that plant miRNAs primarily cause target mRNA cleavage. This assumption, however, is unfounded since the levels of target proteins have not been examined for all plant miRNAs except for miR156/157, miR172, and miR854, for which a role in translational regulation has been established (Aukerman and Sakai 2003; Chen 2004; Arteaga-Vazquez et al. 2006; Gandikota et al. 2007). It is possible that most plant miRNAs also have a role in translational control. It is important that the protein levels of miRNA target genes be examined for multiple miRNAs.

6.4   Function of MicroRNAs

Most of the evolutionarily conserved miRNAs belong to gene families with multiple members. Studies on the miR164 family suggest that members of a gene family can have distinct and partially overlapping functions (Baker et al. 2005; Guo et al. 2005; Sieber et al. 2007). One challenge in the future is to uncover the functional relationship among members of miRNA families.

Most miRNAs also have multiple target genes. What is the regulatory relationship between multiple members of an miRNA gene family and the multiple target genes? Does each miRNA regulate multiple targets? This can only be addressed when a member of the miRNA family can be specifically knocked out to allow an examination of the consequence of the loss of a particular miRNA gene on the expression of each target gene. Although the currently available T-DNA insertion collections of mutant *Arabidopsis* are a valuable resource to find knockouts in specific *MIR* genes, T-DNA insertions at a *MIR* locus may not lead to a complete knockout of the miRNA if the T-DNA insertions are not within the pre-miRNA. Other approaches to obtain a clean deletion of the miRNA sequence or a specific blockade of miRNA function will be complementary approaches that have yet to be developed. To specifically knock out an miRNA gene is the best way to evaluate the biological function of this miRNA gene as opposed to the most commonly adopted method currently, which involves expressing miRNA-resistant versions of a target mRNA. This current approach only reveals the consequence of loss of miRNA-mediated regulation of one of a number of target genes. It also fails to reveal the functional distinction among miRNA family members.

References

Adai A, Johnson C, Mlotshwa S, Archer-Evans S, Manocha V, Vance V, Sundaresan V (2005) Computational prediction of miRNAs in Arabidopsis thaliana. Genome Res 15:78–91

Alefelder S, Patel BK, Eckstein F (1998) Incorporation of terminal phosphorothioates into oligonucleotides. Nucleic Acids Res 26:4983–4988

Allen E, Xie Z, Gustafson AM, Sung GH, Spatafora JW, Carrington JC (2004) Evolution of microRNA genes by inverted duplication of target gene sequences in Arabidopsis thaliana. Nat Genet 36:1282–1290

Arazi T, Talmor-Neiman M, Stav R, Riese M, Huijser P, Baulcombe DC (2005) Cloning and characterization of micro-RNAs from moss. Plant J 43:837–848

Arteaga-Vazquez M, Caballero-Perez J, Vielle-Calzada JP (2006) A family of microRNAs present in plants and animals. Plant Cell 18:3355–3369

Aukerman MJ, Sakai H (2003) Regulation of flowering time and floral organ identity by a microRNA and its APETALA2-like target genes. Plant Cell 15:2730–2741

Axtell MJ, Bartel DP (2005) Antiquity of microRNAs and their targets in land plants. Plant Cell 17:1658–1673

Axtell MJ, Jan C, Rajagopalan R, Bartel DP (2006) A two-hit trigger for siRNA biogenesis in plants. Cell 127:565–577

Baker CC, Sieber P, Wellmer F, Meyerowitz EM (2005) The early extra petals1 mutant uncovers a role for microRNA miR164c in regulating petal number in Arabidopsis. Curr Biol 15:303–315

Bao N, Lye KW, Barton MK (2004) MicroRNA binding sites in Arabidopsis class III HD-ZIP mRNAs are required for methylation of the template chromosome. Dev Cell 7:653–662

Baumberger N, Baulcombe DC (2005) Arabidopsis Argonaute1 is an RNA Slicer that selectively recruits microRNAs and short interfering RNAs. Proc Natl Acad Sci U S A 102:11928–11933

Bohmert K, Camus I, Bellini C, Bouchez D, Caboche M, Benning C (1998) AGO1 defines a novel locus of Arabidopsis controlling leaf development. EMBO J 17:170–180

Bollman KM, Aukerman MJ, Park MY, Hunter C, Berardini TZ, Poethig RS (2003) HASTY, the Arabidopsis ortholog of exportin 5/MSN5, regulates phase change and morphogenesis. Development 130:1493–1504

Bonnet E, Wuyts J, Rouze P, Van de Peer Y (2004) Detection of 91 potential conserved plant microRNAs in Arabidopsis thaliana and Oryza sativa identifies important target genes. Proc Natl Acad Sci U S A 101:11511–11516

Borsani O, Zhu J, Verslues PE, Sunkar R, Zhu JK (2005) Endogenous siRNAs derived from a pair of natural cis-antisense transcripts regulate salt tolerance in Arabidopsis. Cell 123:1279–1291

Boutet S, Vazquez F, Liu J, Beclin C, Fagard M, Gratias A, Morel JB, Crete P, Chen X, Vaucheret H (2003) Arabidopsis HEN1. A genetic link between endogenous miRNA controlling development and siRNA controlling transgene silencing and virus resistance. Curr Biol 13:843–848

Chapman EJ, Prokhnevsky AI, Gopinath K, Dolja VV, Carrington JC (2004) Viral RNA silencing suppressors inhibit the microRNA pathway at an intermediate step. Genes Dev 18:1179–1186

Chen CC, Simard MJ, Tabara H, Brownell DR, McCollough JA, Mello CC (2005) A member of
the polymerase beta nucleotidyltransferase superfamily is required for RNA interference in C.
elegans. Curr Biol 15:378–383

Chen X (2004) A microRNA as a translational repressor of APETALA2 in Arabidopsis flower
development. Science 303:2022–2025

Chen X, Liu J, Cheng Y, Jia D (2002) HEN1 functions pleiotropically in Arabidopsis development
and acts in C function in the flower. Development 129:1085–1094

Dunoyer P, Lecellier CH, Parizotto EA, Himber C, Voinnet O (2004) Probing the microRNA and
small interfering RNA pathways with virus-encoded suppressors of RNA silencing. Plant Cell
16:1235–1250

Ebhardt HA, Thi EP, Wang MB, Unrau PJ (2005) Extensive 3′ modification of plant small RNAs
is modulated by helper component-proteinase expression. Proc Natl Acad Sci U S A
102:13398–13403

Fahlgren N, Howell MD, Kasschau KD, Chapman EJ, Sullivan CM, Cumbie JS, Givan SA, Law
TF, Grant SR, Dangl JL, Carrington JC (2007) High-throughput sequencing of Arabidopsis
microRNAs: evidence for frequent birth and death of MIRNA genes. PLoS ONE 2:e219

Gandikota M, Birkenbihl RP, Hohmann S, Cardon GH, Saedler H, Huijser P (2007) The
miRNA156/157 recognition element in the 3′ UTR of the Arabidopsis SBP box gene SPL3
prevents early flowering by translational inhibition in seedlings. Plant J 49:683–693

Gasciolli V, Mallory AC, Bartel DP, Vaucheret H (2005) Partially redundant functions of
Arabidopsis DICER-like enzymes and a role for DCL4 in producing trans-acting siRNAs. Curr
Biol 15:1494–1500

Grigg SP, Canales C, Hay A, Tsiantis M (2005) SERRATE coordinates shoot meristem function
and leaf axial patterning in Arabidopsis. Nature 437:1022–1026

Guo HS, Xie Q, Fei JF, Chua NH (2005) MicroRNA directs mRNA cleavage of the transcription
factor NAC1 to downregulate auxin signals for Arabidopsis lateral root development. Plant
Cell 17:1376–1386

Han MH, Goud S, Song L, Fedoroff N (2004) The Arabidopsis double-stranded RNA-binding
protein HYL1 plays a role in microRNA-mediated gene regulation. Proc Natl Acad Sci U S A
101:1093–1098

Henderson IR, Zhang X, Lu C, Johnson L, Meyers BC, Green PJ, Jacobsen SE (2006) Dissecting
Arabidopsis thaliana DICER function in small RNA processing, gene silencing and DNA
methylation patterning. Nat Genet 38:721–725

Herr AJ (2005) Pathways through the small RNA world of plants. FEBS Lett 579:5879–5888

Hiraguri A, Itoh R, Kondo N, Nomura Y, Aizawa D, Murai Y, Koiwa H, Seki M, Shinozaki K,
Fukuhara T (2005) Specific interactions between Dicer-like proteins and HYL1/DRB-family
dsRNA-binding proteins in Arabidopsis thaliana. Plant Mol Biol 57:173–188

Hwang HW, Wentzel EA, Mendell JT (2007) A hexanucleotide element directs microRNA
nuclear import. Science 315:97–100

Ibrahim F, Rohr J, Jeong WJ, Hesson J, Cerutti H (2006) Untemplated oligoadenylation promotes
degradation of RISC-cleaved transcripts. Science 314:1893

Jacobsen SE, Running M, Meyerowitz EM (1999) Disruption of an RNA helicase/RNAse III gene
in Arabidopsis causes unregulated cell division in floral meristems. Development
126:5231–5243

Jones-Rhoades MW, Bartel DP (2004) Computational identification of plant microRNAs and their
targets, including a stress-induced miRNA. Mol Cell 14:787–799

Kasschau KD, Fahlgren N, Chapman EJ, Sullivan CM, Cumbie JS, Givan SA, Carrington JC
(2007) Genome-wide profiling and analysis of Arabidopsis siRNAs. PLoS Biol 5:e57

Katiyar-Agarwal S, Morgan R, Dahlbeck D, Borsani O, Villegas A Jr, Zhu JK, Staskawicz BJ, Jin
H (2006) A pathogen-inducible endogenous siRNA in plant immunity. Proc Natl Acad Sci U
S A 103:18002–18007

Khvorova A, Reynolds A, Jayasena SD (2003) Functional siRNAs and miRNAs exhibit strand
bias. Cell 115:209–216

Kim VN (2005) MicroRNA biogenesis: coordinated cropping and dicing. Nat Rev Mol Cell Biol 6:376–385

Kurihara Y, Watanabe Y (2004) Arabidopsis micro-RNA biogenesis through Dicer-like 1 protein functions. Proc Natl Acad Sci U S A 101:12753–12758

Kurihara Y, Takashi Y, Watanabe Y (2006) The interaction between DCL1 and HYL1 is important for efficient and precise processing of pri-miRNA in plant microRNA biogenesis. RNA 12:206–212

Lakatos L, Csorba T, Pantaleo V, Chapman EJ, Carrington JC, Liu YP, Dolja VV, Calvino LF, Lopez-Moya JJ, Burgyan J (2006) Small RNA binding is a common strategy to suppress RNA silencing by several viral suppressors. EMBO J 25:2768–2780

Li J, Yang Z, Yu B, Liu J, Chen X (2005) Methylation protects miRNAs and siRNAs from a 3′-end uridylation activity in Arabidopsis. Curr Biol 15:1501–1507

Liu B, Li P, Li X, Liu C, Cao S, Chu C, Cao X (2005) Loss of function of OsDCL1 affects micro-RNA accumulation and causes developmental defects in rice. Plant Physiol 139:296–305

Liu J, Carmell MA, Rivas FV, Marsden CG, Thomson JM, Song JJ, Hammond SM, Joshua-Tor L, Hannon GJ (2004) Argonaute2 is the catalytic engine of mammalian RNAi. Science 305:1437–1441

Llave C, Kasschau KD, Rector MA, Carrington JC (2002a) Endogenous and silencing-associated small RNAs in plants. Plant Cell 14:1605–1619

Llave C, Xie Z, Kasschau KD, Carrington JC (2002b) Cleavage of Scarecrow-like mRNA targets directed by a class of Arabidopsis miRNA. Science 297:2053–2056

Lobbes D, Rallapalli G, Schmidt DD, Martin C, Clarke J (2006) SERRATE: a new player on the plant microRNA scene. EMBO Rep 7:1052–1058

Lu C, Fedoroff N (2000) A mutation in the Arabidopsis HYL1 gene encoding a dsRNA binding protein affects responses to abscisic acid, auxin, and cytokinin. Plant Cell 12:2351–2366

Lu C, Tej SS, Luo S, Haudenschild CD, Meyers BC, Green PJ (2005) Elucidation of the small RNA component of the transcriptome. Science 309:1567–1569

Lu C, Kulkarni K, Souret FF, MuthuValliappan R, Tej SS, Poethig RS, Henderson IR, Jacobsen SE, Wang W, Green PJ, Meyers BC (2006) MicroRNAs and other small RNAs enriched in the Arabidopsis RNA-dependent RNA polymerase-2 mutant. Genome Res 16:1276–1288

Ma JB, Ye K, Patel DJ (2004) Structural basis for overhang-specific small interfering RNA recognition by the PAZ domain. Nature 429:318–322

Ma JB, Yuan YR, Meister G, Pei Y, Tuschl T, Patel DJ (2005) Structural basis for 5′-end-specific recognition of guide RNA by the A. fulgidus Piwi protein. Nature 434:666–670

Maher C, Stein L, Ware D (2006) Evolution of Arabidopsis microRNA families through duplication events. Genome Res 16:510–519

Matranga C, Tomari Y, Shin C, Bartel DP, Zamore PD (2005) Passenger-strand cleavage facilitates assembly of siRNA into Ago2-containing RNAi enzyme complexes. Cell 123:607–620

McElver J, Tzafrir I, Aux G, Rogers R, Ashby C, Smith K, Thomas C, Schetter A, Zhou Q, Cushman MA, Tossberg J, Nickle T, Levin JZ, Law M, Meinke D, Patton D (2001) Insertional mutagenesis of genes required for seed development in Arabidopsis thaliana. Genetics 159:1751–1763

Megraw M, Baev V, Rusinov V, Jensen ST, Kalantidis K, Hatzigeorgiou AG (2006) MicroRNA promoter element discovery in Arabidopsis. RNA 12:1612–1619

Meister G, Landthaler M, Patkaniowska A, Dorsett Y, Teng G, Tuschl T (2004) Human Argonaute2 mediates RNA cleavage targeted by miRNAs and siRNAs. Mol Cell 15:185–197

Mette MF, van der Winden J, Matzke M, Matzke AJ (2002) Short RNAs can identify new candidate transposable element families in Arabidopsis. Plant Physiol 130:6–9

Miyoshi K, Tsukumo H, Nagami T, Siomi H, Siomi MC (2005) Slicer function of Drosophila Argonautes and its involvement in RISC formation. Genes Dev 19:2837–2848

Molnar A, Schwach F, Studholme DJ, Thuenemann EC, Baulcombe DC (2007) miRNAs control gene expression in the single-cell alga Chlamydomonas reinhardtii. Nature 447:1126–1129

Motamedi MR, Verdel A, Colmenares SU, Gerber SA, Gygi SP, Moazed D (2004) Two RNAi complexes, RITS and RDRC, physically interact and localize to noncoding centromeric RNAs. Cell 119:789–802

Palatnik JF, Allen E, Wu X, Schommer C, Schwab R, Carrington JC, Weigel D (2003) Control of leaf morphogenesis by microRNAs. Nature 425:257–263

Papp I, Mette MF, Aufsatz W, Daxinger L, Schauer SE, Ray A, van der Winden J, Matzke M, Matzke AJ (2003) Evidence for nuclear processing of plant microRNA and short interefering RNA precursors. Plant Physiol 132:1382–1390

Park MY, Wu G, Gonzalez-Sulser A, Vaucheret H, Poethig RS (2005) Nuclear processing and export of microRNAs in Arabidopsis. Proc Natl Acad Sci U S A 102:3691–3696

Park W, Li J, Song R, Messing J, Chen X (2002) CARPEL FACTORY, a Dicer homolog, and HEN1, a novel protein, act in microRNA metabolism in Arabidopsis thaliana. Curr Biol 12:1484–1495

Parker JS, Roe SM, Barford D (2004) Crystal structure of a PIWI protein suggests mechanisms for siRNA recognition and slicer activity. EMBO J 23:4727–4737

Parker JS, Roe SM, Barford D (2005) Structural insights into mRNA recognition from a PIWI domain-siRNA guide complex. Nature 434:663–666

Qi Y, Denli AM, Hannon GJ (2005) Biochemical specialization within Arabidopsis RNA silencing pathways. Mol Cell 19:421–428

Qi Y, He X, Wang XJ, Kohany O, Jurka J, Hannon GJ (2006) Distinct catalytic and non-catalytic roles of Argonaute4 in RNA-directed DNA methylation. Nature 443:1008–1012

Rajagopalan R, Vaucheret H, Trejo J, Bartel DP (2006) A diverse and evolutionarily fluid set of microRNAs in Arabidopsis thaliana. Genes Dev 20:3407–3425

Ray A, Lang JD, Golden T, Ray S (1996) SHORT INTEGUMENT (SIN1), a gene required for ovule development in Arabidopsis, also controls flowering time. Development 122:2631–2638

Reinhart BJ, Weinstein EG, Rhoades MW, Bartel B, Bartel DP (2002) MicroRNAs in plants. Genes Dev 16:1616–1626

Schwab R, Palatnik JF, Riester M, Schommer C, Schmid M, Weigel D (2005) Specific effects of microRNAs on the plant transcriptome. Dev Cell 8:517–527

Schwartz BW, Yeung EC, Meinke DW (1994) Disruption of morphogenesis and transformation of the suspensor in abnormal suspensor mutants of Arabidopsis. Development 120:3235–3245

Schwarz DS, Hutvagner G, Du T, Xu Z, Aronin N, Zamore PD (2003) Asymmetry in the assembly of the RNAi enzyme complex. Cell 115:199–208

Shen B, Goodman HM (2004) Uridine addition after microRNA-directed cleavage. Science 306:997

Sieber P, Wellmer F, Gheyselinck J, Riechmann JL, Meyerowitz EM (2007) Redundancy and specialization among plant microRNAs: role of the MIR164 family in developmental robustness. Development 134:1051–1060

Song JJ, Smith SK, Hannon GJ, Joshua-Tor L (2004) Crystal structure of Argonaute and its implications for RISC slicer activity. Science 305:1434–1437

Souret FF, Kastenmayer JP, Green PJ (2004) AtXRN4 degrades mRNA in Arabidopsis and its substrates include selected miRNA targets. Mol Cell 15:173–183

Tang G, Reinhart BJ, Bartel DP, Zamore PD (2003) A biochemical framework for RNA silencing in plants. Genes Dev 17:49–63

Vaucheret H, Vazquez F, Crete P, Bartel DP (2004) The action of Argonaute1 in the miRNA pathway and its regulation by the miRNA pathway are crucial for plant development. Genes Dev 18:1187–1197

Vazquez F, Gasciolli V, Crete P, Vaucheret H (2004a) The nuclear dsRNA binding protein HYL1 is required for microRNA accumulation and plant development, but not posttranscriptional transgene silencing. Curr Biol 14:346–351

Vazquez F, Vaucheret H, Rajagopalan R, Lepers C, Gasciolli V, Mallory AC, Hilbert JL, Bartel DP, Crete P (2004b) Endogenous trans-acting siRNAs regulate the accumulation of Arabidopsis mRNAs. Mol Cell 16:69–79

Voinnet O (2005) Induction and suppression of RNA silencing: insights from viral infections. Nat Rev Genet 6:206–220

Wang XJ, Reyes JL, Chua NH, Gaasterland T (2004) Prediction and identification of Arabidopsis thaliana microRNAs and their mRNA targets. Genome Biol 5:R65

Williams L, Grigg SP, Xie M, Christensen S, Fletcher JC (2005) Regulation of Arabidopsis shoot apical meristem and lateral organ formation by microRNA miR166 g and its AtHD-ZIP target genes. Development 132:3657–3668

Wu F, Yu L. Cao W, Mao Y, Liu Z, and He Y. (2007) The N-terminal double-stranded RNA binding domains of Arabidopsis HYPONASTIC LEAVES1 are sufficenit for pre-microRNA processing. Plant Cell 19:914–925

Xie Z, Kasschau KD, Carrington JC (2003) Negative feedback regulation of Dicer-Like1 in Arabidopsis by microRNA-guided mRNA degradation. Curr Biol 13:784–789

Xie Z, Johansen LK, Gustafson AM, Kasschau KD, Lellis AD, Zilberman D, Jacobsen SE, Carrington JC (2004) Genetic and functional diversification of small RNA pathways in plants. PLoS Biol 2:E104

Xie Z, Allen E, Fahlgren N, Calamar A, Givan SA, Carrington JC (2005a) Expression of Arabidopsis MIRNA genes. Plant Physiol 138:2145–2154

Xie Z, Allen E, Wilken A, Carrington JC (2005b) DICER-LIKE 4 functions in trans-acting small interfering RNA biogenesis and vegetative phase change in Arabidopsis thaliana. Proc Natl Acad Sci U S A 102:12984–12989

Yang L, Liu Z, Lu F, Dong A, Huang H (2006a) SERRATE is a novel nuclear regulator in primary microRNA processing in Arabidopsis. Plant J 47:841–850

Yang Z, Ebright YW, Yu B, Chen X (2006b) HEN1 recognizes 21–24 nt small RNA duplexes and deposits a methyl group onto the 2′ OH of the 3′ terminal nucleotide. Nucleic Acids Res 34:667–675

Yoshikawa M, Peragine A, Park MY, Poethig RS (2005) A pathway for the biogenesis of trans-acting siRNAs in Arabidopsis. Genes Dev 19:2164–2175

Yu B, Yang Z, Li J, Minakhina S, Yang M, Padgett RW, Steward R, Chen X (2005) Methylation as a crucial step in plant microRNA biogenesis. Science 307:932–935

Yu B, Chapman EJ, Yang Z, Carrington JC, Chen X (2006) Transgenically expressed viral RNA silencing suppressors interfere with microRNA methylation in Arabidopsis. FEBS Lett 580:3117–3120

Zhang X, Yuan YR, Pei Y, Lin SS, Tuschl T, Patel DJ, Chua NH (2006) Cucumber mosaic virus-encoded 2b suppressor inhibits Arabidopsis Argonaute1 cleavage activity to counter plant defense. Genes Dev 20:3255–3268

Zhang X, Henderson IR, Lu C, Green PJ, Jacobsen SE (2007) Role of RNA polymerase IV in plant small RNA metabolism. Proc Natl Acad Sci U S A 104:4536–4541

Zhao T, Li G, Mi S, Li S, Hannon GJ, Wang XJ, Qi Y (2007) A complex system of small RNAs in the unicellular green alga Chlamydomonas reinhardtii. Genes Dev 21:1190–1203

Zilberman D, Cao X, Jacobsen SE (2003) Argonaute4 control of locus-specific siRNA accumulation and DNA and histone methylation. Science 299:716–719

Structure-Function Relationships Among RNA-Dependent RNA Polymerases

Kenneth K.-S. Ng(✉), Jamie J. Arnold, and Craig E. Cameron(✉)

Abstract RNA-dependent RNA polymerases (RdRPs) play key roles in viral transcription and genome replication, as well as epigenetic and post-transcriptional control of cellular gene expression. In this article, we review the crystallographic, biochemical, and molecular genetic data available for viral RdRPs that have led to a detailed description of substrate and cofactor binding, fidelity of nucleotide selection and incorporation, and catalysis. It is likely that the cellular RdRPs will share some of the basic structural and mechanistic principles gleaned from studies of viral

Kenneth K.-S. Ng
Department of Biological Sciences, University of Calgary, 2500 University Drive NW,
Calgary, Alberta, T2N 1N4, Canada
ngk@ucalgary.ca

Craig E. Cameron
Department of Biochemistry and Molecular Biology The Pennsylvania State University,
201 Althouse Laboratory, University Park, PA 16802, USA
cec9@psu.edu

P.J. Paddison and P.K. Vogt (eds.), *RNA Interference.*
Current Topics in Microbiology and Immunology 320.
© Springer-Verlag Berlin Heidelberg 2008

RdRPs. Therefore, studies of the viral RdRP establish a framework for the study of cellular RdRPs, an important yet understudied class of nucleic acid polymerases.

1 Introduction

Under physiological conditions, RNA-dependent RNA polymerases (RdRPs) catalyze the formation of phosphodiester bonds between ribonucleotides in an RNA template-dependent fashion. RdRPs have been found primarily in RNA viruses. In some cases, these enzymes are virion associated; in others, these enzymes are non-structural proteins located in the cytoplasm but, on occasion, are located in the nucleus. In viral systems, the RdRP is responsible for transcription and replication of RNA virus genomes. Given the essential role of the RdRP for virus multiplication, the viral RdRP has been the subject of intensive study for many decades.

More than 30 years ago, RdRP activity was detected in the tissue of numerous plants that were thought to be uninfected (Astier-Manifacier and Cornuet 1971; Astier-Manifacier and Cornuet 1978; Boege and Sänger 1980; Duda et al. 1973). This observation eventually led to the cloning of a gene from tomato thought to be at least a component of this cellular activity of plants, although direct demonstration of RdRP activity associated with the cloned gene product was not possible (Schiebel et al. 1998). Subsequently, it was shown that the plant RdRP gene had homologs in fungi [e.g., QDE-1 in *Neurospora crassa* (Cogoni and Macino 1999)] and nematodes [EGO-1 and RRF genes in *Caenorhabditis elegans* (Smardon et al. 2000)]. In all cases, these genes were shown to be essential for gene silencing events: co-suppression in plants (Mourrain et al. 2000); quelling in *N. crassa* (Cogoni and Macino 1999); and RNA interference (RNAi) in *C. elegans* (Smardon et al. 2000). In particular, the RdRP is implicated in the genesis and/or maintenance of the gene silencing trigger, double-stranded RNA (dsRNA) (Nishikura 2001). Recently, RdRP activity was shown for the QDE-1 gene product, QDE-1p (Makeyev and Bamford 2002), and a structure of this enzyme is imminent (Laurila et al. 2005a). Unfortunately, at this time, the structure-function relationships of this class of RdRPs remain to be defined.

In this article, we will review our current understanding of the structure, function, and mechanism of viral RdRPs. It is likely that the unifying principles and corresponding methods described for viral RdRPs will be useful in guiding studies of cellular RdRPs required for RNAi.

2 RdRP Structures

Three-dimensional structural information is currently available for RdRPs from five families of positive-strand [*Picornaviridae*: poliovirus, human rhinovirus, foot-and-mouth-disease virus (FMDV); *Caliciviridae*: rabbit hemorrhagic disease virus, Norwalk virus; and *Flaviviridae*: hepatitis C virus, bovine viral diarrhea virus] and double-strand (*Cystoviridae*: phage ϕ6 and *Reoviridae*: reovirus) RNA viruses (Table 1). All enzymes share an overall structure that resembles a cupped "right

Table 1 Crystal structures of RdRPs

Virus	PDB	Res. (Å)	Details	Reference(s)
A. Apo and metal-liganded polymerase structures				
PV type 1	1RDR	2.4	Partial structure, non-native N-terminus	Hansen et al. 1997
	1RA6	2.0	Full-length with native N-terminus	Thompson and Peersen 2004
	1RAJ	2.5	68-residue N-terminal truncation	
	1TQL	2.3	G1A N-terminal residue mutant	
HRV–1B	1XR6	2.5	Full-length complex with K^+	Love et al. 2004
HRV–14	1XR5	2.8	Full-length complex with Sm^{3+}	
HRV–16	1XR7	2.3	Full-length native	
	1TP7	2.4	Full-length native with C-terminal His-tag	Appleby et al. 2005
FMDV	1UO9	1.9	Full-length native	Ferrer-Orta et al. 2004
RHDV	1KHV	2.5	Full-length complex with Lu^{3+}	Ng et al. 2002
	1KHW	2.7	Full-length complex with Mn^{2+}	
NV	1SH0	2.2	Full-length native	Ng et al. 2004
	1SH2	2.3		
	1SH3	2.9		
	2B43	2.3	Full-length native	N/A
HCV	1C2P	1.9	21-residue C-terminal truncation	Lesburg et al. 1999
	1CSJ	2.8	55-residue C-terminal truncation	Bressanelli et al. 1999
	1NB4	2.0	21-residue C-terminal truncation+C-terminal His-tag	O'Farrell et al. 2003
	1QUV	2.5	21-residue C-terminal truncation	Ago et al. 1999
BVDV	2CJQ	2.6	Residues 92–672, not domain-swapped	Choi et al. 2006
	1S48	3.0	Residues 92–679, domain-swapped N-terminus	Choi et al. 2004
	1S4F	3.0	Residues 92–674, domain-swapped N-terminus	
Reovirus	1MUK	2.5	Full-length native	Tao et al. 2002
Phage φ6	1HHS	2.0	Full-length complex with Mn^{2+}	Butcher et al. 2001
	1HI8	2.5	Selenomethionine derivative with Mg^{2+}	
	1WAC	3.0	Initiation platform mutant	Laurila et al. 2005b
B. RdRP complexes with NTPs, RNA, and proteins				
PV type 1	1RA7	2.3	GTP complex	Thompson and Peersen 2004
FMDV	1WNE	3.0	Primer-template complex	Ferrer-Orta et al. 2004
	2D7S	3.0	VPg complex	Ferrer-Orta et al. 2006
	2F8E	2.9	VPg-UMP complex	
Reovirus	1MWH	2.5	Cap complex	Tao et al. 2002
	1N1H	2.8	Initiation complex with GTP+template RNA	
	1N38	2.8	Short elongation complex	
	1N35	2.5	Long elongation complex	

(continued)

Table 1 (continued)

Virus	PDB	Res. (Å)	Details	Reference(s)
Phage φ6	1HHT	2.9	RNA template complex	Butcher et al. 2001
	1HI0	3.0	Initiation complex with GTP+template RNA	
	1HI1	3.0	ATP complex	
	1UVI	2.1	Complex with 6 nt RNA	Salgado et al. 2004
	1UVJ	1.9	Complex with 7 nt RNA	
	1UVK	2.4	Dead-end complex	
	1UVL	2.0	Complex with 5 nt RNA, conformation A	
	1UVM	2.0	Complex with 5 nt RNA, conformation B	
	1UVN	3.0	Ca^{2+} inhibition complex+RNA+NTPs	

C. RdRP complexes with inhibitors

HCV	1GX5	1.7	GTP+Mn^{2+} complex	Bressanelli et al. 2002
	1GX6	1.8	UTP+Mn^{2+} complex	
	1NB6	2.6	UTP complex	O'Farrell et al. 2003
	1NB7	2.9	U_4 complex	
	1NHU	2.0	Non-nucleoside inhibitor complexes	Wang et al. 2003
	1NHV	2.9		
	1OS5	2.2	Non-nucleoside inhibitor complex	Love et al. 2003
	1YVF	2.5	Non-nucleoside inhibitor complexes	Pfefferkorn et al. 2005a, b
	1Z4U	2.8		
	1YVX	2.0	Non-nucleoside inhibitor complexes	Biswal et al. 2005
	1YVZ	2.2		
	2AWZ	2.1	Covalent inhibitor complexes	Powers et al. 2006
	2AX0	2.0		
	2AX1	2.1		
	2BRK	2.3	Non-nucleoside inhibitor complexes	Di Marco et al. 2005
	2BRL	2.4		
	2D3U	2.0	Non-nucleoside inhibitor complexes	Biswal et al. 2006
	2D3Z	1.8		
	2D41	2.1		
	2GC8	2.2	Non-nucleoside inhibitor complex	
				Gopalsamy et al. 2006

BVDV, bovine viral diarrhea virus; FMDV, foot-and-mouth disease virus; HCV, hepatitis C virus; HRV, human rhinovirus; N/A, Reference not currently available; NV, norovirus; PDB, Protein Data Bank; PV, poliovirus; Res., maximum resolution limit of diffraction; RHDV, rabbit hemorrhagic disease virus

hand" and contains "fingers," "palm," and "thumb" domains (Fig. 1). This architecture is shared with distantly related DNA-dependent DNA polymerases (DdDPs), DNA-dependent RNA polymerases (DdRPs), and RNA-dependent DNA polymerases (RdDPs or reverse transcriptases). The low level of amino acid sequence identity seen in polymerases from different classes strongly suggests that the structural elements that are conserved in evolutionarily distant species serve important functional roles. In addition to these three central domains, an N-terminal domain that bridges the fingers and thumb domains is found in all RdRPs. In the RdRPs from the *Flaviviridae*,

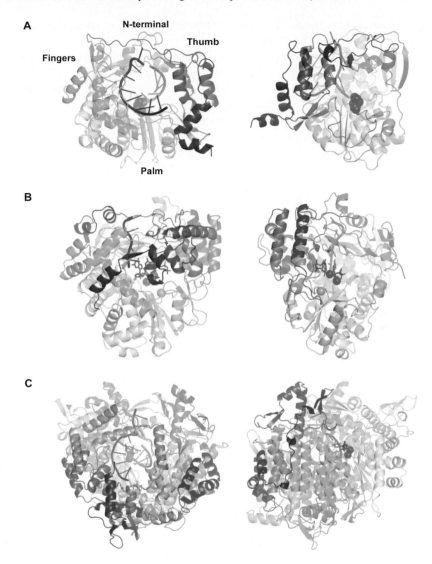

Fig. 1 A-C Overall structures of RdRPs. Ribbon representations of RdRP structures (rainbow coloring with *blue* at the N-terminus and *red* at the C-terminus) bound to RNA template (*black*) and primer (*gray*) strands: **A** FMDV (1WNE) (Ferrer-Orta et al. 2004); **B** Bacteriophage φ6 (1HI0) (Butcher et al. 2001); **C** Reovirus (1N35) (Tao et al. 2002). Two views are presented for each structure, a "front" view down the axis of the RNA-binding, active site cleft (*left panel*) and a "side" or "back" view into the active site. Divalent metal ions at the active site in **B** and **C** are drawn as *magenta spheres*. Asp-338 in motif C of FMDV is drawn in space-filling representation as *magenta spheres* to mark the position of the active site in the absence of bound divalent metal ions

Cystoviridae, and Reoviridae, C-terminal domains that enter or encircle the central cleft of the enzyme are also found.

Six sequence and structural motifs (designated A to F) have been identified in RdRPs (Bruenn 2003; Hansen et al. 1997; Kamer and Argos 1984; O'Reilly and Kao 1998). Most of these motifs are also shared with RdDPs, DdDPs, and DdRPs, indicating the fundamental importance of these structural elements in the enzymatic function of polymerases. Indeed, residues from most of these motifs have been shown to play critical roles in the binding of metal ions, nucleoside triphosphates, and RNA, all of which are critical for the nucleotidyltransferase reaction catalyzed by RdRPs. In the three-dimensional structures of RdRPs, these motifs line the central cavity that is responsible for binding substrates and cofactors, as well as catalyzing the nucleotidyltransferase reaction.

3   Structures of RdRP Complexes

3.1   Divalent Metal Ions

The dependence of polymerase activity upon divalent metal ions was initially demonstrated in early studies of DdDPs, and structural work on a wide range of phosphotransfer enzymes indicates that a basic mechanism involving two metal ions at the active site is a common feature of most if not all DdDPs, DdRPs, RdDPs, and RdRPs (Doublie and Ellenberger 1998; Doublie et al. 1999; Rothwell and Waksman 2005; Steitz 1998). In RdRPs, divalent metal ion dependence was initially demonstrated in poliovirus and subsequently shown to involve several of the most highly conserved residues in all RdRPs (Arnold et al. 1999; Flanegan and Baltimore 1977; Jablonski and Morrow 1995). Mutagenesis studies and crystal structures indicate that metal binding may occur at multiple sites near the active site. Two metal ions [designated A and B, according to Steitz (1998)] appear to be the most important for enzymatic activity. Metal ion A coordinates to the α-phosphate group of the nucleoside triphosphate (NTP) and the 3'-OH of the nascent primer, as well as the side chain carboxylate groups of the two consecutive Asp residues in motif C and the first Asp at the beginning of motif A (Fig. 2). Metal ion B coordinates to the β- and γ-phosphate groups of the NTP, as well as the first two aspartic acid residues of motif A and the first of the two consecutive Asp residues in motif C.

Mutating the Asp residues in motifs A and C that coordinate to the divalent metal ions inactivates or alters the activity of several RdRPs (Arnold et al. 1999; Jablonski and Morrow 1995; Vazquez et al. 2000). In addition, altering the nature of the metal ions by introducing different ions such as Mg^{2+}, Mn^{2+}, Ca^{2+}, and Fe^{2+} affects the polymerase activity of RdRPs in a number of different ways. Properties observed in Mg^{2+} are most consistent with properties observed biologically. The structure of bacteriophage $\phi 6$ RdRP in complex with Ca^{2+} reveals an inactive arrangement of active site residues distinct from that seen in the enzyme bound to Mg^{2+} and Mn^{2+} (Salgado et al. 2004).

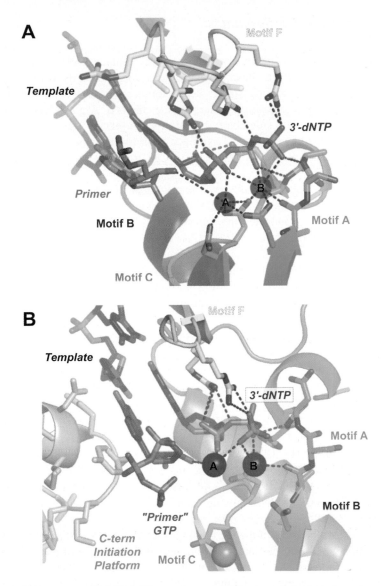

Fig. 2 A, B Structures of E•RNA•NTP complexes. **A** RNA primer-dependent elongation complex formed by reovirus RdRP (1N35) (Tao et al. 2002). **B** Primer-independent (de novo) initiation complex formed by bacteriophage φ6 RdRP (1HI0) (Butcher et al. 2001). Divalent metal ions are drawn as *magenta spheres*. Coordination and hydrogen bonds are drawn as *dashed, red lines*. The 3'-terminal residue of the RNA primer in reovirus RdRP is drawn in *gray* and the two residues of the RNA template that are complementary to the 3'-terminal residue of the RNA primer and the 3'-dNTP are drawn in *black*. The long, 4.5-Å distance between the 3'-OH of the primer and metal ion A is drawn in *magenta* as a *dashed line*

3.2   Nucleoside Triphosphates

The binding of NTPs to RdRPs primarily involves contacts with the triphosphate and sugar moieties, with the base forming interactions primarily with the primer and template (Fig. 2). The triphosphate moiety forms interactions with both divalent metal ions, as well as the positively charged side chains of Arg and Lys residues in motif F. The carboxylate side chain of a highly conserved Asp near the middle of motif A appears to form a critical hydrogen bond for distinguishing the 2′-OH of NTPs from the 2′-H of dNTPs (Arnold and Cameron 2004; Gohara et al. 2004; Gohara et al. 2000).

NTP-binding has also been observed in a number of RdRPs at sites other than the active site. In hepatitis C virus (HCV) and bovine viral diarrhea virus (BVDV) RdRPs, a regulatory guanosine triphosphate (GTP)-binding site has been localized (Bressanelli et al. 2002; Cai et al. 2005; Choi et al. 2006; Choi et al. 2004). In addition, a number of RdRP complexes have been obtained with NTPs in the absence of RNA (Ago et al. 1999; Bressanelli et al. 2002; O'Farrell et al. 2003; Thompson and Peersen 2004). Although the binding modes for NTPs that are observed in these complexes are sometimes similar to the productive mode expected for the phospho-transfer reaction, the absence of base-pairing with the template RNA strand usually leaves the base in a conformation that differs substantially from that expected in the productive mode.

3.3   RNA

At least two distinct modes of RNA binding have been seen in the two major divisions in the RdRP family. In the RdRPs from *Picornaviridae* and *Caliciviridae*, the RNA-binding cleft is approximately 15 Å wide and can fit an A-form RNA duplex, as seen in the FMDV RdRP-RNA complex (Fig. 1A) (Ferrer-Orta et al. 2004) and resembling the mode of DNA binding seen in numerous DdDPs and DdRPs. In contrast, the RdRPs from *Flaviviridae* and *Cystoviridae* contain protein structures that obstruct the cleft, preventing the binding of duplex RNA and providing a plat-form for the assembly of an initiation complex in the absence of an RNA primer (Fig. 1B, 2A; Tao et al. 2002). RNA complexes from these RdRPs reveal a binding cleft that is suited more for binding a single strand of RNA template forming Watson-Crick base pairs with only a short segment of primer RNA (Butcher et al. 2001; O'Farrell et al. 2003). In the reovirus RdRP, a large C-terminal domain is situated in front of the active site cleft without blocking the entry of short RNA primers, thus forming a "cage" around the polymerase active site (Fig. 1C, 2B; Tao et al. 2002). The initiation complex seen in this enzyme is similar to that seen in bacteriophage ϕ6 RdRP, with a priming loop extension of the palm domain forming a platform for dinucleotide synthesis. This loop moves away from the active site to allow for the formation of longer double-strand products, probably in a manner more similar to that expected for the primer-dependent RdRPs.

3.4 Proteins and Higher-Order Complexes

RdRPs have been shown to interact with a number of proteins produced by either the virus or the host, particularly during the initiation of RNA replication. In the *Picornaviridae*, a 22-amino-acid virally encoded initiator protein called VPg (virion protein genome linked) is uridylylated by the RdRP as an initial step in replication (Lee et al. 1977; Nomoto et al. 1977; Paul et al. 1998). The structure of the FMDV RdRP-VPg complex reveals interactions between VPg and the RdRP active-site cleft that position the side-chain hydroxyl group of Tyr 3 in VPg near the α-phosphate moiety of the uridine triphosphate (UTP) cosubstrate (Ferrer-Orta et al. 2006). In combination with mutational studies (Boerner et al. 2005; Lyle et al. 2002; Pathak et al. 2002), this structure reveals a number of residues in the active site cleft involved with the binding of VPg and with the uridylylation reaction involved with the initiation of RNA synthesis.

Higher-order complexes involving proteins and RNA structures are also formed by RdRPs and alternate forms of RdRPs, such as the proteinase-polymerase fusions seen in picornaviruses (Cornell and Semler 2002; Parsley et al. 1999; Ypma-Wong et al. 1988) and caliciviruses (Belliot et al. 2005; Belliot et al. 2003; Kaiser et al. 2006; Sosnovtseva et al. 1999; Wei et al. 2001). Although the formation of such complexes is best understood in the picornaviruses, especially poliovirus, no structural information on these complexes is available at present (Andino et al. 1999; Andino et al. 1993; Andino et al. 1990; Paul et al. 2003). It is likely that higher-order complexes involving RdRPs, other proteins, and RNA play critical roles in the initiation of RNA synthesis, translation, and RNA packaging for most, if not all, RNA viruses (Ortin and Parra 2006).

3.5 Inhibitors

Due to the severe threat to public health posed by HCV, an intensive search for novel antiviral therapies to treat HCV infection has been conducted in the past decade. A wide variety of inhibitors have been identified that target the RdRP from HCV. Most interesting among these have been a series of nonnucleoside inhibitors that appear to bind near the base of the thumb domain to allosterically inhibit polymerase activity, possibly by interfering with a conformational change required for normal catalytic activity (Biswal et al. 2005; Biswal et al. 2006; Dhanak et al. 2002; Di Marco et al. 2005; Gopalsamy et al. 2006; Harper et al. 2005; Love et al. 2003; Tomei et al. 2003; Wang et al. 2003). It is interesting to note that alternate conformational states have been observed in several RdRP structures (Biswal et al. 2005; Choi et al. 2004; Ng et al. 2002), suggesting that important conformational changes may accompany enzymatic catalysis as seen in other classes of polymerases (Doublie et al. 1999; Rothwell and Waksman 2005).

4 Phosphodiester Bond Formation

4.1 Two Metal Ion Mechanism

The chemistry at the active site of all nucleic acid polymerases studied to date is facilitated by a two metal ion mechanism that was proposed by Steitz based on his structural work on the magnesium-dependent exonuclease activity of DNA polymerase I from *Escherichia coli* (Steitz 1993). The model shown in Fig. 3 has been adapted for enzymes with a palm-based active site, which includes the viral RdRP. A magnesium (metal B)-nucleotide complex binds to the active site followed by binding of a second magnesium ion (metal A). The metal designations reflect the occurrence of metal A in some structures in the absence of nucleotide substrate. Metal A is thought to be involved in activation of the 3′-OH for nucleophilic attack by lowering its pK_a value. Metal B orients the β- and γ-phosphates of the nucleotide substrate and stabilizes the negatively charged pentavalent phosphorane transition state (Fig. 4).

The two metal ion mechanism implies that side chains of active site residues do not participate directly in catalysis, only indirectly as ligands for one or more of the magnesium ions (Steitz 1993). However, two proton transfer reactions must occur during the reaction. The 3′-OH nucleophile must be deprotonated and the pyrophosphate (PPi) leaving group must be protonated (Fig. 4). The acceptor and donor for these key proton transfer reactions is not known and is not likely to be solvent given the dearth of ordered solvent in structures of complexes thought to mimic the catalytically active polymerase-nucleic acid-nucleotide complex (Doublie et al. 1998; Franklin et al. 2001; Johnson et al. 2003; Sawaya et al. 1997; Yin and Steitz 2004).

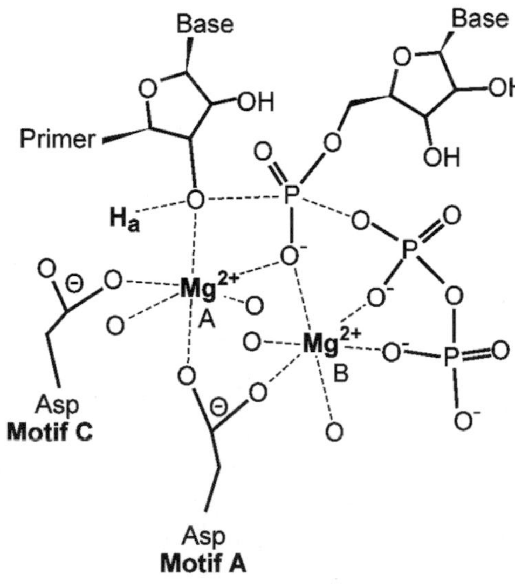

Fig. 3 Two-metal-ion mechanism for nucleotidyl transfer. The nucleoside triphosphate enters the active site with a divalent cation (Mg²⁺, metal B). This metal is coordinated by the β- and γ-phosphates of the nucleotide, by an Asp residue located in structural motif A of all polymerases, and likely water molecules (indicated as oxygen ligands to metal without specific designation). This metal orients the triphosphate in the active site and may contribute to charge neutralization during catalysis. Once the nucleotide is in place, the second divalent cation binds (Mg²⁺, metal A). Metal A is coordinated by the 3′-OH, the α-phosphate, and Asp residues of structural motifs A and C. This metal lowers the pK_a of the 3′-OH facilitating catalysis at physiological pH. (Adapted from Liu and Tsai 2001)

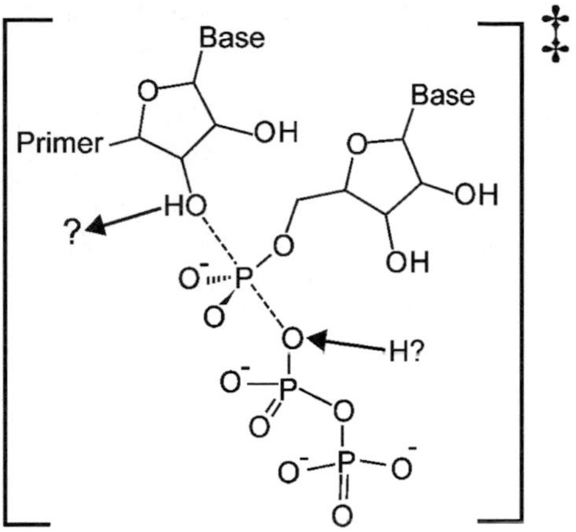

Fig. 4 Pentavalent phosphorane transition state. During the nucleotidyl transfer reaction, two proton transfer reactions must occur. The proton from the 3'-OH nucleophile must be removed; a proton must be donated to the pyrophosphate leaving group. To date there is no information on these steps of the nucleotidyl transfer reaction

4.2   Initiation Vs Elongation

Formally there are two mechanisms for initiation of RNA synthesis: primer independent (de novo) and primer dependent. De novo initiation requires formation of a phosphodiester bond between two ribonucleotides (Fig. 5A). For replication, initiation is templated by the extreme 3'-end of template; however, for transcription, initiation may be templated by internal positions. In Fig. 5A, the 3' nucleotide defining the site of initiation has been designated "n." Residues at the n and n+1 positions of template define the primer (P) and nucleotide (N) binding sites. The 3'-OH of the P-site NTP attacks the α-phosphorous of the N-site NTP to form a dinucleotide. Iterative rounds of incorporation and translocation will ultimately yield a stable elongation complex (Fig. 5B).

De novo initiation generally employs purine nucleotides, often with a preference for GTP at the P-site. With some enzymes, guanosine, guanosine monophosphate (GMP), and guanosine diphosphate (GDP) can substitute for a P-site GTP (Martin and Coleman 1989). Because base-pairing alone is insufficient to stabilize the P-site NTP and the triphosphate is not essential for P-site occupancy, specialized structural elements are employed. For example, in bacteriophage ϕ6, a specialized carboxy-terminal domain presents at least one tyrosine for stacking with the P-site NTP (Butcher et al. 2001). The reovirus polymerase has a specialized loop that serves a similar function (Tao et al. 2002). The dinucleotide product is unstable. As a result, abortive cycling is often observed for polymerases that initiate de novo. Formation of a stable elongation complex generally coincides with formation of an RNA product long enough to form a stable duplex with the template and may require substantial conformational rearrangements of the polymerase (Yin and Steitz 2004).

Enzymes that employ a primer-dependent mechanism for initiation will use either a protein primer or an oligonucleotide of defined origin but random sequence (van Dijk et al. 2004). As discussed in Sect. 3.4, picornaviruses use the tyrosine hydroxyl group of VPg as the nucleophile. VPg binds to the RNA binding pocket of the polymerase independent of the template (Ferrer-Orta et al. 2006).

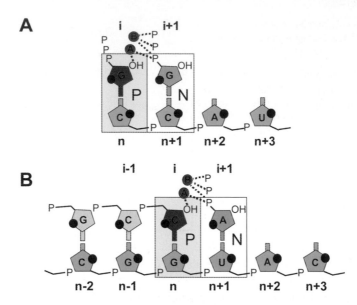

Fig. 5 A, B De novo initiation and elongation complexes. **A** De novo initiation of RNA synthesis involves binding of the initiating nucleotide (GTPi; *red*) at the priming or initiation site (P-site; *green box*) and binding of the first NTP substrate (GTPi+1; *blue*) to the nucleotide binding site (N-site; *white box*). Specific binding sites for divalent cations (*pink circles A and B*) are shown in close proximity to the α-, β-, and γ-phosphates of the first nucleotide substrate. **B** Elongation complex. Nucleotide addition during elongation involves binding of the nascent RNA primer strand, positioning of the 3′-terminal nucleotide in the P-site, and binding of the first NTP substrate (i+1, *blue*) to the nucleotide binding site (N-site; *white box*)

This mechanism has all of the features of a stable elongation complex: limited, if any, abortive cycling and no requirement for large conformational rearrangements.

Transcription by the influenza virus RNA polymerase employs a "cap-snatching" mechanism. Capped mRNAs are cleaved by a subunit of the heterotrimeric polymerase complex to produce capped RNA oligonucleotides (10-15 nt) that are used to prime transcription (van Dijk et al. 2004). The cap is the major determinant for recognition by the endoribonuclease activity of the polymerase complex. The capped RNA product binds stably to the polymerase complex ($t_{1/2}$ ~1 h) (Olsen et al. 1996). The 3′-OH of the terminal nucleotide serves as the nucleophile, with the template being held in the complex independently. Again, this approach provides the advantages of the elongation complex described above. However, this approach can only be used for genome replication if the sequences at the ends of the genome lack information: coding sequence, *cis*-acting elements, etc.

5 Fidelity

RdRPs have often been described as error-prone polymerases. However, it has become increasingly clear that these polymerases are as faithful as replicative DNA polymerases in the absence of their proofreading exonuclease (Castro et al. 2005).

Indeed, biochemical, phenotypic, and direct sequencing experiments have shown that RNA virus polymerases incorporate transition mutations at a frequency of 10^{-5} and transversions mutations at a frequency of 10^{-6}-10^{-7} (Castro et al. 2005). The kinetic and structural bases for fidelity of nucleotide selection is understood best for the RdRP from poliovirus (3Dpol).

5.1 Kinetic Basis

A complete kinetic mechanism for the single nucleotide addition cycle catalyzed by 3Dpol (E) is known. 3Dpol binds to a primer-template substrate (R_n) with a equilibrium dissociation constant in the micromolar range (Arnold and Cameron 2000). This complex isomerizes to form ER_n, a complex that has a half-life on the order of 2-4 h and is competent for binding nucleotide (Arnold and Cameron 2000). As shown in Fig. 6, binding of nucleotide to ER_n yields a complex, ER_nNTP, that undergoes a conformational change to produce a catalytically competent complex ($*ER_nNTP$) (Arnold and Cameron 2004). This conformational change has been suggested to be reorientation of the triphosphate moiety of the incoming NTP into a position suitable for catalysis and coordination of metal A (Arnold et al. 2004). Chemistry occurs ($ER_{n+1}PPi$) followed by translocation with concomitant release of PPi, placing the enzyme in the appropriate register for another round of nucleotide incorporation.

Binding of nucleotides to the ER_n complex is driven by the interaction of the triphosphate with motif F of the enzyme (Arnold and Cameron 2004). As a result,

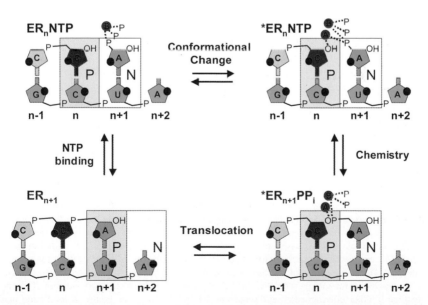

Fig. 6 Elongation cycle. The stages of RNA synthesis can be divided into four steps: nucleotide binding (step 1), a conformational-change step, thought to be orientation of the triphosphate for catalysis (step 2), chemistry (step 3), and translocation (step 4)

nucleotides with an incorrect base or sugar configuration (e.g., 2'-dNTPs) bind as well as the correct nucleotide. However, incorrect nucleotides are incapable of forming a *ER$_n$NTP complex that is stable enough to undergo catalysis (Arnold and Cameron 2004; Arnold et al. 2004). In addition, the rate constant for chemistry is reduced significantly when an incorrect nucleotide is bound (Arnold and Cameron 2004; Arnold et al. 2004).

5.2 Structural Basis

Only one crystal structure is available for an RdRP complex that may represent ER$_n$NTP or *ER$_n$NTP (Tao et al. 2002). However, the conserved nature of palm-based active sites combined with kinetic and thermodynamic analyses of site-directed mutants with nucleotide analogs has led to a structural model for nucleotide selection by 3Dpol that extrapolates well to other classes of nucleic acid polymerases (Gohara et al. 2004). Shown in Fig. 7 is a model for *ER$_n$NTP (Gohara et al. 2004). The orientation of the triphosphate dictates both the stability of this complex and catalytic efficiency. The orientation of the triphosphate requires interaction with conserved structural motif A. Note that one residue of motif A, Asp-238, is located

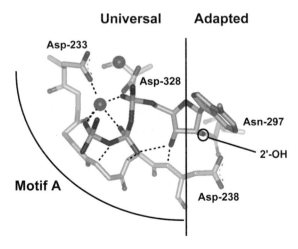

Fig. 7 Structural basis for fidelity. The nucleotide-binding pocket of all nucleic acid polymerases with a canonical "palm"-based active site is highly conserved. The site can be divided into two parts: a region that has "universal" interactions mediated by conserved structural motif A that organize the metals and triphosphate for catalysis, and a region that has "adapted" interactions mediated by conserved structural motif B that dictate whether ribo- or 2'deoxyribonucleotides will be utilized. In the classical polymerase, there is a motif A residue located in the sugar-binding pocket capable of interacting with the motif B residue(s) involved in sugar selection. This motif A residue in other polymerases could represent the link between the nature of the bound nucleotide (correct vs incorrect) to the efficiency of nucleotidyl transfer as described herein for Asp-238 of 3D^{pol}. (Gohara et al. 2004)

in the nucleoside binding pocket. Binding of a nucleotide with an incorrect base or ribose configuration will alter the dynamics or equilibrium position of Asp-238. This perturbation will be communicated to the active site by changes in the positions of the other motif A residues, placing the triphosphate in a suboptimal orientation and leading to a destabilized *ER$_n$NTP complex with reduced catalytic efficiency.

6 RdRPs of RNAi

Very little is known about the structure, function, and mechanism of the RdRPs of RNAi. The most conserved region, based on sequence alignments, is shown in Fig. 8 and represents, at best, 20% of the protein (Huang et al. 2003). The DxDGD motif has been shown to be essential for RdRP activity (Makeyev and Bamford 2002) and is reminiscent of the metal-binding GDD motif (motif C) of the viral RdRPs. The enzyme clearly has a requirement for divalent cation (Makeyev and Bamford 2002). Studies of the enzyme from *N. crassa* have suggested that the enzyme lacks template specificity and uses a de novo initiation mechanism, initiating both from the end and perhaps from internal positions (Makeyev and Bamford 2002). When initiating from an end, long products can be produced (Makeyev and Bamford 2002), consistent with the observation of transitive silencing in related systems (Sijen et al. 2001). The primary product of the reaction is single-stranded RNA on the order of 20 nt in length, a size appropriate for direct incorporation into the RISC complex (Sijen et al. 2001).

7 Concluding Remarks

Our current understanding of viral RdRPs has required the capacity to apply molecular genetic, biochemical, and structural approaches. Analysis of cellular RdRPs has not reached this stage but is well on its way. *N. crassa* is clearly an

```
tomato   RSRIFIPN--GRTMMGCLDESRTLEYGQVFVQFTGAG-HGEFSDDLHPFNNSRSTNSNFILKGNVVVAKNPCL
QDE-1    KLNIRVGR--SAYIYMIADFWGVLEENEVHVGFSSK-----FRDEEESFTLLSDC--------DVLVARSPAH
EGO-1    KEQIPIPCDLGRSMLGVVDETGRLQYGQIFVQYTKN-----LALKLPPKNAARQV-----LTGTVLLTKNPCI
RRF-1    KEQIQIPSELGRSMLGVVDETGRLQYGQIFVQYTKN-----YKKKLPPRDSNNKVHGSEIVTGTVLLTKNPCI
SDE1     KSRIFVTS--GRWLMGCLDEAGILEHGQCFIQVSKPSIENCFSKHGSRFKETKKDL--EVVKGYVAIAKNPCL
RrpA     KCHIEIKD--SRMLLGVCDPTNSLPPNTVFVQLEEE-------DE-DDDDDGRKYE--KVIEGLVMVIKNPCT

tomato   HPGDIRVLKAVNVRALHHMVDCVVFPQKGKRPHPNECSGSDLDGDIYFVCWDQDMIPP-RQVQPMEYP-PAPS
QDE-1    FPSDIQRVRAVFKPELHSLKDVIIFSTKGDVPLAKKLSGGDYDGDMAWVCWDPEIVDGFVNAEMPLEPDLSRY
EGO-1    VAGDVRIFEAVDIPELHHMCDVVVFPQHGPRPHPDEMAGSDLDGDEYSIIWDQQLLLD-KNEDPYDFTSEKQK
RRF-1    VPGDVRIFEAVDIPELHHMCDVVVFPQHGPRPHPDEMAGSDLDGDEYSVIWDQELLLE-RNEEPFDFAVEKIK
SDE1     HPGDVRILEAVDVPQLHHMYDCLIFPQKGDRPHTNEASGSDLDGDLYFVAWDQKLIPPNRKSYPAMHYDAAEE
RrpA     HPGDVRYLKAVDNIRLRHLRNVLVFSTKGDVPNFKEISGSDLDGDRYFFCYDKSLIGNRSESETAYLVVETVS
```

Fig. 8 Alignment of conserved regions of RNAi RdRPs. Comparison of putative RdRP amino acid sequence from different organisms including tomato plant, *Neurospora (QDE-1)*, *C. elegans (EGO-1, RRF-1)*, *Arabidopsis (SDE1)*, and *Dictyostelium discoideum (RrpA)*. Amino acids in *red* indicate conserved residues in all sequences in the alignment. Those in *blue* and *green* indicate conservative substitutions and semi-conservative substitutions, respectively

organism amenable to molecular genetics and a biochemical system is available for the RdRP from this organism. Importantly, a structure is imminent. Note added in proof: The crystal structure of the QDE-1, a cell-encoded RdRP from *N. crassa* was recently reported (Salgado et al. 2006). The publication reporting this structure is, These major advances in the *N. crassa* system will undoubtedly have a major impact on progress in other systems.

Acknowledgements The authors would like to thank Professor Matthias Götte (McGill University) for providing the templates for Figs. 5 and 6. K.K.S.N. is a Scholar of the Alberta Heritage Foundation for Medical Research and a New Investigator of the Canadian Institutes for Health Research (CIHR). His laboratory is supported by grants from the CIHR, Natural Sciences and Engineering Research Council of Canada, Canadian Foundation for Innovation and the Alberta Ingenuity Centre for Carbohydrate Science. C.E.C. is recipient of an Established Investigator Award from the American Heart Association (0340028N) and his lab is supported by grants from the National Institutes of Health (AI045818, AI053531, AI054776).

References

Ago H, Adachi T, Yoshida A, Yamamoto M, Habuka N, Yatsunami K, Miyano M (1999) Crystal structure of the RNA-dependent RNA polymerase of hepatitis C virus. Structure Fold Des 7:1417-1426

Andino R, Rieckhof GE, Baltimore D (1990) A functional ribonucleoprotein complex forms around the 5′ end of poliovirus RNA. Cell 63:369-380

Andino R, Rieckhof GE, Achacoso PL, Baltimore D (1993) Poliovirus RNA synthesis utilizes an RNP complex formed around the 5′-end of viral RNA. EMBO J 12:3587-3598

Andino R, Boddeker N, Silvera D, Gamarnik AV (1999) Intracellular determinants of picornavirus replication. Trends Microbiol 7:76-82

Appleby TC, Luecke H, Shim JH, Wu JZ, Cheney IW, Zhong W, Vogeley L, Hong Z, Yao N (2005) Crystal structure of complete rhinovirus RNA polymerase suggests front loading of protein primer. J Virol 79:277-288

Arnold JJ, Cameron CE (2000) Poliovirus RNA-dependent RNA polymerase [3D(pol)]. Assembly of stable, elongation-competent complexes by using a symmetrical primer-template substrate (sym/sub). J Biol Chem 275:5329-5336

Arnold JJ, Cameron CE (2004) Poliovirus RNA-dependent RNA polymerase (3Dpol): pre-steady-state kinetic analysis of ribonucleotide incorporation in the presence of Mg^{2+}. Biochemistry 43:5126-5137

Arnold JJ, Ghosh SK, Cameron CE (1999) Poliovirus RNA-dependent RNA polymerase [3D(pol)]. Divalent cation modulation of primer, template, and nucleotide selection. J Biol Chem 274:37060-37069

Arnold JJ, Gohara DW, Cameron CE (2004) Poliovirus RNA-dependent RNA polymerase (3Dpol): pre-steady-state kinetic analysis of ribonucleotide incorporation in the presence of Mn^{2+}. Biochemistry 43:5138-5148

Astier-Manifacier S, Cornuet P (1971) RNA-dependent RNA polymerase in Chinese cabbage. Biochim Biophys Acta 232:484-493

Astier-Manifacier S, Cornuet P (1978) Purification and molecular weight of an RNA-dependant RNA polymerase from Brassicae oleracea var. Botrytis (in French). C R Acad Sci Hebd Seances Acad Sci D 287:1043-1046

Belliot G, Sosnovtsev SV, Mitra T, Hammer C, Garfield M, Green KY (2003) In vitro proteolytic processing of the MD145 norovirus ORF1 nonstructural polyprotein yields stable precursors and products similar to those detected in calicivirus-infected cells. J Virol 77:10957-10974

Belliot G, Sosnovtsev SV, Chang KO, Babu V, Uche U, Arnold JJ, Cameron CE, Green KY (2005) Norovirus proteinase-polymerase and polymerase are both active forms of RNA-dependent RNA polymerase. J Virol 79:2393-2403

Biswal BK, Cherney MM, Wang M, Chan L, Yannopoulos CG, Bilimoria D, Nicolas O, Bedard J, James MN (2005) Crystal structures of the RNA-dependent RNA polymerase genotype 2a of hepatitis C virus reveal two conformations and suggest mechanisms of inhibition by non-nucleoside inhibitors. J Biol Chem 280:18202-18210

Biswal BK, Wang M, Cherney MM, Chan L, Yannopoulos CG, Bilimoria D, Bedard J, James MN (2006) Non-nucleoside inhibitors binding to hepatitis C virus NS5B polymerase reveal a novel mechanism of inhibition. J Mol Biol 361:33-45

Boege F, Sänger HL (1980) RNA-dependent RNA polymerase from healthy tomato leaf tissue. FEBS Lett 121:91-96

Boerner JE, Lyle JM, Daijogo S, Semler BL, Schultz SC, Kirkegaard K, Richards OC (2005) Allosteric effects of ligands and mutations on poliovirus RNA-dependent RNA polymerase. J Virol 79:7803-7811

Bressanelli S, Tomei L, Roussel A, Incitti I, Vitale RL, Mathieu M, De Francesco R, Rey FA (1999) Crystal structure of the RNA-dependent RNA polymerase of hepatitis C virus. Proc Natl Acad Sci U S A 96:13034-13039

Bressanelli S, Tomei L, Rey FA, De Francesco R (2002) Structural analysis of the hepatitis C virus RNA polymerase in complex with ribonucleotides. J Virol 76:3482-3492

Bruenn JA (2003) A structural and primary sequence comparison of the viral RNA-dependent RNA polymerases. Nucleic Acids Res 31:1821-1829

Butcher SJ, Grimes JM, Makeyev EV, Bamford DH, Stuart DI (2001) A mechanism for initiating RNA-dependent RNA polymerization. Nature 410:235-240

Cai Z, Yi M, Zhang C, Luo G (2005) Mutagenesis analysis of the rGTP-specific binding site of hepatitis C virus RNA-dependent RNA polymerase. J Virol 79:11607-11617

Castro C, Arnold JJ, Cameron CE (2005) Incorporation fidelity of the viral RNA-dependent RNA polymerase: a kinetic, thermodynamic and structural perspective. Virus Res 107:141-149

Choi KH, Groarke JM, Young DC, Kuhn RJ, Smith JL, Pevear DC, Rossmann MG (2004) The structure of the RNA-dependent RNA polymerase from bovine viral diarrhea virus establishes the role of GTP in de novo initiation. Proc Natl Acad Sci U S A 101:4425-4430

Choi KH, Gallei A, Becher P, Rossmann MG (2006) The structure of bovine viral diarrhea virus RNA-dependent RNA polymerase and its amino-terminal domain. Structure 14:1107-1113

Cogoni C, Macino G (1999) Gene silencing in Neurospora crassa requires a protein homologous to RNA-dependent RNA polymerase. Nature 399:166-169

Cornell CT, Semler BL (2002) Subdomain specific functions of the RNA polymerase region of poliovirus 3CD polypeptide. Virology 298:200-213

Dhanak D, Duffy KJ, Johnston VK, Lin-Goerke J, Darcy M, Shaw AN, Gu B, Silverman C, Gates AT, Nonnemacher MR, Earnshaw DL, Casper DJ, Kaura A, Baker A, Greenwood C, Gutshall LL, Maley D, DelVecchio A, Macarron R, Hofmann GA, Alnoah Z, Cheng HY, Chan G, Khandekar S, Keenan RM, Sarisky RT (2002) Identification and biological characterization of heterocyclic inhibitors of the hepatitis C virus RNA-dependent RNA polymerase. J Biol Chem 277:38322-38327

Di Marco S, Volpari C, Tomei L, Altamura S, Harper S, Narjes F, Koch U, Rowley M, De Francesco R, Migliaccio G, Carfi A (2005) Interdomain communication in hepatitis C virus polymerase abolished by small molecule inhibitors bound to a novel allosteric site. J Biol Chem 280:29765-29770

Doublie S, Ellenberger T (1998) The mechanism of action of T7 DNA polymerase. Curr Opin Struct Biol 8:704-712

Doublie S, Tabor S, Long AM, Richardson CC, Ellenberger T (1998) Crystal structure of a bacteriophage T7 DNA replication complex at 2.2 Å resolution. Nature 391:251-258

Doublie S, Sawaya MR, Ellenberger T (1999) An open and closed case for all polymerases. Structure 7:R31-R35

Duda CT, Zaitlin M, Siegel A (1973) In vitro synthesis of double-stranded RNA by an enzyme system isolated from tobacco leaves. Biochim Biophys Acta 319:62-71

Ferrer-Orta C, Arias A, Perez-Luque R, Escarmis C, Domingo E, Verdaguer N (2004) Structure of foot-and-mouth disease virus RNA-dependent RNA polymerase and its complex with a template-primer RNA. J Biol Chem 279:47212-47221

Ferrer-Orta C, Arias A, Agudo R, Perez-Luque R, Escarmis C, Domingo E, Verdaguer N (2006) The structure of a protein primer-polymerase complex in the initiation of genome replication. EMBO J 25:880-888

Flanegan JB, Baltimore D (1977) Poliovirus-specific primer-dependent RNA polymerase able to copy poly(A). Proc Natl Acad Sci U S A 74:3677-3680

Franklin MC, Wang J, Steitz TA (2001) Structure of the replicating complex of a pol alpha family DNA polymerase. Cell 105:657-667

Gohara DW, Crotty S, Arnold JJ, Yoder JD, Andino R, Cameron CE (2000) Poliovirus RNA-dependent RNA polymerase (3Dpol): structural, biochemical, and biological analysis of conserved structural motifs A and B. J Biol Chem 275:25523-25532

Gohara DW, Arnold JJ, Cameron CE (2004) Poliovirus RNA-dependent RNA polymerase (3Dpol): kinetic, thermodynamic, and structural analysis of ribonucleotide selection. Biochemistry 43:5149-5158

Gopalsamy A, Chopra R, Lim K, Ciszewski G, Shi M, Curran KJ, Sukits SF, Svenson K, Bard J, Ellingboe JW, Agarwal A, Krishnamurthy G, Howe AY, Orlowski M, Feld B, O'Connell J, Mansour TS (2006) Discovery of proline sulfonamides as potent and selective hepatitis C virus NS5b polymerase inhibitors. Evidence for a new NS5b polymerase binding site. J Med Chem 49:3052-3055

Hansen JL, Long AM, Schultz SC (1997) Structure of the RNA-dependent RNA polymerase of poliovirus. Structure 5:1109-1122

Harper S, Avolio S, Pacini B, Di Filippo M, Altamura S, Tomei L, Paonessa G, Di Marco S, Carfi A, Giuliano C, Padron J, Bonelli F, Migliaccio G, De Francesco R, Laufer R, Rowley M, Narjes F (2005) Potent inhibitors of subgenomic hepatitis C virus RNA replication through optimization of indole-N-acetamide allosteric inhibitors of the viral NS5B polymerase. J Med Chem 48:4547-4557

Huang L, Gledhill J, Cameron CE (2003) RNA-dependent RNA polymerase in gene silencing. In: Hannon GJ (ed) RNAi: a guide to gene silencing. Cold Spring Harbor Laboratory Press, Cold Spring Harbor, pp 175-203

Jablonski SA, Morrow CD (1995) Mutation of the aspartic acid residues of the GDD sequence motif of poliovirus RNA-dependent RNA polymerase results in enzymes with altered metal ion requirements for activity. J Virol 69:1532-1539

Johnson SJ, Taylor JS, Beese LS (2003) Processive DNA synthesis observed in a polymerase crystal suggests a mechanism for the prevention of frameshift mutations. Proc Natl Acad Sci U S A 100:3895-3900

Kaiser WJ, Chaudhry Y, Sosnovtsev SV, Goodfellow IG (2006) Analysis of protein-protein interactions in the feline calicivirus replication complex. J Gen Virol 87:363-368

Kamer G, Argos P (1984) Primary structural comparison of RNA-dependent polymerases from plant, animal and bacterial viruses. Nucleic Acids Res 12:7269-7282

Laurila MR, Salgado PS, Makeyev EV, Nettelship J, Stuart DI, Grimes JM, Bamford DH (2005a) Gene silencing pathway RNA-dependent RNA polymerase of Neurospora crassa: yeast expression and crystallization of selenomethionated QDE-1 protein. J Struct Biol 149:111-115

Laurila MR, Salgado PS, Stuart DI, Grimes JM, Bamford DH (2005b) Back-priming mode of phi6 RNA-dependent RNA polymerase. J Gen Virol 86:521-526

Lee YF, Nomoto A, Detjen BM, Wimmer E (1977) A protein covalently linked to poliovirus genome RNA. Proc Natl Acad Sci U S A 74:59-63

Lesburg CA, Cable MB, Ferrari E, Hong Z, Mannarino AF, Weber PC (1999) Crystal structure of the RNA-dependent RNA polymerase from hepatitis C virus reveals a fully encircled active site. Nat Struct Biol 6:937-943

Liu J, Tsai MD (2001) DNA polymerase beta: pre-steady-state kinetic analyses of dATP alpha S stereoselectivity and alteration of the stereoselectivity by various metal ions and by site-directed mutagenesis. Biochemistry 40:9014-9022

Love RA, Parge HE, Yu X, Hickey MJ, Diehl W, Gao J, Wriggers H, Ekker A, Wang L, Thomson JA, Dragovich PS, Fuhrman SA (2003) Crystallographic identification of a noncompetitive inhibitor binding site on the hepatitis C virus NS5B RNA polymerase enzyme. J Virol 77:7575-7581

Love RA, Maegley KA, Yu X, Ferre RA, Lingardo LK, Diehl W, Parge HE, Dragovich PS, Fuhrman SA (2004) The crystal structure of the RNA-dependent RNA polymerase from human rhinovirus: a dual function target for common cold antiviral therapy. Structure 12:1533-1544

Lyle JM, Clewell A, Richmond K, Richards OC, Hope DA, Schultz SC, Kirkegaard K (2002) Similar structural basis for membrane localization and protein priming by an RNA-dependent RNA polymerase. J Biol Chem 277:16324-16331

Makeyev EV, Bamford DH (2002) Cellular RNA-dependent RNA polymerase involved in post-transcriptional gene silencing has two distinct activity modes. Mol Cell 10:1417-1427

Martin CT, Coleman JE (1989) T7 RNA polymerase does not interact with the 5'-phosphate of the initiating nucleotide. Biochemistry 28:2760-2762

Mourrain P, Beclin C, Elmayan T, Feuerbach F, Godon C, Morel JB, Jouette D, Lacombe AM, Nikic S, Picault N, Remoue K, Sanial M, Vo TA, Vaucheret H (2000) Arabidopsis SGS2 and SGS3 genes are required for posttranscriptional gene silencing and natural virus resistance. Cell 101:533-542

Ng KK, Cherney MM, Vazquez AL, Machin A, Alonso JM, Parra F, James MN (2002) Crystal structures of active and inactive conformations of a caliciviral RNA-dependent RNA polymerase. J Biol Chem 277:1381-1387

Ng KK, Pendas-Franco N, Rojo J, Boga JA, Machin A, Alonso JM, Parra F (2004) Crystal structure of Norwalk virus polymerase reveals the carboxyl terminus in the active site cleft. J Biol Chem 279:16638-16645

Nishikura K (2001) A short primer on RNAi: RNA-directed RNA polymerase acts as a key catalyst. Cell 107:415-418

Nomoto A, Detjen B, Pozzatti R, Wimmer E (1977) The location of the polio genome protein in viral RNAs and its implication for RNA synthesis. Nature 268:208-213

O'Farrell D, Trowbridge R, Rowlands D, Jager J (2003) Substrate complexes of hepatitis C virus RNA polymerase (HC-J4): structural evidence for nucleotide import and de-novo initiation. J Mol Biol 326:1025-1035

O'Reilly EK, Kao CC (1998) Analysis of RNA-dependent RNA polymerase structure and function as guided by known polymerase structures and computer predictions of secondary structure. Virology 252:287-303

Olsen DB, Benseler F, Cole JL, Stahlhut MW, Dempski RE, Darke PL, Kuo LC (1996) Elucidation of basic mechanistic and kinetic properties of influenza endonuclease using chemically synthesized RNAs. J Biol Chem 271:7435-7439

Ortin J, Parra F (2006) Structure and function of RNA replication. Annu Rev Microbiol 60:305-326

Parsley TB, Cornell CT, Semler BL (1999) Modulation of the RNA binding and protein processing activities of poliovirus polypeptide 3CD by the viral RNA polymerase domain. J Biol Chem 274:12867-12876

Pathak HB, Ghosh SK, Roberts AW, Sharma SD, Yoder JD, Arnold JJ, Gohara DW, Barton DJ, Paul AV, Cameron CE (2002) Structure-function relationships of the RNA-dependent RNA polymerase from poliovirus (3Dpol). A surface of the primary oligomerization domain functions in capsid precursor processing and VPg uridylylation. J Biol Chem 277:31551-31562

Paul AV, van Boom JH, Filippov D, Wimmer E (1998) Protein-primed RNA synthesis by purified poliovirus RNA polymerase. Nature 393:280-284

Paul AV, Peters J, Mugavero J, Yin J, van Boom JH, Wimmer E (2003) Biochemical and genetic studies of the VPg uridylylation reaction catalyzed by the RNA polymerase of poliovirus. J Virol 77:891-904

Pfefferkorn JA, Greene ML, Nugent RA, Gross RJ, Mitchell MA, Finzel BC, Harris MS, Wells PA, Shelly JA, Anstadt RA, Kilkuskie RE, Kopta LA, Schwende FJ (2005a) Inhibitors of HCV NS5B polymerase. Part 1. Evaluation of the southern region of (2Z)-2-(benzoylamino)-3-(5-phenyl-2-furyl)acrylic acid. Bioorg Med Chem Lett 15:2481-2486

Pfefferkorn JA, Nugent R, Gross RJ, Greene M, Mitchell MA, Reding MT, Funk LA, Anderson R, Wells PA, Shelly JA, Anstadt R, Finzel BC, Harris MS, Kilkuskie RE, Kopta LA, Schwende FJ (2005b) Inhibitors of HCV NS5B polymerase. Part 2. Evaluation of the northern region of (2Z)-2-benzoylamino-3-(4-phenoxy-phenyl)-acrylic acid. Bioorg Med Chem Lett 15:2812-2818

Powers JP, Piper DE, Li Y, Mayorga V, Anzola J, Chen JM, Jaen JC, Lee G, Liu J, Peterson MG, Tonn GR, Ye Q, Walker NP, Wang Z (2006) SAR and mode of action of novel non-nucleoside inhibitors of hepatitis C NS5b RNA polymerase. J Med Chem 49:1034-1046

Rothwell PJ, Waksman G (2005) Structure and mechanism of DNA polymerases. Adv Protein Chem 71:401-440

Salgado PS, Makeyev EV, Butcher SJ, Bamford DH, Stuart DI, Grimes JM (2004) The structural basis for RNA specificity and Ca^{2+} inhibition of an RNA-dependent RNA polymerase. Structure 12:307-316

Salgado P, Koivunen MRL, Makeyev EV, Bamford DH, Stuart DI, Grimes JM (2006) The structure of an RNAi polymerase links RNA silencing and transcription, PLoS Biology 4(12):e434

Sawaya MR, Prasad R, Wilson SH, Kraut J, Pelletier H (1997) Crystal structures of human DNA polymerase beta complexed with gapped and nicked DNA: evidence for an induced fit mechanism. Biochemistry 36:11205-11215

Schiebel W, Pelissier T, Riedel L, Thalmeir S, Schiebel R, Kempe D, Lottspeich F, Sanger HL, Wassenegger M (1998) Isolation of an RNA-directed RNA polymerase-specific cDNA clone from tomato. Plant Cell 10:2087-2101

Sijen T, Fleenor J, Simmer F, Thijssen KL, Parrish S, Timmons L, Plasterk RH, Fire A (2001) On the role of RNA amplification in dsRNA-triggered gene silencing. Cell 107:465-476

Smardon A, Spoerke JM, Stacey SC, Klein ME, Mackin N, Maine EM (2000) EGO-1 is related to RNA-directed RNA polymerase and functions in germ-line development and RNA interference in C. elegans. Curr Biol 10:169-178

Sosnovtseva SA, Sosnovtsev SV, Green KY (1999) Mapping of the feline calicivirus proteinase responsible for autocatalytic processing of the nonstructural polyprotein and identification of a stable proteinase-polymerase precursor protein. J Virol 73:6626-6633

Steitz TA (1993) DNA- and RNA-dependent DNA polymerases. Curr Opin Struct Biol 3:31-38

Steitz TA (1998) A mechanism for all polymerases. Nature 391:231-232

Tao Y, Farsetta DL, Nibert ML, Harrison SC (2002) RNA synthesis in a cage-structural studies of reovirus polymerase lambda3. Cell 111:733-745

Thompson AA, Peersen OB (2004) Structural basis for proteolysis-dependent activation of the poliovirus RNA-dependent RNA polymerase. EMBO J 23:3462-3471

Tomei L, Altamura S, Bartholomew L, Biroccio A, Ceccacci A, Pacini L, Narjes F, Gennari N, Bisbocci M, Incitti I, Orsatti L, Harper S, Stansfield I, Rowley M, De Francesco R, Migliaccio G (2003) Mechanism of action and antiviral activity of benzimidazole-based allosteric inhibitors of the hepatitis C virus RNA-dependent RNA polymerase. J Virol 77:13225-13231

van Dijk AA, Makeyev EV, Bamford DH (2004) Initiation of viral RNA-dependent RNA polymerization. J Gen Virol 85:1077-1093

Vazquez AL, Alonso JM, Parra F (2000) Mutation analysis of the GDD sequence motif of a calicivirus RNA-dependent RNA polymerase. J Virol 74:3888-3891

Wang M, Ng KK, Cherney MM, Chan L, Yannopoulos CG, Bedard J, Morin N, Nguyen-Ba N, Bethell RC, James MN (2003) Non-nucleoside analogue inhibitors bind to an allosteric site on HCV NS5B polymerase: crystal structures and mechanism of inhibition. J Biol Chem 278:9489-9495

Wei L, Huhn JS, Mory A, Pathak HB, Sosnovtsev SV, Green KY, Cameron CE (2001) Proteinase-polymerase precursor as the active form of feline calicivirus RNA-dependent RNA polymerase. J Virol 75:1211-1219

Yin YW, Steitz TA (2004) The structural mechanism of translocation and helicase activity in T7 RNA polymerase. Cell 116:393-404

Ypma-Wong MF, Dewalt PG, Johnson VH, Lamb JG, Semler BL (1988) Protein 3CD is the major poliovirus proteinase responsible for cleavage of the P1 capsid precursor. Virology 166:265-270

RNAi-Mediated Chromatin Silencing in Fission Yeast

Sharon A. White(✉) and Robin C. Allshire

Abstract In the fission yeast *Schizosaccharomyces pombe*, the RNAi pathway plays an important role in the formation and maintenance of heterochromatin. Heterochromatin, or silent chromatin, is an epigenetically inherited attribute of eukaryotic chromosomes which is required for gene regulation, chromosome segregation and maintenance of genome stability. In *S. pombe*, heterochromatin forms on related repetitive DNA sequences at specific loci. These repetitive sequences, in concert with the RNAi machinery, are thought to attract several proteins including

Sharon A. White
Welcome Trust Centre for Cell Biology, Institute of Cell Biology, The University of Edinburgh, Edinburgh, EH9 3JR Scotland, UK,
Sharon.A.White@ed.ac.uk

P.J. Paddison and P.K. Vogt (eds.), *RNA Interference.*
Current Topics in Microbiology and Immunology 320.
© Springer-Verlag Berlin Heidelberg 2008

chromatin-modifying enzymes which act to promote heterochromatin formation. The purification of complexes participating in heterochromatin formation has allowed us to begin to analyse in detail the processes involved. In the future this will help us to understand how the RNAi machinery acts to induce the chromatin modifications which lead to heterochromatin assembly in fission yeast.

1 Overview

The term RNA interference (RNAi) encompasses many related processes in different organisms such as quelling in fungi, co-suppression in plants or RNA knock-down in metazoa (Agrawal et al. 2003; Hannon 2002). In the fission yeast *Schizosaccharomyces pombe*, RNAi has an important function in the formation of heterochromatin at discrete chromosomal loci; centromeres, telomeres, the mating-type locus and ribosomal DNA (rDNA). Outside of these regions, it is not known whether RNAi contributes directly to the regulation of specific genes. RNAi can direct specific chromatin modification in fission yeast and this plays a vital role in transcriptional gene silencing (TGS) at centromeres, telomeres and the mating-type locus by suppressing the production of non-coding transcripts. RNAi can also act post-transcriptionally to silence genes (PTGS) by instigating the sequence-specific degradation of RNA transcripts without affecting transcription of the template itself.

To understand how RNAi contributes to heterochromatin formation it is first necessary to understand the biology of heterochromatin in fission yeast. RNAi-mediated heterochromatin formation is particularly important at centromeres, where it is required to attract a high density of cohesin to hold sister chromatids in tight physical cohesion until their segregation at anaphase. Understanding the processes which contribute to chromosome segregation and the chromatin structures underlying centromere integrity is important as the resulting cellular defects, both in *S. pombe* and in more complex eukaryotes, can cause genomic instability. Chromosome loss or gain as a consequence aberrant centromere function can drive aneuploidy and tumour formation and ultimately lead to a reduction in organism viability (Hassold and Hunt 2001; Wassmann and Benezra 2001).

In this chapter the role of RNAi in forming chromatin structures at specific loci in fission yeast will be described. We will discuss the various protein components and complexes involved and their possible role in directing chromatin modification which allows heterochromatin formation at these specific locations.

1.1 Fission Yeast

S. pombe provides an excellent model organism for the dissection of molecular events involved in chromosome structure and function due to its genetic tractability and comparatively small genome size. *S. pombe* has 4,979 protein-coding genes contained within 13.8 Mb. The genome is divided between three chromosomes;

chromosome I is 5.7 Mb, chromosome II is 4.6 Mb and chromosome III is 3.5 Mb (Wood et al. 2002). *S. pombe* is a unicellular archiascomycete fungus which shares many biological characteristics with more complex eukaryotes. For this reason it has been used with great success to study several cellular processes including cell-cycle control and DNA repair and recombination, as well RNAi-mediated hetero-chromatin formation and chromosome segregation (Egel 2004).

1.2   Active and Silent Chromatin Differ

Eukaryotic genomes are packaged into higher-order chromatin structures which can be simply described as two functionally and structurally distinct regions of the genome termed heterochromatin (silent chromatin) and euchromatin (active chroma-tin) (Richards and Elgin 2002). Higher-order chromatin structure, besides merely packaging the huge mass of chromosomal DNA into the relatively small nucleus, is essential for many processes in the cell ranging from gene regulation to accurate chromosome segregation during mitosis and meiosis. Euchromatin is traditionally associated with regions of transcriptional activity, including most active genes. In contrast, heterochromatin is a highly specialised structure which remains condensed throughout the whole cell cycle and was thought to be transcriptionally inactive by virtue of its inaccessibility to transcription factors. This transcriptionally inactive state is also imposed on genes placed within heterochromatic regions. The 'off' or 'silent' state requires specific chromatin modifications which allow its duplication and propagation through mitotic and meiotic divisions (Richards and Elgin 2002). Heterochromatin has a vital role in maintaining the structural integrity of specific chromosomal regions; it is essential to sustain stable structures at defined regions of repetitive DNA such as centromeres, telomeres and transposable elements. Recombination is known to be repressed across centromeres and the silent mating-type loci in fission yeast (Nielsen and Egel 1989; Niwa et al. 1989). It is likely that silent chromatin structures inhibit the potentially detrimental effects of homologous recombination between repetitive elements on different chromosomes.

2   The Organisation of Fission Yeast Centromeres

Large blocks of heterochromatin are prevalent at the centromere regions of many eukaryotes. In metazoa, large arrays of repetitive DNA of up to several megabase pairs are packaged as heterochromatin at centromeres. The structure of *S. pombe* centromeres is somewhat similar to that of more complex eukaryotes in that they are also relatively large, repetitive and complex structures which occupy 35–110 kb (Steiner et al. 1993; Takahashi et al. 1992). This is in contrast to the comparatively simple point centromeres of the budding yeast *Saccharomyces cerevisiae* which are only 125 bp (Cleveland et al. 2003; Sullivan et al. 2001). Fission yeast kinetochores bind 2–4 microtubules at mitosis (Ding et al. 1993). This is again more reminiscent of the multiple microtubule interactions to each kinetochore in metazoa than the single microtubule attachment observed in budding yeast (Winey et al. 1995). *S. pombe* centromeres are composed of a unique central core (*cc*) of 4–7 kb which is flanked by the innermost repeats (*imr*L/R) and the outer repeats on which centromeric heterochromatin forms (Steiner et al. 1993; Takahashi et al. 1992; Allshire et al. 1995; Partridge et al. 2000; Fig. 1). Together the central core and *imr* repeats make up the central domain and are packaged in a centromere-specific form of chromatin containing the histone H3 variant Cnp1 (the CENP-A homologue in fission yeast), which replaces histone H3 (Takahashi et al. 2000). This central domain has an unusual chromatin structure as partial digestion with micrococcal nuclease produces a smeared pattern rather than the typical ladder pattern (Polizzi and Clarke 1991; Takahashi et al. 1992). Genes are also silenced when placed in this central domain, but the factors involved are distinct from those that affect heterochromatin formation on the outer repeats (Allshire et al. 1994, 1995; Ekwall et al. 1996; Partridge et al. 2000; Pidoux et al. 2003). Thus, this central domain is functionally and structurally distinct from the heterochromatic outer repeat regions (Allshire et al. 1995; Partridge et al. 2000). The central core itself is essential for centromere activity, but alone it is not sufficient to assemble an active centromere. Studies using minichromosomes have demonstrated that at least part of the heterochromatic outer repeat, in combination with central domain sequences, is essential to allow the de novo formation of active centromeres (Baum et al. 1994; Ngan and Clarke 1997; Takahashi et al. 1992).

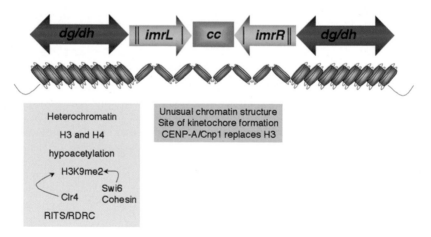

Fig. 1 Centromere organisation in fission yeast. The central core (*cc*) is flanked by inverted innermost repeats (*imr*) the sequence of which is unique to each centromere. Together *cc* and *imr* form the central domain, which is the site of kinetochore formation, and in this region most histone H3 is replaced by the H3 variant Cnp1 (mammalian CENP-A). The central domain is flanked by arrays of inverted repeats, the number and organisation of which vary at each centromere although the sequence is similar. These outer repeat regions (*dg/dh*) are packaged as heterochromatin in which lysine residues in the N-terminal tails of histones H3 and H4 are hypoacetylated. H3 is dimethylated on lysine 9 (H3K9me2) by the histone methyltransferase Clr4. This H3K9me2 recruits the chromo domain protein Swi6, which causes heterochromatin to spread and is required for the association of the cohesin complex. Both the RITS and RDRC complexes are known to associate with the centromeric outer repeats. *Dark blue vertical lines* denote the position of tRNA gene clusters

The outer repeats (*otr*) themselves are composed of two elements, known as the *dh* and *dg* (or K and L) repeats, which are arranged differently with respect to each other at each centromere (Steiner et al. 1993; Takahashi et al. 1992). Because these repeats are packaged into heterochromatin, expression levels of marker genes (*ade6⁺* and *ura4⁺*, for example) inserted at sites across the outer repeats are subject to variable repression or expression, resulting in phenotypic variegation, and this has allowed the development of screens to identify many factors involved in heterochromatin and hence centromere structure and function (Allshire et al. 1995; Ekwall et al. 1999).

2.1 Distinct Boundaries Demarcate Specific Domains Within and Around Fission Yeast Centromeres

The transition from outer repeat heterochromatin to central domain CENP-A^{cnp1} chromatin coincides with the presence of 2–4 tRNA genes (Kuhn et al. 1991; Steiner et al. 1993; Takahashi et al. 1991, 1992). For example, two tRNA genes are found at the boundaries between the *imr* and *otr* repeats at centromere 1. In addition, tRNA genes are present at five of the six extremities of the three centromeres between the *otr* and surrounding euchromatin, the exception occurring at the right side of centromere 1(Fig. 1). Strong DNase hypersensitive sites coincide with the tRNA genes in the *imrL/R* of centromere 1, and it had been suspected that these tRNA genes might act to separate outer repeat heterochromatin from the CENP-A^{cnp1} chromatin of the central domain (Partridge et al. 2000; Takahashi et al. 1992, 2000). Genome-wide analysis has confirmed that heterochromatin is absent inside of the 2–4 tRNA genes clustered at the *cc/otr* boundary. The transition between outer repeat heterochromatin and adjacent euchromatin also coincides with the presence of tRNA genes, TfIIIC binding sites or other elements which may act as boundaries (Cam and Grewal 2004; Noma et al. 2006). A recent study also demonstrated that the tRNA^{Ala} found at the boundary between the central domain and outer repeats at centromere 1 is transcribed and is required to restrict heterochromatin to its normal location. Inactivation of this transcriptionally active tRNA permits heterochromatin to spill into the *imr* sequences. However, deletion of the other tRNA^{Glu} gene, only 424 bp away from tRNA^{Ala}, had a very weak effect. Attempts to simultaneously delete both the tRNA^{Glu} and tRNA^{Ala} failed, indicating perhaps that these tRNA genes act together to provide an important function at the centromere (Scott et al. 2006).

3 Methylated Histone H3 Binds Swi6 to Form Heterochromatin

The definition of heterochromatin is documented as a cytologically visible region of condensed chromatin. More recently it has become possible to analyse heterochromatin at a molecular level and identify the proteins and histone modifications associated with these regions (Richards and Elgin 2002). It is now commonly accepted that heterochromatin can also be defined as regions which display low levels of histone acetylation and are associated with the methylation of histone H3 on lysine 9 (H3K9me) and binding of chromo domain proteins related to *Drosophila* and mammalian heterochromatin protein 1 such as Swi6 in *S. pombe*. The specific methylation of H3 on lysine 9 creates a binding site for Swi6 allowing it to bind histone H3 via its chromodomain (Bannister et al. 2001). Swi6, like HP1, dimerises via its chromo shadow domain and this may create an interaction surface for the recruitment of other proteins (Cowieson et al. 2000). Methylation of lysine 9 in fission yeast is mediated by the conserved histone methyltransferase Clr4 (Suv39 in *Drosophila* and mammals). Clr4 has been shown to be required for the association of Swi6 with outer repeat heterochromatin at centromeres, the mating-type locus and telomeres (Ekwall et al. 1996; Nakayama et al. 2001; Partridge et al. 2000). Strains expressing histone H3 that lack lysine 9 are defective in silencing and Swi6 localisation. This underscores the importance of lysine 9 of H3 and its methylation by Clr4 in recruiting Swi6 (Mellone et al. 2003).

Clr4 is the only orthologue of Suv39 in fission yeast. These histone methyltransferases can catalyse mono-, di- and tri-methylation of lysine 9 of histone H3. In *S. pombe* most H3K9 methylation appears to be dimethyl, although mono- and tri-methyl states have been detected (Yamada et al. 2005). In the absence of Clr4 all H3K9 methylation is lost, and thus Clr4 is probably the only enzyme responsible for this modification. Like its Suv39 orthologues, Clr4 contains a chromo and a SET domain. It is the conserved SET domain of Clr4 that is responsible for the H3K9 methyltransferase activity, and mutations in this domain affect the levels of H3K9 methylation at centromeres and the mating-type locus (Nakayama et al. 2001; Rea et al. 2000). Perhaps surprisingly the genes encoding Clr4 and Swi6 are not essential, thus aiding analyses of these proteins in fission yeast. However, loss of Clr4 or Swi6 function results in defective silent chromatin at centromeres, telomeres and the mating-type locus (Allshire et al. 1995; Ekwall and Ruusala 1994; Klar and Bonaduce 1991; Lorentz et al. 1994; Thon et al. 1994).

3.1 Histone Deacetylation Acts to Allow H3K9 Methylation

It is known that histone methyltransferases are unable to methylate target lysine residues that are acetylated, and therefore histone deacetylases (HDACs) are required to allow methylation (Rea et al. 2000). Within regions of heterochromatin the lysine residues in the tails of histones H3 and H4 exhibit low acetylation levels, and this hypoacetylated state is important for the integrity of heterochromatin. Transient inhibition of HDACs using trichostatin A (TSA) induced hyperacetylation of histone H3 and H4 on the outer repeats, resulting in derepression of marker genes, loss of Swi6 localisation and defective chromosome segregation (Ekwall et al. 1997). This expressed state was found to be heritable through several generations even in the absence of TSA. It is likely that this forced hyperacetylation blocked methylation of lysine 9 by Clr4, thereby causing loss of H3 lysine 9 methylation and thus propagation of the expressed state. Deacetylation of H3 and H4 is therefore essential for the formation of intact heterochromatin and associated functions.

Several HDACs—Sir2, Clr3, and Clr6—are involved in heterochromatin formation. *Clr6* is an essential gene, with broad substrate specificity (Bjerling et al. 2002; Nakayama et al. 2003; Wiren et al. 2005), Sir2 specifically deacetylates H3K9 and H4K16 residues and is required for H3K9 methylation (Shankaranarayana et al. 2003; Wiren et al. 2005). Clr3 specifically deacetylates H3K14 and it is required to recruit the histone methyltransferase Clr4 (Bjerling et al. 2002; Nakayama et al. 2001; Wiren et al. 2005). It has been proposed that Clr3 may stabilise histone H3K9 methylation by prohibiting histone modifications associated with active transcription, thereby discouraging RNA polymerase II (RNAPII) association with regions of heterochromatin (Yamada et al. 2005).

4 The Role of Heterochromatin at Specific Chromosomal Loci

The loss of Clr4 or Swi6 and other components results in defective silencing of marker genes inserted in the heterochromatin formed over the outer repeats at centromeres, the mating-type locus and adjacent to telomeres. Reduced silencing arises due to a reduction in Clr4-dependent H3K9 methylation (H3K9me) and subsequent loss of Swi6 association and localisation (Ekwall et al. 1996; Nakayama et al. 2001; Partridge et al. 2000). What are the consequences for the cellular functions and viability?

4.1 Centromeric Heterochromatin

Cells with defective heterochromatin display increased rates of chromosome loss and an elevated frequency of lagging chromosomes on late anaphase spindles (Allshire et al. 1995; Ekwall et al. 1995, 1996). Consequently, mutants are sensitive to microtubule destabilising drugs such as thiabendazole. This indicates that loss of heterochromatin from centromeres affects centromere function. These defects arise because Swi6 is somehow required to recruit the cohesin complex over the outer repeats. The cohesin complex is required for tight physical cohesion of sister chromatids. In the absence of Swi6 (and Clr4), subunits of cohesin (Rad21 and Psc3) dissociate from centromeric outer repeats, and cohesion at centromeres, but not chromosome arms, is lost (Bernard and Allshire 2002; Bernard et al. 2001; Nonaka et al. 2002). Thus, any mutations affecting the formation of heterochromatin at centromeres ultimately lead to defective chromosome segregation. Fission yeast cells that lack centromeric heterochromatin remain viable because cohesion along chromosome arms is unaffected and is sufficient to sustain reasonable levels of chromosome segregation in an organism with just three chromosomes. Consistent with this, cells with a mild lesion in the Rad21 cohesin subunit require Swi6/heterochromatin for viability (Bernard et al. 2001).

4.2 Telomeric Heterochromatin

The role of heterochromatin at other chromosomal regions in *S. pombe* is perhaps not quite as apparent as at centromeres. Blocks of heterochromatin are found over regions of approximately 40 kb adjacent to each telomere (Kanoh et al. 2005; Nimmo et al. 1994, 1998; Fig. 2). This telomeric heterochromatin is possibly required in some way to prevent end-to-end fusion, to protect chromosome ends from enzymatic degradation or to prevent homologous recombination between telomere repeats at the ends of different chromosomes (Ferreira et al. 2004; Mandell et al. 2005; Sadaie et al. 2003). It is known that telomeres are clustered at the nuclear periphery in mitotically dividing cells (Funabiki et al. 1993) whereas during meiotic prophase they gather together at the spindle pole body to aid pairing

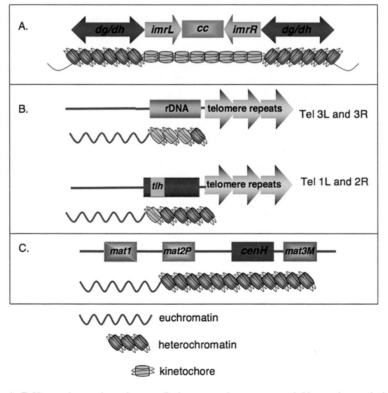

Fig. 2 A, B Heterochromatic regions on fission yeast chromosomes. **A** Heterochromatin is associated with the outer repeat regions of fission yeast centromeres. The central core (*cc*) is flanked by the inner inverted repeats (*imr*) and the heterochromatic outer repeats (*otr* or *dg/dh*). **B** Only telomeres on chromosome 3 contain rDNA repeats. Subtelomeric regions on chromosomes 1 and 2 contain telomere-linked helicase genes (*tlh*) with homology to *dg/dh* centromeric repeats. The sequencing of telomeres is not yet complete and available sequences have not yet been assigned to specific chromosome ends due to high similarity. **C** At the mating-type locus heterochromatin spans around 20 kb covering *mat2-P, cenH* and *mat3-M*

of homologous chromosomes and recombination (Chikashige et al. 1994; Cooper et al. 1998; Nimmo et al. 1998). When telomeric heterochromatin is impaired telomere length is unaffected, but telomere clustering is disrupted to some extent (Ekwall et al. 1996; Hall et al. 2003; Tuzon et al. 2004). This demonstrates a possible role for telomeric heterochromatin in maintaining proper chromosomal organisation within the nucleus. Disruption of telomeric heterochromatin also causes derepression of genes within the subtelomeric repeats and also of marker genes inserted adjacent to telomeric regions (Allshire et al. 1995; Hansen et al. 2006; Kanoh et al. 2005; Mandell et al. 2005; Nimmo et al. 1998).

4.3   Heterochromatin at the Mating-Type Locus

Heterochromatin also plays an important role in regulating mating-type switching. The fission yeast mating-type locus contains three mating-type cassettes, *mat1* (either *P* or *M*), *mat2-P* and *mat3-M* over approximately 30 kb region on chromosome 2 (Egel 2004; Klar 1992). Depending on whether *P* or *M* information is found at *mat1*, cells preferentially recombine either *mat2-P* (in a *mat1-M* cell) or *mat3-M* (in a *mat1-P* cell) with *mat1* in a process known as switching. *mat1* is transcriptionally active but *mat2-P* and *mat3-M* are maintained in a silent state (Fig. 2). The mating-type of a haploid cell is determined by the exchange between *P* and *M* information at the *mat1* locus. Heterochromatin is required to maintain the 20-kb region containing *mat2-P* and *mat3-M* in a silent state as expression of both causes haploid cells to undergo an aberrant meiosis which is usually lethal when it occurs in haploid cells (Thon et al. 2005). The *cenH* region between *mat2* and *mat3* has 96% homology to *dh* elements at centromeres. *cenH* is required for efficient silencing and switching as replacement of this region by a marker gene causes variegated expression (Grewal and Klar 1997). As at centromeres, Swi6 also attracts cohesin to *mat2–mat3*, and mutations in cohesin subunits lead to defective mating-type switching (Nonaka et al. 2002). Furthermore, analyses suggest that heterochromatin influences long-range chromatin interactions between *mat1* and the silent mating-type cassettes to determine the direction of the switching event (Jia et al. 2004b).

From the above discussion it is clear that in fission yeast heterochromatin is required to form stable structures at distinct chromosomal loci in order to contribute to the normal function of these regions.

5   RNAi Components Are Required for Heterochromatin Integrity

Heterochromatin forms on related repetitive sequences at fission yeast centromeres, the mating-type locus and adjacent to telomeres. Although not fully understood, it had seemed most likely that the formation of this silent chromatin was driven by this repetitive DNA and specific DNA binding proteins which would attract HDACs and methylases to promote binding of Swi6 and other proteins. However, it is now apparent that the RNAi machinery is required for the assembly and maintenance of heterochromatin in fission yeast. Like Clr4 and Swi6, deletion of RNAi components was found to result in defective heterochromatin formation and chromosome missegregation (Hall et al. 2003; Volpe et al. 2002, 2003).

It is ironic that despite centromeres having been previously thought of as transcriptionally silent regions, the *dg/dh* repeats themselves were found to produce convergently transcribed non-coding RNA transcripts. These transcripts accumulate in many mutants involved in heterochromatin formation and in mutants lacking RNAi components (Volpe et al. 2002, 2003). Non-coding transcripts have also been shown to originate from the mating-type locus and sequences adjacent to telomeres (Kanoh et al. 2005; Mandell et al. 2005; Noma et al. 2004). Thus, at these regions transcription itself contributes to the transcriptionally silent state. In wild-type cells these transcripts are made but are continually processed. Moreover, small interfering RNAs (siRNAs) identical in sequence to the *dg/dh* region have been identified (Cam and Grewal 2004; Reinhart and Bartel 2002).

The discovery of two key complexes, the RNA-induced initiation of transcriptional gene silencing complex (RITS), which appears to be the main RNAi effector complex, and the RNA-directed RNA polymerase complex (RDRC) have provided further insights into the mechanisms of RNAi-mediated heterochromatin formation in fission yeast (Motamedi et al. 2004; Noma et al. 2004; Verdel et al. 2004). These findings demonstrate that the formation of heterochromatin is much more complex than first imagined.

Many organisms contain several genes encoding Dicer and Argonaute homologues, thereby complicating analyses of the RNAi pathway. Fission yeast has an advantage in that it only possesses a single gene encoding each of the key proteins required for RNAi, and these are not essential for cell viability. In several other organisms, the effector complex RISC (RNA-induced silencing complex) containing Argonaute and guide siRNAs is known to target homologous mRNAs and inhibit their expression by either blocking translation or mediating their degradation (Agrawal et al. 2003; Hannon 2002). In fission yeast, Dicer (Dcr1) is the ribonuclease which cleaves dsRNA into approx. 22- to 25-nt double-stranded siRNAs, and Argonaute (Ago1) is a component of the RITS effector which directly binds these siRNA molecules. These siRNAs act to guide RITS to homologous target RNAs, and it appears to act only in the nucleus to bring about modification of homologous chromatin and transcriptional silencing.

A general model of events is now widely accepted whereby non-coding RNA transcripts derived from repetitive DNA sequences form a double-stranded RNA (dsRNA) template. This dsRNA is processed by Dicer into siRNAs. These siRNAs are incorporated into the RITS RNAi effector complex to target homologous RNAs and induce heterochromatin assembly (Motamedi et al. 2004; Noma et al. 2004; Sugiyama et al. 2005). In fission yeast, siRNA production must somehow bring about the recruitment of HDACs and the histone methylase Clr4 to methylate H3 on lysine 9 allowing Swi6 binding and heterochromatin formation on homologous

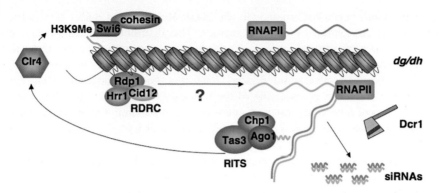

Fig. 3 An overview of RNAi-induced heterochromatin formation in fission yeast. The outer repeats are transcribed by RNA polymerase II. These non-coding transcripts are assumed to provide a dsRNA substrate for Dcr1 perhaps by annealing or through the action of Rdp1. Cleavage of dsRNA by Dcr1 produces siRNAs which are incorporated into the RITS complex. This somehow recruits the histone methyltransferase Clr4 which dimethylates histone H3 on lysine 9. This in turn creates a binding site for Swi6 and Chp1. The exact role of RDRC is unclear, but Rdp1 associates with the outer repeats (?). Swi6 is required to maintain a high density of the cohesin complex and thus cohesion between sister chromatids

dg/dh repeats (Fig. 3). In plants it has also been shown that the RNAi pathway can feedback onto homologous chromatin so as to induce modifications such as DNA methylation, another mark of silent chromatin (Mathieu and Bender 2004; Matzke and Birchler 2005). However, DNA methylation has not been detected in fission yeast (Wilkinson et al. 1995).

Both RITS and RDRC components can be detected on centromeric outer repeats (Motamedi et al. 2004; Noma et al. 2004; Sugiyama et al. 2005; Verdel et al. 2004). While RITS must utilise siRNAs to somehow home in on homologous sequences, RDRC may play a role in providing the source of dsRNA for siRNA generation by Dcr1. However, the exact function of RDRC remains to be resolved. Furthermore, recent studies have identified factors involved in ubiquitination, sumoylation, and RNAPII transcription as affecting RNAi-mediated heterochromatin formation.

5.1 Non-coding Transcripts and siRNAs Are Produced from Silent Loci

Although overlapping non-coding transcripts derived from *dg/dh* repeats at centromeres can be detected, it is not known how the initiating dsRNA that provides the template for siRNA production is formed. It seems reasonable to assume that these centromeric transcripts are the source of a dsRNA substrate that is processed by Dcr1 to produce homologous siRNAs. The first few siRNAs identified were homologous to the centromeric *dh* element, but comprehensive sequence analyses of siRNA associated with RITS identified siRNAs homologous to both the *dh* and *dg* centromeric repeats (Cam and Grewal 2004; Reinhart and Bartel 2002). These siRNAs are concentrated in specific regions. This distribution could reflect variation in the density of transcripts from certain regions or in the way the transcripts are converted to dsRNA. This remains to be investigated further as the transcripts arising from heterochromatic regions have not been characterised in detail. However, comprehensive mapping of these transcripts is challenging because the arrangement of repeats at each centromere varies. In addition, the sequence similarity of *dg* and *dh* elements makes it difficult to distinguish repeats from each centromere and other regions of heterochromatin.

RNAs homologous to centromere repeats may be produced by transcription; however, Rdp1 has been shown to be able to synthesise RNA from an RNA template (Motamedi et al. 2004; Sugiyama et al. 2005). This activity of Rdp1 could be required to produce a complementary second strand using primary centromeric non-coding RNA transcripts as a template (Volpe et al. 2002). Apart from siRNA derived from the centromeric outer repeat *dg/dh* elements, siRNAs were also identified which are homologous to unique inverted repeat elements found at the outer boundaries on centromere 1 and 3, the region of centromere homology (*cenH*) at the mating-type locus, the sub-telomeric *cenH*-like sequences, rDNA and also a few from the *imr* region of centromere 1 (Cam and Grewal 2004). Since these siRNAs were associated with RITS, this suggests that all of these sequences can be targeted for RNAi-induced heterochromatin formation.

5.2   RITS: The Effector Complex

The RITS comprises three proteins: Ago1, Chp1 and Tas3. The complex also contains siRNAs which directly bind Ago1 and presumably guide the complex to homologous target RNAs (Fig. 3). In other organisms, the effector complex RISC containing Argonaute and guide siRNAs is known to target homologous mRNAs and inhibit their expression by either binding the mature mRNA and blocking their translation or by inducing their degradation by virtue of the 'slicer' endonuclease activity inherent in some Argonaute proteins (Agrawal et al. 2003; Baumberger and Baulcombe 2005; Hannon 2002; Liu et al. 2004; Miyoshi et al. 2005; Rivas et al. 2005). The incorporation of siRNA into *Drosophila* or mammalian RISC requires a loading complex containing Dcr1 (Preall and Sontheimer 2005). siRNAs are loaded as a duplex and one strand is cleaved by Argonaute leaving behind a single 'guide' strand which confers target specificity (Matranga et al. 2005; Miyoshi et al. 2005; Preall and Sontheimer 2005). In fission yeast it is not known how siRNAs are loaded into RITS or whether Ago1 displays this endonuclease activity.

Like Swi6, the Chp1 subunit of RITS contains a chromo domain and this chromo domain has also been shown to bind histone H3 when methylated on lysine 9 (Partridge et al. 2002). However, Chp1 not only binds to H3K9me2 but, as part of the RITS complex, it is required to target this modification to sequences homologous to the siRNA carried by RITS (Partridge et al. 2002; Verdel et al. 2004). The fact that Chp1 also binds target chromatin when methylated on lysine 9 implies a physical link between Chp1/RITS and its chromosomal targets, and that binding of RITS to chromatin via RNAi reinforces transcriptional silencing. After the initial unknown events that nucleate a patch of heterochromatin, Chp1 could be required to stabilise the interaction of RITS with heterochromatin. Therefore, the binding of the RITS components themselves may contribute to heterochromatin integrity by being loaded *in cis* with siRNA generated from any RNA synthesised in the vicinity. Consistent with this, each of the individual RITS components is required for complete methylation of H3K9me2 and Swi6 association with marker gene insertions at centromeres (Verdel et al. 2004; Noma et al. 2004). Surprisingly, all RITS components are also required for siRNA generation, again indicating that a feedback mechanism operates between chromatin modification and siRNA generation (Noma et al. 2004). RITS components do not always act together; for example, Ago1 alone is required for the post-transcriptional repression of a transgene via expression of an exogenous dsRNA hairpin but Tas3 and Chp1 are not (Sigova et al. 2004). This makes sense since only the single Argonaute protein in fission yeast can be responsible for the targeting of nascent and mature transcripts. The function of Tas3 is unknown but like Chp1 it is located mainly in the nucleus (Noma et al. 2004).

Chp1, and presumably other RNAi components, is required for the establishment of heterochromatin at centromeres, mating-type locus and telomeres (Sadaie et al. 2004). In the absence of RNAi, H3K9 methylation is reduced but it is not completely abolished from repetitive sequences at these locations. Swi6 and a related chromo domain protein, Chp2, are required to maintain this residual H3K9 methylation at centromeres and the mating-type locus in the absence of Chp1. Thus, it appears that chromo domain proteins contribute in several ways to heterochromatin formation in fission yeast. Chp1 appears to be a key player, since it is required for full methylation of histone H3K9, it associates with chromatin only when it is methylated on lysine 9 and it is required for the production of the siRNA that allow it and H3K9me to be targeted to homologous chromatin. Because of these inherent interdependencies, the order of events that trigger RNAi-mediated heterochromatin formation is difficult to determine.

This interdependency is further highlighted by the fact that all components of RITS associate with regions of heterochromatin and that this is also dependent on Clr4 and Dcr1 (Cam and Grewal 2004; Noma et al. 2004). As with Chp1, the production of siRNAs and their incorporation into RITS are required for the association of Ago1 and Tas3 with centromeric heterochromatin. All RITS components, however, remain associated with the mating-type locus in cells lacking Dcr1 and thus siRNA (Jia et al. 2004a; Noma et al. 2004). In addition, in the absence of Ago1, Tas3 and Chp1 can still interact, and both proteins still associate with the mating-type locus and telomeres but not centromeres (Petrie et al. 2005). This may indicate an RNAi-independent role for these proteins at these regions or could simply reflect the ability of Chp1 to methylate H3K9 after targeting. This also suggests that RITS is required for the maintenance of heterochromatin at centromeres but not at other loci.

Exactly how the RITS complex loaded with siRNAs recognises homologous targets to induce the specific chromatin modifications that lead to heterochromatin formation at these locations is unknown and requires further scrutiny. It is possible that siRNAs recognise homologous chromatin by targeting homologous nascent transcripts still associated with chromatin templates in an RNA–RNA-mediated interaction. Equally, RITS-associated siRNAs could somehow bind or interact with homologous DNA sequences to induce the modification of nearby chromatin. Evidence to date points towards an RNA–RNA interaction as the RITS complex has been shown to associate with non-coding centromere RNA transcripts but only when Dcr1 is present in the cell (Motamedi et al. 2004). Consistent with this, tethering Tas3, and consequently RITS, to a normal euchromatic transcript (*ura4*) allows production of *ura4*-homologous siRNAs, lysine 9 methylation of H3 on the *ura4+* gene and silencing (Buhler et al. 2006). This suggests that nascent transcripts can be converted to dsRNA at their site of production allowing Dcr1 to act *in cis* to form siRNAs which are directly loaded into RITS to allow chromatin modification. This artificial RNA-tethered RITS version of heterochromatin requires Dcr1, all RITS and RDRC components, and Clr4. It is also possible that mature centromere and other transcripts are exported to the cytoplasm for processing to siRNA where these are then loaded into Ago1 to form RITS on their journey back to the nucleus.

5.3   RDRC: RNA-Directed RNA Polymerase Complex

The RITS complex has been shown to physically interact with the RDRC. The components of RDRC are also required for the integrity of silent chromatin. RDRC is composed of Rdp1, Hrr1 and Cid12. Rdp1 is an RNA-dependent RNA polymerase, Hrr1 is a putative RNA helicase, and Cid12 is a putative poly(A) polymerase (Motamedi et al. 2004). As with the RITS complex, each of the components of RDRC is required for siRNA generation, complete H3K9 methylation of heterochromatic loci, and Swi6 association with heterochromatic loci (Motamedi et al. 2004; Sugiyama et al. 2005). The association of RDRC components with RITS subunits is also dependent on Dcr1 and Clr4 and the catalytic activity of Rdp1 itself (Motamedi et al. 2004; Sugiyama et al. 2005). Thus, both RDRC and RITS appear to be dependent on one another for their association with heterochromatic loci and the formation of silent chromatin. The dependency of RITS on RDRC holds steadfast even when silent chromatin is induced by tethering Tas3/RITS to euchromatic *ura4* transcripts (Buhler et al. 2006). Thus, the generation of dsRNA substrate, the processing of dsRNA to siRNA, loading of siRNAs into RISC and subsequent targeting of chromatin are all intimately linked. This also suggests that Rdp1 is part of a self-enforcing RNAi feedback loop that couples siRNA production and heterochromatin formation (Buhler et al. 2006; Noma et al. 2004; Sugiyama et al. 2005).

In vitro analyses indicate that Rdp1 can act as an RNA-dependent RNA polymerase in that it can synthesise RNA from a single-stranded RNA substrate in the presence or absence of a complementary primer. Mutations which destroy this activity cause phenotypes equivalent to those observed in cells lacking RNAi (Motamedi et al. 2004; Sugiyama et al. 2005). Hence the ability of Rdp1 to synthesise complementary RNA is essential for the production of centromeric siRNA and heterochromatin formation. It remains unclear why Rdp1 is so important for RNAi-mediated chromatin modification in fission yeast, as other eukaryotes such as *Drosophila* and mammals do not encode an RNA-dependent RNA polymerase but still have an active RNAi pathway. In plants, RNA-dependent RNA polymerase is required for transgene silencing, but not for silencing mediated by viruses. This suggests that exogenous viruses are capable of synthesising sufficient dsRNA to bypass the need for RdRP activity (Dalmay et al. 2000). In the filamentous fungi *Neurospora crassa* and *Aspergillus nidulans* the requirement of RdRP for robust RNA-dependent silencing is variable (Catalanotto et al. 2002; Hammond and Keller 2005). Fission yeast seems to be extremely dependent on Rdp1 for RNAi-mediated silencing since in its absence, although centromeric transcripts are still produced, no siRNAs are detected. The observation that Rdp1 associates with centromeric chromatin and transcripts is compatible with a model where Rdp1 acts on nascent transcripts to synthesise dsRNA leading to the production of the initial siRNAs (Motamedi et al. 2004; Sugiyama et al. 2005; Volpe et al. 2002). Alternatively, Rdp1 may utilise pre-existing rare primary siRNAs, formed by Dcr1-mediated cleavage of annealed centromere transcripts, to prime synthesis of additional dsRNA and amplify the signal. However, Rdp1 is also required for a form of PTGS in *S. pombe* triggered by the expression of an exogenous hairpin RNA (Sigova et al. 2004). In this case siRNAs are presumably not limiting, as with plant viruses, so it is not entirely clear why Rdp1 is required.

The role of Hrr1 is unknown, but it has significant similarity to (1) DEAD box helicases such as Smg2 in *Caenorhabditis elegans*, which acts in the nonsense-mediated decay pathway as well as RNAi, and (2) Sde3 in plants, which is required for RNAi-mediated transgene silencing (Dalmay et al. 2001; Domeier et al. 2000). It is conceivable that Hrr1 is required to unwind siRNA duplexes prior to loading into RISC or it might act upon dsRNA providing single-stranded RNA templates for Rdp1 (Motamedi et al. 2004). The role of Cid12 is also unknown; it is possible that it binds the 3 end of transcripts producing a poly(A) tract that somehow primes RNA synthesis by Rdp1. In *C. elegans* a related putative poly(A) polymerase, RDE-3, has also been shown to be required for efficient RNAi and siRNA production (Chen et al. 2005). Polyadenylation by proteins such as Cid12 might also play a role in RNA degradation since the addition of short poly(A) tracts is known to attract the exosome and degrade RNAs (Anderson 2005). Cid12 may be required for the specific degradation of non-coding transcripts originating from regions of heterochromatin either for regulation or to somehow aid the provision of a template for Rdp1. The details of how these activities act on endogenous transcripts to execute efficient siRNA production and silencing remains to be determined.

5.4   Transcription of Centromere Repeats and Silencing Requires RNAPII

Transcripts from the mating-type locus and from the centromere are polyadenylated (Djupedal et al. 2005). This is a well-known hallmark of mature transcripts produced by RNAPII (Birse et al. 1997). However, it is possible that this polyadenylation is due to the putative activity of Cid12 rather than that normally associated with termination of RNAPII transcription. RNAPII itself is enriched at heterochromatic loci, which reinforces the idea that it is responsible for the transcription of these regions (Fig. 3; Cam and Grewal 2004; Kato et al. 2005). Consistent with this, a specific mutation in the second largest subunit of RNAPII, Rpb2, causes loss of silent chromatin from outer repeat regions of centromeres regulating the expression of normally silent marker genes. Interestingly mutation of Rpb2 causes a reduction in H3K9me2, accumulation of centromere transcripts and loss of siRNA homologous to centromere repeats. General transcription does not appear to be affected in Rpb2 mutant cells, so the loss of heterochromatin is probably due to a defect in processing non-coding centromere transcripts to siRNAs (Kato et al. 2005). A specific role for RNAPII in the production of non-coding centromeric transcripts is also supported by the finding that a mutation in the small RNAPII subunit Rpb7 results in loss of centromeric siRNA-defective heterochromatin formation at centromeres (Djupedal et al. 2005). However, Rpb7 mutation causes decreased transcription of the centromeric repeats indicating that Rpb7 has a specific role in promoting transcription of centromere repeats under conditions where general transcription of euchromatic genes appears normal. Thus, in Rpb7-mutant cells no RNA substrate is made; therefore no siRNAs are formed. It is unclear how the Rpb2 mutant affects heterochromatin formation. One possibility is that when the RITS complex and RDRC engage a nascent transcript associated with RNAPII on its template there is an interaction between RITS/RDRC and RNAPII subunits. Once stabilised, such interactions might promote RNA production by Rdp1 and the recruitment of chromatin-modifying activities. Such interactions between RNAi components and RNAPII may be disrupted in the Rpb2 mutant.

5.5   The Histone Methyltransferase Clr4 Affects siRNA Production and Associates with Rik1

The RNAi pathway is required for full methylation of H3K9 on homologous chromatin and thus Clr4 would be expected to act downstream of the RNAi components. Clr4 is essential to create the H3K9me2 binding site for the chromo domain proteins Chp1, Chp2, Swi6 and possibly Clr4 itself (Bannister et al. 2001; Partridge et al. 2002; Sadaie et al. 2004). Surprisingly, Clr4 is also required to produce centromeric siRNAs, which accounts for why RITS and RDRC are delocalised in its absence (Noma et al. 2004; Sugiyama et al. 2005). The complete role of Clr4 in the RNAi pathway is difficult to understand mainly due to the inherent feedback in the process and thus our inability to decipher the initiating events that lead to heterochromatin formation. However, it is clear that Clr4 plays a central role since the methylation of H3K9 is required to allow binding of key components.

In most cases, loss of any component involved in heterochromatin formation results in at least a significant reduction in, if not a complete loss of, H3K9 methylation. However, it is still unknown how Clr4 itself is recruited via RNAi to form heterochromatic loci. It had been demonstrated that Clr4 interacts with Rik1 (Sadaie et al. 2004). As with other components, Rik1 is known to be required for silencing, H3K9 methylation, Swi6 association/localisation and production of centromeric siRNAs (Allshire et al. 1995; Egel et al. 1989; Ekwall et al. 1996; Ekwall and Ruusala 1994; Hong et al. 2005; Horn et al. 2005; Jia et al. 2005; Li et al. 2005; Partridge et al. 2000). The Rik1 protein contains a -propeller domain with similarity to a cleavage specificity and polyadenylation factor (CPSF-A) which may be involved in RNA binding (Neuwald and Poleksic 2000). It has been proposed that Rik1 could act to guide Clr4 to its target regions (Jia et al. 2005; Li et al. 2005).

5.6 Rik1 and Clr4 Interact in a Complex Which Has E3 Ubiquitin Ligase Activity

Rik1 is related to DNA damage binding protein 1 (DDB1), a component of an E3 ligase complex in plants (Yanagawa et al. 2004). Recent analyses have demonstrated that Rik1 co-purifies and associates with several other proteins; Raf1 (also known as Dos1, Cmc1 and Clr8), Raf2 (or Dos2/Cmc2/Clr7), the E3 ubiquitin ligase subunits Cul4 and Pip1, the small ubiquitin like protein Nedd8 and the histones H2B and H4 (Fig. 4). Deletion of the genes encoding Raf1, Raf2 or Pcu4 perturbs heterochromatin formation at centromeres, telomeres and at the mating-type locus (Hong et al. 2005; Horn et al. 2005; Jia et al. 2005; Li et al. 2005; Thon et al. 2005). Levels of H3K9 methylation are substantially reduced at centromeres and at the mating-type locus while a modification normally associated with expressed genes, methylation of H3K4, increases. As with other mutants affecting H3K9 methylation and RNAi the generation centromeric siRNAs is abolished and chromosome segregation is defective.

Ubiquitin is a small regulatory protein that can be covalently attached to substrate proteins and is another post-translational modification which, like acetylation and methylation, occurs on lysine residues (Hershko and Ciechanover 1998). Polyubiquitination (the addition of chains of ubiquitin) is a multi-step pathway that ultimately targets proteins for degradation via the proteasome (Hershko and Ciechanover 1998). Monoubiquitination, the addition of a single ubiquitin molecule to a substrate, is involved in protein regulation. Histones H2A and H2B are known to be monoubiquitinated and in *S. cerevisiae* ubiquitination of H2B K120 is required for methylation of H3 on K4 and K79 (Osley 2004). Rik1, Raf2 and Clr4 purifications were demonstrated to have E3 ubiquitin ligase activity in vitro (Horn et al. 2005). The in vivo substrates for this ubiquitination are unknown; however, the fact that H2B and H4 co-purify with Clr4 and Rik1 may indicate that ubiquitination of histones is involved in heterochromatin formation (Hong et al. 2005; Horn et al. 2005; Fig. 4). A related complex from human cells (Cul4–DDB1–Roc1) has recently been shown to ubiquitinate histones H3 and H4 on several lysines in vivo and in vitro (Wang et al. 2006). Given that Pcu4 and Rik1, fission yeast homologues of Cul4 and DDB1, are required for methylation of H3 on K9 and associate with the H3K9 methyltransferase

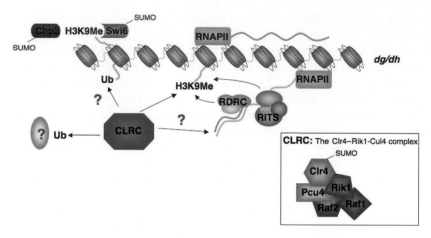

Fig. 4 Possible interactions between RNAi, chromatin modifiers and chromatin. RNAPII transcripts could provide a platform to recruit RDRC and RITS. RDRC may be involved in the production of dsRNA which is required for siRNA production, RITS association and subsequent H3K9me2. Thus, RNAi H3K9 methylation and the formation of intact heterochromatin appear to be locked in a closed loop where loss of any one component leads to the collapse of RNAi-induced heterochromatin formation. Loading of siRNAs into Ago1 allows RITS to be guided to homologous nascent transcripts, which recruits Clr4 and formation of heterochromatin. The Clr4–Rik1–Cul4 complex (CLRC) contains Rik1, Raf1 and Raf2, which are also required for H3K9 dimethylation. CLRC also contains an E3 ubiquitin ligase, Cul4, which could be responsible for the modification and/or turnover of histones or of another unknown factor involved in RNAi-induced heterochromatin formation (*?*). Swi6, Chp2 and Clr4 are known to be sumoylated in vivo. The significance of this is unclear but could be involved in protein targeting

Clr4, it is conceivable that ubiquitination of histones by the Rik1 complex promotes H3K9 methylation. Ubiquitination of H3/H4 might destabilise nucleosomes and force exchange with new H3 which is then methylated on H3K9 by Clr4 during the replacement process. Alternatively, ubiquitination of H3/H4 may induce conformational changes in nucleosomes presenting the H3 tail and lysine 9 to Clr4 for methylation.

5.7 Sumoylation Is Required for Heterochromatin Integrity

Small ubiquitin-related modifer (SUMO) is a small peptide that is also conjugated to specific target lysine residues in a manner similar to ubiquitin. SUMO may act to prevent other modifications on lysines such as acetylation, methylation and ubiquitination. Many regulators of transcription are known to be sumoylated, and in general this promotes transcriptional repression by interactions with HDACs (Gill 2005). Intriguingly all four histones have also been shown to be sumoylated in *S. cerevisiae*, and this appears to act to oppose ubiquitination and acetylation and inhibit transcription (Nathan et al. 2006). Sumoylation is also involved in maintaining heterochromatin stability in fission yeast (Shin et al. 2005). Deletion of the gene encoding SUMO (*Pmt3*) causes defective silencing at centromeres and at the mating-type locus but had no effect at telomeres. In addition, a SUMO-conjugating enzyme has been shown to interact with Chp2 and also to be associated with regions of heterochromatin perhaps through interactions with Swi6 or Clr4. Swi6, Clr4 and Chp2 are sumoylated in vivo, and defective sumoylation of either Swi6 or Chp2 impairs silencing (Shin et al. 2005).

The involvement of ubiquitination and sumoylation in heterochromatin formation in fission yeast are relatively new discoveries. These modifications may act to promote or inhibit specific protein–protein interactions and/or other modification in a variety of ways. Apart from promoting repressive modification of histones, it is perhaps possible that RNAPII is ubiquitinated and/or sumoylated in response to RNAi, allowing RNAPII and its nascent transcript to be efficiently engaged by RNAi components. RITS, RDRC, Clr4 and Swi6 might also be regulated by post-translational modification during transcription and cell cycles.

6 RNAi Is Dispensable at the Mating-Type Locus and Telomeres

Components of the RNAi pathway are required to direct heterochromatin assembly at specific regions. At centromeres it is apparent that the RNAi pathway is necessary for the formation and maintenance of silent chromatin although some features, such as residual H3K9 methylation and Swi6 localisation, remain even after inactivation of RNAi. In contrast, RNAi is required to establish heterochromatin at the mating-type locus but is dispensable for its maintenance. Transcription of the *cenH* element residing between *mat2* and *mat3* attracts the RNAi machinery to nucleate heterochromatin formation in a similar fashion to that seen at centromeres (Hall et al. 2002). However, unlike at centromeres, the silent state is propagated in the absence of active RNAi. This is due to an alternative pathway involving Atf1 and Pcr1, two members of the stress-activated ATF/CREB protein family, which act in an RNAi-independent manner to tether heterochromatin components to the mating-type locus. When either of the genes encoding Atf1 or Pcr1 is deleted in combination with RNAi components, heterochromatin is completely abolished. This suggests that the two pathways act in parallel and that Atf1 and Pcr1 act to retain specific factors such as Clr4 and hence Swi6 once they have been delivered to the locus by the RNAi machinery (Jia et al. 2004a; Kim et al. 2004). Interestingly both Atf1 and Pcr1 physically interact with Swi6. In addition, Atf1 associates with the Clr6 HDAC, while Clr4 can bind both Atf1 and Pcr1 in vitro (Jia et al. 2004a; Kim et al. 2004). This supports the idea that these DNA binding proteins act to maintain the silent state at the mating-type locus in the absence of RNAi.

A distinct process also occurs at telomeres where Taz1, a telomere terminal repeat DNA binding protein, is able to establish heterochromatin independently from the RNAi machinery (Allshire et al. 1995; Kanoh et al. 2005; Nimmo et al. 1998). RNAi components are also required for normal clustering of telomeres at the nuclear periphery in interphase cells (Hall et al. 2003). Telomere length remains normal in cells lacking genes required for RNAi-mediated heterochromatin formation (Ekwall et al. 1996; Hall et al. 2003). Although Clr4 and Rik1 are required for Swi6 localisation and silencing at telomeres, Swi6 localisation and silencing is retained in cells lacking Dcr1, Ago1 or Rdp1 (Allshire et al. 1995; Hall et al. 2003). This RNAi-independent form of silencing at telomeres is due to a redundant pathway where the terminal telomere repeats themselves can recruit Clr4 via Taz1 bound to terminal telomere repeats (Allshire 1995; Cooper et al. 1997; Kanoh et al. 2005). Loss of Taz 1 causes the terminal repeats at telomeres to elongate and leads to loss of silencing, but Swi6 remains localised due to the maintenance of heterochromatin on telomere-associated repeats (Cooper et al. 1997; Kanoh et al. 2005; Nimmo et al. 1998).

6.1   RNAi Acts at rDNA and Other Loci

In fission yeast approximately 100 copies of the 5.8S, 18S and 25S ribosomal RNA genes are tandemly arranged as 10.4-kb repeats occupying approx. 1,000 kb adjacent to telomeres on chromosome 3 and are transcribed by RNA polymerase I in the nucleolus. When RNAPII-transcribed marker genes are placed the rDNA they are transcriptionally silenced in a process that requires Clr4, Chp2, Swi6 and, to a lesser extent, Chp1 (Thon and Verhein-Hansen 2000). Genome-wide heterochromatin and euchromatin profiling confirmed that in addition to centromeres, telomeres and the mating-type loci, heterochromatin is also found associated with rDNA, and siRNA homologous to rDNA can be detected (Cam and Grewal 2004). H3K9 methylation and Ago1, but not Rdp1, was found to be associated with particular regions of rDNA repeats. Moreover, H3K9 methylation, Swi6, RITS components, and Rdp1 were found to associate with a silenced RNAPII marker gene inserted within rDNA. H3K9 methylation and Swi6 association with this gene requires Chp1, Dcr1 and Clr4. The rDNA arrays themselves were found to be subject to increased inter-repeat recombination, indicating that this heterochromatin contributes to the mitotic stability of rDNA arrays by suppressing recombination. In other organisms it is known that only a proportion of ribosomal repeats are actively transcribed (Dammann et al. 1993, 1995). It is possible that this RNAi-mediated heterochromatin also acts to regulate the number of active rRNA genes.

In these genome-wide studies, a number of other chromosomal loci were also highlighted as being potential sites of heterochromatin formation by their relatively high levels of H3K9 methylation in mitotically dividing cells. These islands of heterochromatin mainly corresponded to genes which are only expressed in meiosis (Cam and Grewal 2004). Therefore, heterochromatin may be required to maintain repression of these genes in vegetative cultures but it is unknown if RNAi is required to direct H3K9 methylation to these loci. Regardless, it is possible that RNAi is involved in endogenous gene regulation in fission yeast as it is in *Drosophila* and plants (Aravin et al. 2001; Chan et al. 2004).

In many organisms the expression of a synthetic dsRNA homologous to an endogenous gene can target homologous RNA resulting in degradation of that RNA and in some cases modification of DNA/chromatin at the homologous locus (Agrawal et al. 2003; Hannon 2002). In fission yeast the expression of an exogenous dsRNA hairpin can induce the production of siRNAs homologous to green fluorescent protein (GFP), allowing some silencing of a GFP transgene (Sigova et al. 2004). This was shown to require the presence of Clr4, Rdp1, Dcr1 and Ago1 but not Swi6, Tas3 or Chp1. However, the level of on-going transcription from the transgene does not appear to be affected, indicating that this silencing must be due to post-transcriptional processing of the GFP transcript by RNAi. Further investigation of such silencing is required, as in this GFP system both target GFP transcripts and homologous siRNAs are thought to be very highly expressed compared to the apparent lower levels of naturally occurring centromere transcripts and siRNAs. Strong transcription of the target or too much siRNA could interfere with, rather than promote, RNAi-mediated heterochromatin formation at an artificial locus. It is also unknown if these hairpin-derived GFP siRNAs are incorporated into the RITS complex. Nonetheless, such artificial assays provide a useful tool to further investigate defects in mutants affecting RNAi-mediated heterochromatin formation and offer some clue as to where and how specific proteins may act in the process. Other assays utilising tricks to direct the RNAi machinery to particular loci such as ectopic silencing via repeats placed in euchromatin or tethering components to RNA or DNA at euchromatic loci should also allow further insights into the mechanism of RNA-mediated heterochromatin assembly (Buhler et al. 2006; Hall et al. 2002; Partridge et al. 2002).

7 Perspectives

The past 5 years have been a fast-moving period in terms of developing our understanding of RNAi-mediated heterochromatin formation in fission yeast. Most of the genes involved have homologues in more complex eukaryotes, and it appears that many of the processes involved are conserved to differing degrees in different organisms. The initial discovery that the RNAi pathway directly contributes to heterochromatin formation and function in fission yeast was surprising. However, it is now clear that small RNAs direct chromatin and DNA modifications in a number of systems. Despite the identification of the RITS, RDRC and Rik1/Clr4 complexes, our knowledge of how non-coding transcripts are processed to bring about chromatin modifications and heterochromatin assembly is still rudimentary. For instance, we do not know how RDRC contributes to RNA processing and siRNA production, or how the key histone methyltransferase Clr4 or HDACs are recruited by RNAi factors to bring about methylation of histone H3 on lysine 9 on chromatin homologous to siRNA borne by RITS to occur. Dissection of the process is hampered by the fact the entire RNAi-mediated heterochromatin assembly pathway appears to collapse upon any intervention. New, more subtle assays will be required to work out the intricate details of how endogenous transcripts from repetitive DNA elements are processed to siRNAs and how these siRNAs direct chromatin modification to induce silent chromatin assembly.

Acknowledgements S.A.W. and R.C.A. would like to thank members of the Allshire lab for useful discussion and advice on the text. R.C.A. is a Wellcome Trust Principal Research Fellow and a member of the Epigenome Network of Excellence. Our research is funded by the Wellcome Trust.

References

Agrawal N, Dasaradhi PV, Mohmmed A, Malhotra P, Bhatnagar RK, Mukherjee SK (2003) RNA interference: biology, mechanism, and applications. Microbiol Mol Biol Rev 67:657–685

Allshire RC (1995) Elements of chromosome structure and function in fission yeast. Semin Cell Biol 6:55–64

Allshire RC, Javerzat JP, Redhead NJ, Cranston G (1994) Position effect variegation at fission yeast centromeres. Cell 76:157–169

Allshire RC, Nimmo ER, Ekwall K, Javerzat JP, Cranston G (1995) Mutations derepressing silent centromeric domains in fission yeast disrupt chromosome segregation. Genes Dev 9:218–233

Anderson JT (2005) RNA turnover: unexpected consequences of being tailed. Curr Biol 15: R635–R638

Aravin AA, Naumova NM, Tulin AV, Vagin VV, Rozovsky YM, Gvozdev VA (2001) Double-stranded RNA-mediated silencing of genomic tandem repeats and transposable elements in the D. melanogaster germline. Curr Biol 11:1017–1027

Bannister AJ, Zegerman P, Partridge JF, Miska EA, Thomas JO, Allshire RC, Kouzarides T (2001) Selective recognition of methylated lysine 9 on histone H3 by the HP1 chromo domain. Nature 410:120–124

Baum M, Ngan VK, Clarke L (1994) The centromeric K-type repeat and the central core are together sufficient to establish a functional Schizosaccharomyces pombe centromere. Mol Biol Cell 5:747–761

Baumberger N, Baulcombe DC (2005) Arabidopsis ARGONAUTE1 is an RNA Slicer that selectively recruits microRNAs and short interfering RNAs. Proc Natl Acad Sci U S A 102:11928–11933

Bernard P, Allshire R (2002) Centromeres become unstuck without heterochromatin. Trends Cell Biol 12:419–424

Bernard P, Maure JF, Partridge JF, Genier S, Javerzat JP, Allshire RC (2001) Requirement of heterochromatin for cohesion at centromeres. Science 294:2539–2542

Bjerling P, Silverstein RA, Thon G, Caudy A, Grewal S, Ekwall K (2002) Functional divergence between histone deacetylases in fission yeast by distinct cellular localization and in vivo specificity. Mol Cell Biol 22:2170–2181

Buhler M, Verdel A, Moazed D (2006) Tethering RITS to a nascent transcript initiates RNAi- and heterochromatin-dependent gene silencing. Cell 125:873–886

Cam H, Grewal SI (2004) RNA interference and epigenetic control of heterochromatin assembly in fission yeast. Cold Spring Harb Symp Quant Biol 69:419–427

Catalanotto C, Azzalin G, Macino G, Cogoni C (2002) Involvement of small RNAs and role of the qde genes in the gene silencing pathway in Neurospora. Genes Dev 16:790–795

Chan SW, Zilberman D, Xie Z, Johansen LK, Carrington JC, Jacobsen SE (2004) RNA silencing genes control de novo DNA methylation. Science 303:1336

Chen CC, Simard MJ, Tabara H, Brownell DR, McCollough JA, Mello CC (2005) A member of the polymerase beta nucleotidyltransferase superfamily is required for RNA interference in C. elegans. Curr Biol 15:378–383

Chikashige Y, Ding DQ, Funabiki H, Haraguchi T, Mashiko S, Yanagida M, Hiraoka Y (1994) Telomere-led premeiotic chromosome movement in fission yeast. Science 264:270–273

Cleveland DW, Mao Y, Sullivan KF (2003) Centromeres and kinetochores: from epigenetics to mitotic checkpoint signaling. Cell 112:407–421

Cooper JP, Nimmo ER, Allshire RC, Cech TR (1997) Regulation of telomere length and function by a Myb-domain protein in fission yeast. Nature 385:744–747

Cooper JP, Watanabe Y, Nurse P (1998) Fission yeast Taz1 protein is required for meiotic telomere clustering and recombination. Nature 392:828–831

Cowieson NP, Partridge JF, Allshire RC, McLaughlin PJ (2000) Dimerisation of a chromo shadow domain and distinctions from the chromodomain as revealed by structural analysis. Curr Biol 10:517–525

Dalmay T, Hamilton A, Rudd S, Angell S, Baulcombe DC (2000) An RNA-dependent RNA polymerase gene in Arabidopsis is required for posttranscriptional gene silencing mediated by a transgene but not by a virus. Cell 101:543–553

Dalmay T, Horsefield R, Braunstein TH, Baulcombe DC (2001) SDE3 encodes an RNA helicase required for post-transcriptional gene silencing in Arabidopsis. EMBO J 20:2069–2078

Dammann R, Lucchini R, Koller T, Sogo JM (1993) Chromatin structures and transcription of rDNA in yeast Saccharomyces cerevisiae. Nucleic Acids Res 21:2331–2338

Dammann R, Lucchini R, Koller T, Sogo JM (1995) Transcription in the yeast rRNA gene locus: distribution of the active gene copies and chromatin structure of their flanking regulatory sequences. Mol Cell Biol 15:5294–5303

Ding R, McDonald KL, McIntosh JR (1993) Three-dimensional reconstruction and analysis of mitotic spindles from the yeast, Schizosaccharomyces pombe. J Cell Biol 120:141–151

Djupedal I, Portoso M, Spahr H, Bonilla C, Gustafsson CM, Allshire RC, Ekwall K (2005) RNA Pol II subunit Rpb7 promotes centromeric transcription and RNAi-directed chromatin silencing. Genes Dev 19:2301–2306

Domeier ME, Morse DP, Knight SW, Portereiko M, Bass BL, Mango SE (2000) A link between RNA interference and nonsense-mediated decay in Caenorhabditis elegans. Science 289:1928–1931

Egel R (2004) The molecular biology of Schizosaccharomyces pombe: genetics, genomics and beyond. Springer, Berlin Heidelberg New York

Egel R, Willer M, Nielsen O (1989) Unblocking of meiotic crossing-over between the silent mating-type cassettes of fission yeast, conditioned by the recessive, pleiotropic mutant rik1. Curr Genet 14:407–410

Ekwall K, Ruusala T (1994) Mutations in rik1, clr2, clr3 and clr4 genes asymmetrically derepress the silent mating-type loci in fission yeast. Genetics 136:53–64

Ekwall K, Javerzat JP, Lorentz A, Schmidt H, Cranston G, Allshire R (1995) The chromodomain protein Swi6: a key component at fission yeast centromeres. Science 269:1429–1431

Ekwall K, Nimmo ER, Javerzat JP, Borgstrom B, Egel R, Cranston G, Allshire R (1996) Mutations in the fission yeast silencing factors clr4+ and rik1+ disrupt the localisation of the chromo domain protein Swi6p and impair centromere function. J Cell Sci 109:2637–2648

Ekwall K, Olsson T, Turner BM, Cranston G, Allshire RC (1997) Transient inhibition of histone deacetylation alters the structural and functional imprint at fission yeast centromeres. Cell 91:1021–1032

Ekwall K, Cranston G, Allshire RC (1999) Fission yeast mutants that alleviate transcriptional silencing in centromeric flanking repeats and disrupt chromosome segregation. Genetics 153:1153–1169

Ferreira MG, Miller KM, Cooper JP (2004) Indecent exposure: when telomeres become uncapped. Mol Cell 13:7–18

Funabiki H, Hagan I, Uzawa S, Yanagida M (1993) Cell cycle-dependent specific positioning and clustering of centromeres and telomeres in fission yeast. J Cell Biol 121:961–976

Gill G (2005) Something about SUMO inhibits transcription. Curr Opin Genet Dev 15:536–541

Grewal SI, Klar AJ (1997) A recombinationally repressed region between mat2 and mat3 loci shares homology to centromeric repeats and regulates directionality of mating-type switching in fission yeast. Genetics 146:1221–1238

Hall IM, Shankaranarayana GD, Noma K, Ayoub N, Cohen A, Grewal SI (2002) Establishment and maintenance of a heterochromatin domain. Science 297:2232–2237

Hall IM, Noma K, Grewal SI (2003) RNA interference machinery regulates chromosome dynamics during mitosis and meiosis in fission yeast. Proc Natl Acad Sci U S A 100:193–198

Hammond TM, Keller NP (2005) RNA silencing in Aspergillus nidulans is independent of RNA-dependent RNA polymerases. Genetics 169:607–617

Hannon GJ (2002) RNA interference. Nature 418:244–251

Hansen KR, Ibarra PT, Thon G (2006) Evolutionary-conserved telomere-linked helicase genes of fission yeast are repressed by silencing factors, RNAi components and the telomere-binding protein Taz1. Nucleic Acids Res 34:78–88

Hassold T, Hunt P (2001) To err (meiotically) is human: the genesis of human aneuploidy. Nat Rev Genet 2:280–291

Hershko A, Ciechanover A (1998) The ubiquitin system. Annu Rev Biochem 67:425–479

Hong EE, Villen J, Moazed D (2005) A Cullin E3 ubiquitin ligase complex associates with Rik1 and the Clr4 histone H3-K9 methyltransferase and is required for RNAi-mediated heterochromatin formation. RNA Biol 2:106–111

Horn PJ, Bastie JN, Peterson CL (2005) A Rik1-associated, cullin-dependent E3 ubiquitin ligase is essential for heterochromatin formation. Genes Dev 19:1705–1714

Jia S, Noma K, Grewal SI (2004a) RNAi-independent heterochromatin nucleation by the stress-activated ATF/CREB family proteins. Science 304:1971–1976

Jia S, Yamada T, Grewal SI (2004b) Heterochromatin regulates cell type-specific long-range chromatin interactions essential for directed recombination. Cell 119:469–480

Jia S, Kobayashi R, Grewal SI (2005) Ubiquitin ligase component Cul4 associates with Clr4 histone methyltransferase to assemble heterochromatin. Nat Cell Biol 7:1007–1013

Kanoh J, Sadaie M, Urano T, Ishikawa F (2005) Telomere binding protein Taz1 establishes Swi6 heterochromatin independently of RNAi at telomeres. Curr Biol 15:1808–1819

Kato H, Goto DB, Martienssen RA, Urano T, Furukawa K, Murakami Y (2005) RNA polymerase II is required for RNAi-dependent heterochromatin assembly. Science 309:467–469

Kim HS, Choi ES, Shin JA, Jang YK, Park SD (2004) Regulation of Swi6/HP1-dependent heterochromatin assembly by cooperation of components of the mitogen-activated protein kinase pathway and a histone deacetylase Clr6. J Biol Chem 279:42850–42859

Klar AJ (1992) Developmental choices in mating-type interconversion in fission yeast. Trends Genet 8:208–213

Klar AJ, Bonaduce MJ (1991) swi6, a gene required for mating-type switching, prohibits meiotic recombination in the mat2-mat3 "cold spot" of fission yeast. Genetics 129:1033–1042

Kuhn RM, Clarke L, Carbon J (1991) Clustered tRNA genes in Schizosaccharomyces pombe centromeric DNA sequence repeats. Proc Natl Acad Sci U S A 88:1306–1310

Li F, Goto DB, Zaratiegui M, Tang X, Martienssen R, Cande WZ (2005) Two novel proteins, dos1 and dos2, interact with rik1 to regulate heterochromatic RNA interference and histone modification. Curr Biol 15:1448–1457

Liu J, Carmell MA, Rivas FV, Marsden CG, Thomson JM, Song JJ, Hammond SM, Joshua-Tor L, Hannon GJ (2004) Argonaute2 is the catalytic engine of mammalian RNAi. Science 305:1437–1441

Lorentz A, Ostermann K, Fleck O, Schmidt H (1994) Switching gene swi6, involved in repression of silent mating-type loci in fission yeast, encodes a homologue of chromatin-associated proteins from Drosophila and mammals. Gene 143:139–143

Mandell JG, Bahler J, Volpe TA, Martienssen RA, Cech TR (2005) Global expression changes resulting from loss of telomeric DNA in fission yeast. Genome Biol 6:R1

Mathieu O, Bender J (2004) RNA-directed DNA methylation. J Cell Sci 117:4881–4888

Matranga C, Tomari Y, Shin C, Bartel DP, Zamore PD (2005) Passenger-strand cleavage facilitates assembly of siRNA into Ago2-containing RNAi enzyme complexes. Cell 123:607–620

Matzke MA, Birchler JA (2005) RNAi-mediated pathways in the nucleus. Nat Rev Genet 6:24–35

Mellone BG, Ball L, Suka N, Grunstein MR, Partridge JF, Allshire RC (2003) Centromere silencing and function in fission yeast is governed by the amino terminus of histone H3. Curr Biol 13:1748–1757

Miyoshi K, Tsukumo H, Nagami T, Siomi H, Siomi MC (2005) Slicer function of Drosophila Argonautes and its involvement in RISC formation. Genes Dev 19:2837–2848

Motamedi MR, Verdel A, Colmenares SU, Gerber SA, Gygi SP, Moazed D (2004) Two RNAi complexes, RITS and RDRC, physically interact and localize to noncoding centromeric RNAs. Cell 119:789–802

Nakayama J, Rice JC, Strahl BD, Allis CD, Grewal SI (2001) Role of histone H3 lysine 9 methylation in epigenetic control of heterochromatin assembly. Science 292:110–113

Nakayama J, Xiao G, Noma K, Malikzay A, Bjerling P, Ekwall K, Kobayashi R, Grewal SI (2003) Alp13, an MRG family protein, is a component of fission yeast Clr6 histone deacetylase required for genomic integrity. EMBO J 22:2776–2787

Nathan D, Ingvarsdottir K, Sterner DE, Bylebyl GR, Dokmanovic M, Dorsey JA, Whelan KA, Kršmanovic M, Lane WS, Meluh PB, Johnson ES, Berger SL (2006) Histone sumoylation is a negative regulator in Saccharomyces cerevisiae and shows dynamic interplay with positive-acting histone modifications. Genes Dev 20:966–976

Neuwald AF, Poleksic A (2000) PSI-BLAST searches using hidden markov models of structural repeats: prediction of an unusual sliding DNA clamp and of beta-propellers in UV-damaged DNA-binding protein. Nucleic Acids Res 28:3570–3580

Ngan VK, Clarke L (1997) The centromere enhancer mediates centromere activation in Schizosaccharomyces pombe. Mol Cell Biol 17:3305–3314

Nielsen O, Egel R (1989) Mapping the double-strand breaks at the mating-type locus in fission yeast by genomic sequencing. EMBO J 8:269–276

Nimmo ER, Cranston G, Allshire RC (1994) Telomere-associated chromosome breakage in fission yeast results in variegated expression of adjacent genes. EMBO J 13:3801–3811

Nimmo ER, Pidoux AL, Perry PE, Allshire RC (1998) Defective meiosis in telomere-silencing mutants of Schizosaccharomyces pombe. Nature 392:825–828

Niwa O, Matsumoto T, Chikashige Y, Yanagida M (1989) Characterization of Schizosaccharomyces pombe minichromosome deletion derivatives and a functional allocation of their centromere. EMBO J 8:3045–3052

Noma K, Sugiyama T, Cam H, Verdel A, Zofall M, Jia S, Moazed D, Grewal SI (2004) RITS acts in cis to promote RNA interference-mediated transcriptional and post-transcriptional silencing. Nat Genet 36:1174–1180

Noma K, Cam HP, Maraia RJ, Grewal SI (2006) A role for TFIIIC transcription factor complex in genome organization. Cell 125:859–872

Nonaka N, Kitajima T, Yokobayashi S, Xiao G, Yamamoto M, Grewal SI, Watanabe Y (2002) Recruitment of cohesin to heterochromatic regions by Swi6/HP1 in fission yeast. Nat Cell Biol 4:89–93

Osley MA (2004) H2B ubiquitylation: the end is in sight. Biochim Biophys Acta 1677:74–78

Partridge JF, Borgstrom B, Allshire RC (2000) Distinct protein interaction domains and protein spreading in a complex centromere. Genes Dev 14:783–791

Partridge JF, Scott KS, Bannister AJ, Kouzarides T, Allshire RC (2002) cis-Acting DNA from fission yeast centromeres mediates histone H3 methylation and recruitment of silencing factors and cohesin to an ectopic site. Curr Biol 12:1652–1660

Petrie VJ, Wuitschick JD, Givens CD, Kosinski AM, Partridge JF (2005) RNA interference (RNAi)-dependent and RNAi-independent association of the Chp1 chromodomain protein with distinct heterochromatic loci in fission yeast. Mol Cell Biol 25:2331–2346

Pidoux AL, Richardson W, Allshire RC (2003) Sim4: a novel fission yeast kinetochore protein required for centromeric silencing and chromosome segregation. J Cell Biol 161:295–307

Polizzi C, Clarke L (1991) The chromatin structure of centromeres from fission yeast: differentiation of the central core that correlates with function. J Cell Biol 112:191–201

Preall JB, Sontheimer EJ (2005) RNAi: RISC gets loaded. Cell 123:543–545

Rea S, Eisenhaber F, O'Carroll D, Strahl BD, Sun ZW, Schmid M, Opravil S, Mechtler K, Ponting CP, Allis CD, Jenuwein T (2000) Regulation of chromatin structure by site-specific histone H3 methyltransferases. Nature 406:593–599

Reinhart BJ, Bartel DP (2002) Small RNAs correspond to centromere heterochromatic repeats. Science 297:1831

Richards EJ, Elgin SC (2002) Epigenetic codes for heterochromatin formation and silencing: rounding up the usual suspects. Cell 108:489–500

Rivas FV, Tolia NH, Song JJ, Aragon JP, Liu J, Hannon GJ, Joshua-Tor L (2005) Purified Argonaute2 and an siRNA form recombinant human RISC. Nat Struct Mol Biol 12:340–349

Sadaie M, Naito T, Ishikawa F (2003) Stable inheritance of telomere chromatin structure and function in the absence of telomeric repeats. Genes Dev 17:2271–2282

Sadaie M, Iida T, Urano T, Nakayama J (2004) A chromodomain protein, Chp1, is required for the establishment of heterochromatin in fission yeast. EMBO J 23:3825–3835

Scott KC, Merrett SL, Willard HF (2006) A heterochromatin barrier partitions the fission yeast centromere into discrete chromatin domains. Curr Biol 16:119–129

Shankaranarayana GD, Motamedi MR, Moazed D, Grewal SI (2003) Sir2 regulates histone H3 lysine 9 methylation and heterochromatin assembly in fission yeast. Curr Biol 13:1240–1246

Shin JA, Choi ES, Kim HS, Ho JC, Watts FZ, Park SD, Jang YK (2005) SUMO modification is involved in the maintenance of heterochromatin stability in fission yeast. Mol Cell 19:817–828

Sigova A, Rhind N, Zamore PD (2004) A single Argonaute protein mediates both transcriptional and posttranscriptional silencing in Schizosaccharomyces pombe. Genes Dev 18:2359–2367

Steiner NC, Hahnenberger KM, Clarke L (1993) Centromeres of the fission yeast Schizosaccharomyces pombe are highly variable genetic loci. Mol Cell Biol 13:4578–4587

Sugiyama T, Cam H, Verdel A, Moazed D, Grewal SI (2005) RNA-dependent RNA polymerase is an essential component of a self-enforcing loop coupling heterochromatin assembly to siRNA production. Proc Natl Acad Sci U S A 102:152–157

Sullivan BA, Blower MD, Karpen GH (2001) Determining centromere identity: cyclical stories and forking paths. Nat Rev Genet 2:584–596

Takahashi K, Murakami S, Chikashige Y, Niwa O, Yanagida M (1991) A large number of tRNA genes are symmetrically located in fission yeast centromeres. J Mol Biol 218:13–17

Takahashi K, Murakami S, Chikashige Y, Funabiki H, Niwa O, Yanagida M (1992) A low copy number central sequence with strict symmetry and unusual chromatin structure in fission yeast centromere. Mol Biol Cell 3:819–835

Takahashi K, Chen ES, Yanagida M (2000) Requirement of Mis6 centromere connector for localizing a CENP-A-like protein in fission yeast. Science 288:2215–2219

Thon G, Verhein-Hansen J (2000) Four chromo-domain proteins of Schizosaccharomyces pombe differentially repress transcription at various chromosomal locations. Genetics 155:551–568

Thon G, Cohen A, Klar AJ (1994) Three additional linkage groups that repress transcription and meiotic recombination in the mating-type region of Schizosaccharomyces pombe. Genetics 138:29–38

Thon G, Hansen KR, Altes SP, Sidhu D, Singh G, Verhein-Hansen J, Bonaduce MJ, Klar AJ (2005) The Clr7 and Clr8 directionality factors and the Pcu4 cullin mediate heterochromatin formation in the fission yeast Schizosaccharomyces pombe. Genetics 171:1583–1595

Tuzon CT, Borgstrom B, Weilguny D, Egel R, Cooper JP, Nielsen O (2004) The fission yeast heterochromatin protein Rik1 is required for telomere clustering during meiosis. J Cell Biol 165:759–765

Verdel A, Jia S, Gerber S, Sugiyama T, Gygi S, Grewal SI, Moazed D (2004) RNAi-mediated targeting of heterochromatin by the RITS complex. Science 303:672–676

Volpe T, Schramke V, Hamilton GL, White SA, Teng G, Martienssen RA, Allshire RC (2003) RNA interference is required for normal centromere function in fission yeast. Chromosome Res 11:137–146

Volpe TA, Kidner C, Hall IM, Teng G, Grewal SI, Martienssen RA (2002) Regulation of heterochromatic silencing and histone H3 lysine-9 methylation by RNAi. Science 297:1833–1837

Wang H, Zhai L, Xu J, Joo HY, Jackson S, Erdjument-Bromage H, Tempst P, Xiong Y, Zhang Y (2006) Histone H3 and H4 ubiquitylation by the CUL4-DDB-ROC1 ubiquitin ligase facilitates cellular response to DNA damage. Mol Cell 22:383–394

Wassmann K, Benezra R (2001) Mitotic checkpoints: from yeast to cancer. Curr Opin Genet Dev 11:83–90

Wilkinson CR, Bartlett R, Nurse P, Bird AP (1995) The fission yeast gene pmt1+ encodes a DNA methyltransferase homologue. Nucleic Acids Res 23:203–210

Winey M, Mamay CL, O'Toole ET, Mastronarde DN, Giddings TH Jr, McDonald KL, McIntosh JR (1995) Three-dimensional ultrastructural analysis of the Saccharomyces cerevisiae mitotic spindle. J Cell Biol 129:1601–1615

Wiren M, Silverstein RA, Sinha I, Walfridsson J, Lee HM, Laurenson P, Pillus L, Robyr D, Grunstein M, Ekwall K (2005) Genomewide analysis of nucleosome density histone acetylation and HDAC function in fission yeast. EMBO J 24:2906–2918

Wood V, Gwilliam R, Rajandream MA, Lyne M, Lyne R, Stewart A, Sgouros J, Peat N, Hayles J, Baker S, Basham D, Bowman S, Brooks K, Brown D, Brown S, Chillingworth T, Churcher C, Collins M, Connor R, Cronin A, Davis P, Feltwell T, Fraser A, Gentles S, Goble A, Hamlin N, Harris D, Hidalgo J, Hodgson G, Holroyd S, Hornsby T, Howarth S, Huckle EJ, Hunt S, Jagels K, James K, Jones L, Jones M, Leather S, McDonald S, McLean J, Mooney P, Moule S, Mungall K, Murphy L, Niblett D, Odell C, Oliver K, O'Neil S, Pearson D, Quail MA, Rabbinowitsch E, Rutherford K, Rutter S, Saunders D, Seeger K, Sharp S, Skelton J, Simmonds M, Squares R, Squares S, Stevens K, Taylor K, Taylor RG, Tivey A, Walsh S, Warren T, Whitehead S, Woodward J, Volckaert G, Aert R, Robben J, Grymonprez B, Weltjens I, Vanstreels E, Rieger M, Schafer M, Muller-Auer S, Gabel C, Fuchs M, Dusterhoft A, Fritzc C, Holzer E, Moestl D, Hilbert H, Borzym K, Langer I, Beck A, Lehrach H, Reinhardt R, Pohl TM, Eger P, Zimmermann W, Wedler H, Wambutt R, Purnelle B, Goffeau A, Cadieu E, Dreano S, Gloux S, Lelaure V, Mottier S, Galibert F, Aves SJ, Xiang Z, Hunt C, Moore K, Hurst SM, Lucas M, Rochet M, Gaillardin C, Tallada VA, Garzon A, Thode G, Daga RR, Cruzado L, Jimenez J, Sanchez M, del Rey F, Benito J, Dominguez A, Revuelta JL, Moreno S, Armstrong J, Forsburg SL, Cerutti L, Lowe T, McCombie WR, Paulsen I, Potashkin J, Shpakovski GV, Ussery D, Barrell BG, Nurse P (2002) The genome sequence of Schizosaccharomyces pombe. Nature 415:871–880

Yamada T, Fischle W, Sugiyama T, Allis CD, Grewal SI (2005) The nucleation and maintenance of heterochromatin by a histone deacetylase in fission yeast. Mol Cell 20:173–185

Yanagawa Y, Sullivan JA, Komatsu S, Gusmaroli G, Suzuki G, Yin J, Ishibashi T, Saijo Y, Rubio V, Kimura S, Wang J, Deng XW (2004) Arabidopsis COP10 forms a complex with DDB1 and DET1 in vivo and enhances the activity of ubiquitin conjugating enzymes. Genes Dev 18:2172–2181

A Role for RNAi in Heterochromatin Formation in *Drosophila*

Nicole C. Riddle and Sarah C.R. Elgin(✉)

Abstract Heterochromatin is a specialized form of DNA packaging that results in a transcriptionally inactive conformation. While much progress has been made in characterizing the heterochromatin structure biochemically and via its effects on genes and transgenes, very little is known about how heterochromatin formation is initiated. Recent evidence from the yeast *Saccharomyces pombe* suggests the involvement of the RNA interference (RNAi) machinery in heterochromatin formation, and in particular in the targeting of the heterochromatin machinery to specific sites in the genome. In this article, we review the evidence for an involvement of RNAi in heterochromatin formation in the model system *Drosophila melanogaster*. It appears that while there are numerous threads that connect heterochromatin formation and gene silencing with the RNAi pathways in *Drosophila*, a direct role for RNAi in particular in the targeting of heterochromatin formation is still lacking.

Abbreviations aa: Amino acids; Adh: Alcohol dehydrogenase; ATP: Adenine triphosphate; ChIP: Chromatin immunoprecipitation; dsRNA: Double-stranded RNA; E(var): Enhancer of variegation; H3K4: Histone 3 lysine 4; H3K9me: Histone 3

Sarah C.R. Elgin
Department of Biology, Washington University, One Brookings Dr., Campus Box 1137St. Louis, MO 63130, USA
selgin@biology.wustl.edu

P.J. Paddison and P.K. Vogt (eds.), *RNA Interference.*
Current Topics in Microbiology and Immunology 320.
© Springer-Verlag Berlin Heidelberg 2008

methylated at lysine 9; HDAC: Histone deacetylase; HP1: Heterochromatin protein 1; I-RNA: Iosine-containing RNA; LTR: Long terminal repeat; miRNA: microRNA; MNase: Micrococcal nuclease; mRNA: Messenger RNA; PEV: Position effect variegation; rasiRNA: Repeat associated small interfering RNA; RISC: RNA-induced silencing complex; RITS: RNA-induced transcriptional silencing; RNAi: RNA interference; siRNA: Small interfering RNA; Su(var) Suppressor of variegation; TSN: Tudor SN; VIG: Vasa intronic gene; ADAR: Adenosine deaminase

1   Definition of Heterochromatin

Cytologically, the genome can be divided roughly into two categories, heterochromatin and euchromatin, based on the mode of chromatin packaging. Heterochromatin was originally defined as the nuclear material that remains deeply stained (i.e., heteropycnotic) by nucleic-acid specific dyes as the cell cycle progresses from metaphase to interphase (Heitz 1928). In general, heterochromatin is associated with pericentric and telomeric regions of chromosomes. Subsequent studies of this material have expanded the definition of heterochromatin to include a cluster of characteristics, each applicable in most, but not all cases. For example, heterochromatic regions consist predominantly of repetitious DNA, including satellite DNA and remnants of transposable elements. While these regions contain substantially fewer genes than euchromatin, in *Drosophila* they are not completely devoid of genes. Interestingly, those genes that are present appear to depend on the heterochromatic environment for optimal expression (Hearn et al. 1991; Lu et al. 2000). In addition, heterochromatic regions are more densely packaged, replicate late in S phase, and show extremely low or no meiotic recombination (Ashburner et al. 2005; Weiler and Wakimoto 1995).

Two key observations, namely X inactivation and position effect variegation (PEV), have linked formation of the condensed heterochromatic state with the inactivation of genes normally active in a euchromatic environment. X chromosome inactivation affects one of the two X chromosomes in female mammals, silencing the majority of genes on that chromosome. The inactive X cforms the Barr body, readily observed in stained nuclei as a heteropycnotic domain (reviewed in Lyon 1999). While the initial decision of which X chromosome to inactivate appears to be random, once the decision is made, it is clonally inherited. X inactivation unequivocally demonstrates the effects of altered chromatin structure on gene expression and confirms the general association of heterochromatin with a silent state.

PEV arises from a rearrangement of chromosomes that places a normally active euchromatic gene adjacent to a breakpoint within the heterochromatin. This rearrangement causes silencing of genes adjacent to the breakpoint in a variegating pattern, apparently as a consequence of a clonally inherited decision similar to X inactivation (see Fig. 1). PEV occurs in many organisms but has been studied most intensively in the fruit fly *Drosophila melanogaster*, where genes required for eye or body pigmentation (*white* and *yellow* respectively) provide convenient markers for the study of PEV (reviewed in Weiler and Wakimoto 1995). Larval polytene chromosomes of individuals carrying such a rearrangement show that the genomic

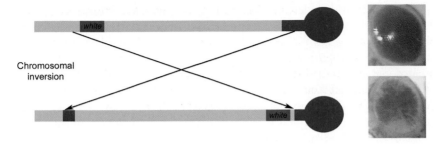

Fig. 1 Position effect variegation. In the original configuration of the *Drosophila* X chromosome shown in the *top* of the illustration, the *white* gene (*red box*) is far from the centromeric heterochromatin (*dark blue* area on the *right side* of the chromosome diagram). *White* is strongly expressed, leading to a fully red eye, as seen in the photograph on the *right*. If a chromosomal inversion places the *white* gene close to a breakpoint in the centromeric heterochromatin (as illustrated in the *bottom* part of the figure), the *white* gene can be silenced and no longer expressed. As this silencing is stochastic, and only occurs in a subset of cells, a mottled red pattern is observed in the eye (photograph on the *bottom right*)

region containing the marker gene is indeed packaged in a dense, heterochromatic form; however, this type of packaging is restricted to cells in which the gene is actually silenced (Zhimulev et al. 1986). Both this finding and mammalian X chromosome inactivation strongly support the connection between an altered chromatin state, chromatin packaging, and gene silencing. In *Drosophila*, PEV is a commonly used assay in heterochromatin studies, and it will feature prominently in this review.

Given a variegating phenotype, it is relatively simple to select for second site mutations that alter the phenotype, leading to reduced or increased levels of silencing [designated as *Su(var)* or *E(var)* alleles respectively]. Extensive screens in *Drosophila* have led to the characterization of over 30 such loci, with many more mutations identified, estimated to represent a total of ca. 150 genes (see Schotta et al. 2003). Heterochromatin protein 1 (HP1) was one of the first *Su(var)*-encoded proteins identified and characterized. Originally, HP1 was identified in a cytological screen using monoclonal antibodies generated against tightly binding nuclear proteins. HP1 is predominantly associated with the pericentric heterochromatin, telomeres, the small fourth chromosome (considered entirely heterochromatic by several of the above criteria), and some sites along the chromosome arms (James and Elgin 1986). A cloned version of the gene was used to identify its chromosomal position; sequencing of known *Su(var)* alleles mapping to this site confirmed that a mutation in the gene encoding HP1, *Su(var)2-5*, leads to a loss of silencing (Eissenberg et al. 1990, 1992). Several genes identified by *Su(var)* mutations code for proteins that play a structural role in heterochromatin, while others encode enzymes that are required to shift the histone modification state (Wallrath 1998). These enzymes include both those required to remove modification marks associated with the active state (for example HDAC1, coded for by *rpd3*) and those required to add modification marks associated with the inactive state [for example, the histone H3 lysine 9 methyltransferase, coded for by *Su(var)3-9*] (reviewed in Grewal and Elgin 2002).

Studies of PEV have demonstrated that genes closer to the breakpoint (i.e., the heterochromatin mass) have a higher probability of being silenced, while this probability is less for genes further removed. This finding suggests one fundamental characteristic of heterochromatin: this form of packaging can spread along the chromosome. It appears that heterochromatin formation is initiated at multiple sites within a domain and then spreads by a self-assembly process until either a barrier is encountered or the process fails due to depletion of necessary structural components (Locke et al. 1988). This hypothesis is supported by the observation that the dosage of several heterochromatin proteins has "antipodal" effects on the level of gene expression. For example, while loss of one copy of *Su(var)2-5* (HP1) leads to a loss of silencing, the presence of an extra copy of the gene results in increased silencing of a heterochromatic *white* reporter gene (Locke et al. 1988). Similar results have been obtained using the genes encoding HP2 (Shaffer et al. 2006), SU(VAR)3-7 (Spierer et al. 2005), and SU(VAR)3-9 (Schotta et al. 2003), suggesting that they all play a structural role in heterochromatin formation.

A potential mechanism for heterochromatin spreading has been suggested based on the interactions of HP1. HP1 is a small protein (212 aa in *D. melanogaster*) with two conserved domains, an N-terminal "chromodomain" and a related C-terminal "chromoshadow" domain. The protein dimerizes through the chromoshadow domain. This domain also interacts with several other proteins, including the three mentioned above, HP2, SU(VAR)3-7, and SU(VAR)3-9. It was first reported in mammals that the HP1 chromodomain binds specifically to histone H3 modified by methylation at lysine 9 (H3K9me2/3; Bannister et al. 2001; Lachner et al. 2001). This finding was the key observation leading to a model for the spreading of heterochromatin silencing along the chromosome observed in PEV. Because HP1 can recognize both the specific histone modification (H3K9me2/3) and bind the modifying enzyme [SU(VAR)3-9, a histone H3K9 methyltransferase], the modification can be propagated, regenerated, and potentially inherited as an epigenetic mark (see Fig. 2). Overall, the effects of the two chromatin modifiers HP1 and SU(VAR)3-9 are tightly linked, which is further demonstrated by the finding that the localization of HP1 and SU(VAR)3-9 to pericentric heterochromatin is mutually dependent (Schotta et al. 2002). While the interaction of SU(VAR)3-9 and HP1 provides a model for propagating a heterochromatic nucleosome organization, it remains unclear how this process is targeted to appropriate regions of the genome.

While PEV was originally discovered as a result of a chromosomal rearrangement, the above biochemical studies suggest that insertion of a reporter gene into a heterochromatic environment by transposition could also result in a variegating phenotype. As in the case of chromosome rearrangements, gene silencing would occur due to the spreading of the repressive chromatin structure (over the reporter gene). This hypothesis has been confirmed by numerous experiments using *Drosophila* (Wallrath and Elgin 1995), yeast (Allshire et al. 1994; Gottschling et al. 1990), and mammals (Festenstein et al. 1999). This approach has allowed the investigation of the chromatin structure of reporter genes in various chromatin environments. Using *Drosophila* embryos, micrococcal nuclease (MNase) digestion experiments have shown that the nucleosome spacing associated with a silenced

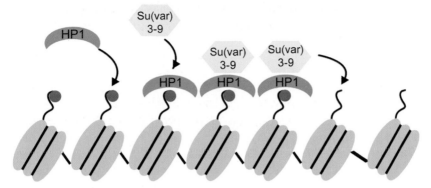

Fig. 2 Spreading of heterochromatin. Due to the fact that HP1, one of the key structural components of heterochromatin, can recognize H3K9me as well as recruit SU(VAR)3-9, the histone methyl transferase generating this modification, once initiated, heterochromatin can spread as shown in the diagram. Nucleosomes are shown in *light blue*, with the DNA represented in *black*. For each nucleosome, one histone H3 tail is shown, which can be modified by methylation at K9 (*purple circle*). If H3K9me is present, HP1 (*blue*) can bind to it. In turn, SU(VAR)3-9 (*yellow*) can bind to nucleosome-bound HP1. SU(VAR)3-9 can methylate the adjacent H3 at K9, propagating the spread of heterochromatin. In addition, the transition from euchromatin to heterochromatin is facilitated by the concomitant removal of active marks such as histone acetylation, for example, by the RDP3 histone deacetylase (not shown; Carrozza et al. 2005; Keogh et al. 2005). Many other chromosomal proteins contribute to maintaining a stable chromatin structure

(heterochromatic) reporter is much more regular than the spacing found for euchromatic insertion sites, with smaller MNase cleavage targets (Sun et al. 2001; Wallrath and Elgin 1995). The promoters of silenced transgenes also exhibit a loss of DNase I hypersensitive sites (DH sites; nucleosome-free regions commonly found at the 5′ ends of genes and at other regulatory sites) and are more resistant to DNase I digestion in general (Cryderman et al. 1999; Sun et al. 2001). Loss of DH sites has been shown to be dependent on the presence of HP1. The changes in nucleosome spacing, and the implied denser chromatin structure, may well contribute to a loss of accessibility, preventing RNA polymerase II from recognizing and/or accessing the reporter genes (Cryderman et al. 1999).

The studies cited above helped to define heterochromatin, albeit imperfectly, and have led to a better biochemical understanding of the chromatin packaging that can lead to gene silencing. However, they leave open the question of how heterochromatin formation is targeted in the cell nucleus. How is the decision made to inactivate certain regions of the genome by this mechanism, and leave others accessible for expression? One possible mechanism might be via proteins that bind specific target DNA sequences. Such proteins have been identified. For example, D1 is an AT-hook protein that binds to AT-rich satellite DNA in *Drosophila*, mutations of which cause suppression of w^{m4} variegation (Aulner et al. 2002). This type of binding, however, seems an unlikely mechanism for targeting heterochromatin formation to transposable elements, for example, which are more variable. Results from recent studies in *S. pombe* and plants indicate that RNA interference (RNAi) is used to target gene silencing in these organisms. These findings provided an impetus to ask whether or not a similar RNAi system might operate in *Drosophila*.

2   Biochemistry of RNAi

The earliest evidence for the existence of the RNAi pathway was uncovered by studies of gene silencing in plants, where it was noted that the introduction of multiple transgene copies often led to posttranscriptional gene silencing (Jorgensen et al. 1996; Matzke et al. 1989; Napoli et al. 1990; van der Krol et al. 1990). Eventually, double-stranded RNA (dsRNA) was implicated in this process (by experiments carried out in plants and worms) and shown to be able to induce silencing of genes with homologous sequences (Fire et al. 1998; Metzlaff et al. 1997). In particular, small RNA species were found to be involved in mediating the control of gene expression from transgenes as well as from endogenous gene copies (Hamilton and Baulcombe 1999). Soon it was recognized that the RNAi pathway could provide a common mechanism for a number of disparate gene silencing phenomena, including both transcriptional and posttranscriptional cases.

Posttranscriptional silencing is thought to occur via the action of the RNA-induced silencing complex (RISC). While more recent evidence suggests that there are most likely a number of functionally differentiated RISCs, the complex originally purified from *Drosophila* tissue culture cells contains the following protein components: AGO2, an Argonaute family protein; TudorSN, a putative endonuclease (TSN); VIG, the product of *vasa intronic gene*; and FXR, the *Drosophila* homolog of the fragile X mental retardation protein (Caudy et al. 2002; Hammond et al. 2001). To induce silencing, dsRNA is recognized by a Dicer protein, which cleaves the dsRNA into 21- to 23-nucleotide (nt) small interfering RNA (siRNA). One siRNA strand remains associated with the Dicer protein and subsequently is loaded into the RISC complex, making contact with the other RISC components. The siRNA, which is an integral part of the active RISC, targets the complex to endogenous mRNA transcripts of complementary sequence. The mRNA molecules identified by this process are then cut and degraded by the endonucleolytic activity of RISC (in the case of *Drosophila*, the AGO2 subunit). Thus, the combined action of a Dicer and RISC leads to posttranscriptional silencing of genes with homology to dsRNA due to the degradation of their mRNA. Alternatively, Dicer-derived siRNAs can lead to posttranscriptional gene silencing by causing translational inhibition of homologous mRNAs. (For details on both of these processes, please see the other chapters in this volume or the recent review by Sontheimer 2005.)

A second protein complex that participates in transcriptional gene silencing has been isolated in yeast (*S. pombe*). This complex shows structural similarity to RISC and is named RNA-induced transcriptional silencing (RITS) complex. It contains CHP1 (a chromodomain protein, and a structural element of heterochromatin), TAS3 (a protein of unknown function), and like RISC, an Argonaute class protein, AGO1, as well as siRNAs (Verdel et al. 2004). Similar to the siRNA found in RISC, the siRNA component of the RITS complex is generated by a Dicer protein (Verdel et al. 2004). In the RITS complex, siRNAs serve to guide the complex to potentially heterochromatic locations in the genome based on sequence homology. Once localized, the RITS complex interacts with histone modifying enzymes such as CLR4 (the H3K9 methyltransferase), and SWI6, the yeast HP1 homolog (Motamedi et al. 2004; Noma et al. 2004). Through the recruitment of heterochromatin associated proteins, and possibly chromatin remodeling factors, RITS can induce heterochromatin formation. An RNA-dependent RNA polymerase (RPD1/RDR1) is involved in this pathway in addition to the RITS components (Sugiyama et al. 2005). RPD1 amplifies the siRNA response by generating additional dsRNA from nascent transcripts, which can subsequently feed into the pathway after being processed by a Dicer, thus reinforcing the transcriptional gene silencing. It is a rather curious feature of this process that it appears that transcription, presumably at low levels, is thus used to ensure gene silencing.

Proteins that are part of the RNAi pathway have been identified in *Drosophila*, in part due to their sequence similarity to known proteins in other model systems (see Table 1 for a summary). The *Drosophila* genome encodes two Dicer proteins (Bernstein et al. 2001): DCR-1, which is predominantly responsible for the generation of microRNAs (miRNAs, small RNA species, derived from endogenous

Table 1 RNAi pathway genes in *Drosophila melanogaster*. A "Yes" in the TEs column indicates that mutations in this gene affect transposable element silencing. Entries in the PEV column indicate the effect mutations in this gene have on PEV. References for the data summarized in this table are given in the text

Gene	Function	TEs	PEV?
Dcr–1	Dicer protein, preferentially miRNA processing	ND	ND
Dcr–2	Dicer protein, preferentially siRNA processing, viral RNA processing	ND	ND
Ago1	Argonaute protein, miRNA processing	Yes	ND
Ago2	Argonaute protein, siRNA processing, viral RNA processing	Yes	Suppresses
Ago3	Argonaute protein, unknown function	ND	ND
Piwi	Argonaute protein, heterochromatin formation, viral RNA processing	Yes	Suppresses
Aubergine	Argonaute protein	Yes	Suppresses
Homeless/Spindle-E	RNA helicase; heterochromatin formation	Yes	Suppresses
Armitage	RNA helicase; RISC maturation; stellate silencing	ND	ND
Rm62/Lip	RNA helicase; heterochromatin formation	Yes	Suppresses
R2D2	dsRNA binding protein, siRNA processing, viral RNA processing	ND	ND
Drosha	miRNA processing	Yes	ND
Loquacious/R3D1	dsRNA binding protein, miRNA processing, *Stellate*	ND	ND
Tudor-SN	Endonuclease, component of RISC	ND	ND
FMR1	Fragile X Protein orthologue, component of RISC	ND	ND
VIG	*Vasa intronic gene* product, component of RISC, viral RNA processing	ND	ND

ND, not determined

hairpin transcripts, that function in developmental gene regulation), and DCR-2, which mainly generates siRNAs (Lee et al. 2004). There are five Argonaute proteins, AGO1, AGO2, AGO3, PIWI, and AUBERGINE (AUB). Similar to the subfunctionalization seen with the Dicer proteins, one Argonaute protein, AGO1, is primarily involved in the processing of miRNAs, while a second family member, AGO2, is chiefly responsible for the processing of siRNAs. However, recent data indicate that this division of labor is not complete, as both AGO1 and AGO2 can degrade mRNA targets (Miyoshi et al. 2005; Okamura et al. 2004). AUB and PIWI have been implicated in transposon silencing and appear to be involved in heterochromatin formation as well (Kalmykova et al. 2005; Pal-Bhadra et al. 2004; Reiss et al. 2004). AGO3 seems to be more similar in function to PIWI and AUB than to AGO1 or AGO2 (Brennecke et al. 2007). Three candidate RNA helicases are also part of the RNAi pathway in *Drosophila*: SPN-E (aka HOMELESS) and RM62 (aka LIP) are involved in heterochromatin formation (Csink et al. 1994; Pal-Bhadra et al. 2004), while ARMITAGE (ARMI) is required for RISC maturation (Tomari et al. 2004). Besides these three classes of proteins, the *Drosophila* RISC from S2 cells, which has been studied in detail, also includes VIG, TSN, and FMR1 (Caudy et al. 2002). While the Argonaute and Dicer proteins are essential for siRNA processing, it is possible that VIG, TSN, and FMR1 are only present in one or a few specialized RISCs. An additional protein class in the RNAi pathway is dsRNA binding proteins, which in *Drosophila* include R2D2, which transiently binds the siRNA duplex (Liu et al. 2003) and LOQUACIOUS (LOQS) (Forstemann et al. 2005; Saito et al. 2005). In contrast to yeast and plants, *Drosophila* appears to lack an RNA-dependent RNA polymerase activity, based on similarity searches against public databases of the published genome sequence. The absence of this activity is supported by the observation that targeting of a particular exon for posttranscriptional gene silencing does not lead to the formation of upstream degradation sites (Celotto and Graveley 2002; Roignant et al. 2003).

The following model has emerged for RNAi in *Drosophila* based on the genes present in the *Drosophila* genome and the experimental data available (see Fig. 3). In the case of siRNAs, the RNAi pathway is initiated by a long double-stranded RNA, which is recognized by the Dicer protein DCR-2. DCR-2 cleaves the double-stranded RNA into siRNAs. R2D2 (a double-stranded RNA binding protein homologous to RDE4 from *C. elegans*) binds to the DCR-2-bound double-stranded siRNA, and additional proteins are recruited to form the RISC-loading complex. R2D2 and the unnecessary siRNA strand (passenger strand) leave the complex. AGO2, VIG, TSN, and FMR1 are among the proteins recruited to form RISC with the bound siRNA, which serves as the agent for targeting specific mRNAs for degradation. Parallel to the processing of siRNAs is the pathway handling miRNAs, derived from endogenous hairpin RNA. In this case, DROSHA and DCR-1 process the hairpin RNA into fragments of approx. 21 nt (Lee et al. 2003). These fragments are incorporated into a protein complex containing AGO1, which targets homologous mRNAs for translational inhibition, sequestration, and/or degradation, thus contributing to developmental gene control. LOQS is a double-stranded RNA binding protein that is required for the processing of miRNAs (Jiang et al. 2005; Saito et al.

2005). It is unclear to what extent the siRNA and miRNA pathways intersect, specifically to what degree the components of one pathway can substitute for components of the other. These pathways each have distinct components, but also share
some components, and further work is needed to gauge the amount of crosstalk
between them (Murchison and Hannon 2004). A pathway for processing dsRNA to
target repetitious sequences for transcriptional gene silencing can be postulated;
however, we do not know the source of the initiating RNA (whether from a hairpin,
long double-stranded transcript, or the complementation of a single strand transcript), and are only beginning to identify components (see also Fig. 3).

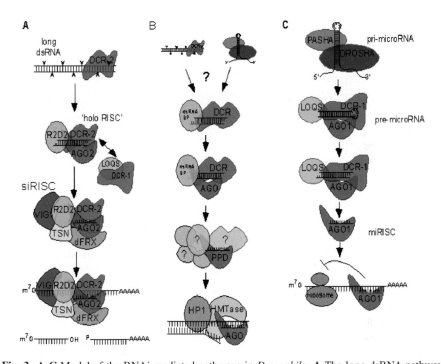

Fig. 3 A-C Model of the RNAi-mediated pathways in *Drosophila*. **A** The long dsRNA pathway
primarily uses DCR-2 to generate siRNAs that are incorporated into AGO2-containing HoloRISC.
DCR-1-LOQS have some role in this pathway as well. siRNA-bound AGO2 interacts with target
RNAs and cleaves them. **B** Hypothetical pathway leading to heterochromatin formation. Long
dsRNA molecules, or alternatively hairpin RNAs, are processed into siRNAs. They are then recognized by a double-stranded RNA binding protein and incorporated into a RISC-like complex, which
might include a double-stranded RNA binding protein, a Dicer protein, as well as an Argonaute
family member. Incorporated into a targeting complex, the siRNA serves to target specific regions
of the genome for heterochromatin formation and recruits chromatin-modifying enzymes such as
histone methyltransferases. Eventually, heterochromatin-associated proteins such as heterochromatin protein 1 are recruited as well. *PPD*, Paz-PIWI domain protein. Note that the source of the critical small RNAs could also be the recently observed piRNAs, which are abundant in germline (for
a recent review see Lin 2007). **C** MicroRNA pathway, where long primary-mircroRNAs are cleaved
by DROSHA/PASHA to generate pre-microRNAs, which are further cleaved by DCR-1/LOQS to
generate ~22-nt microRNA duplexes. These are then loaded into AGO1-containing miRISC, which
inhibits translation by binding to complementary sequences in the 3′-UTR of corresponding
mRNAs. (Adapted from Leuschner et al. 2005 and Gregory et al. 2005)

3   Links Between RNAi and Heterochromatin

Several observations linking gene silencing with altered chromatin structure also suggest a connection to RNAi. Most important in establishing this connection have been studies of cosuppression and of transcriptional gene silencing involving transposable elements. "Cosuppression" denotes the observation that multiple copies of the same gene, including both endogenous and transgenic copies, in a dispersed (not tandem) configuration, exhibit a decrease (suppression) in gene expression with increased gene dosage. This phenomenon was described initially in plants (Napoli et al. 1990). In *Drosophila*, the first described case of cosuppression involved a transgene consisting of the *white* promoter fused to an *Adh* reporter gene (Pal-Bhadra et al. 1997). Quantitative Northern analysis demonstrated that mRNA levels were reduced in homozygous flies (with two copies of the transgene) compared to heterozygous individuals (with one copy). In general, multiple transgene copies resulted in a form of gene silencing that was dependent on proteins encoded by the *Polycomb* group of genes (Pal-Bhadra et al. 1997). This finding suggests that the silencing might occur at the transcriptional level. In addition to *white-Adh* transgenes, the full-length *Adh* gene can participate in this copy number-dependent silencing as well. However, silencing of the full-length *Adh* copies is posttranscriptional. A role for the RNAi pathway was confirmed by the detection of siRNAs from the *Adh* locus and the finding that silencing was disrupted by mutations in the Argonaute family member *piwi* (Pal-Bhadra et al. 2002).

One possible explanation for the silencing observed might be found in the nature of the transgenes. The various constructs were introduced into *Drosophila* using *P* element-mediated transformation and contain the ends of a *P* element transposon. As will be discussed in more detail later in this review, transposable elements are often silenced at the level of transcription. It is possible that the *P* element remnants associated with the transgene are able to recruit the machinery responsible for gene silencing; this does not explain, however, the difference in silencing mechanisms observed between the *w-Adh* and the full-length *Adh* constructs.

Interestingly, the Argonaute family member *piwi*, which is known to affect post-transcriptional silencing phenomena, also has a strong effect on transcriptional silencing of the *white-Adh* reporter gene construct. This impact of *piwi* was demonstrated in an experimental system that included the *w-Adh* reporter gene construct, the endogenous *Adh* gene, and a construct combining the *Adh* promoter with the coding region of *white* named *Adh-w*. In this system, the addition of *w-Adh* copies results in transcriptional silencing of *Adh-w* in a manner that is dependent on the presence of the endogenous *Adh* gene. When the *piwi* mutation was introduced into the background carrying these transgenes, it did not affect the transcriptional silencing of *w-Adh/Adh*. In contrast, based on eye color observations (*white*) and Northern blot analysis (*white*), it was shown that the loss of *piwi* resulted in a partial restoration of expression from the *Adh-w* transgene, which had also originally been transcriptionally silenced. Thus, in *piwi* mutants, transcriptional silencing can be alleviated in certain cases, a finding that links the RNAi pathway to transcriptional gene silencing using the Polycomb proteins (Pal-Bhadra et al. 2002).

Additional evidence for such a link has been uncovered in experiments with the Polycomb response element (PRE)-containing regulatory element *FAB-7*. The PREs recruit Polycomb complexes, thus contributing to silencing. Using immunostaining techniques, DCR-2, AGO1, and PIWI were shown to colocalize with Polycomb bodies in interphase diploid nuclei. The three RNAi proteins are not necessary for the recruitment of Polycomb complexes to *FAB-7*; however, mutants in these genes were deficient in the long-range chromosome interactions that are precipitated by *FAB-7* elements (Grimaud et al. 2006). While the available data at this point do not provide clear evidence for a specific mode of action for the RNAi pathway in Polycomb-mediated silencing, it appears clear that the two processes are linked at a minimum through shared protein components.

Another silencing phenomenon, reminiscent of cosuppression, has been seen in studies of hybrid dysgenesis. Hybrid dysgenesis is observed in *Drosophila* when males harboring certain transposable elements are crossed to females lacking them. In the offspring of such crosses, high levels of transposition and sterility are detected. These effects are due to the reactivation of the novel transposable element and can be prevented by exposing the "naïve" strain that lacks the transposon to any portion of the element (Ashburner et al. 2005). The fact that expression of any portion of the element can maintain silencing after the cross is reminiscent of the silencing properties of the *w-Adh* construct mentioned in the previous section. In addition, small RNA species matching the transposable element have been shown to play a role in subsequent repression of the transposable element (Blumenstiel and Hartl 2005). Finally, certain aspects of hybrid dysgenesis also are impacted by the dosage of *Su(var)3-9*, which encodes an H3K9 methyltransferase (Dimitri et al. 2005), and *Su(var)2-5*, which encodes HP1 (Marin et al. 2000; Ronsseray et al. 1996). Both loci are critical for heterochromatin formation.

While hybrid dysgenesis overall is still poorly understood, and in fact might represent more than one distinct phenomenon, the current data suggest that dysgenesis is the consequence of mobilization of a repetitious element due to a shift from the element's silent state to an active state. The presence of siRNAs matching the reactivated transposable element provides a clear link to the RNAi pathway. Because some forms of hybrid dysgenesis are also impacted by mutations in the structural components of heterochromatin, they provide a link between heterochromatin formation and the RNAi machinery, suggesting that targeted heterochromatin formation is normally used to silence the transposable elements.

Studies of the regulation of transposable elements provide additional evidence for a link between the RNAi pathway, gene silencing, and heterochromatin formation. In *Drosophila*, the *gypsy* retrotransposon usually is silenced to prevent its transposition. Many copies reside in heterochromatic areas of the genome. Northern blot analysis shows the presence of siRNAs derived from *gypsy* elements. In addition, the silencing of *gypsy* elements is dependent on the presence of a functional copy of *piwi* (Sarot et al. 2004). Lack of a functional *piwi* allele can cause increased transposition of two other transposable elements, *copia* and *mgd1*, in the male germline, indicating that *piwi* is required for transposon silencing in that instance as well (Kalmykova et al. 2005). However, it is currently unknown whether the silencing observed is transcriptional or posttranscriptional. It is also possible that the mechanism involves a combination of both, as a functional *piwi* product and siRNAs have been associated with both types of silencing in the *w-Adh* and *Adh* studies mentioned above.

Investigations into the regulation of other *Drosophila* transposons also testify to the relationship between the RNAi pathway and heterochromatin formation. One case of *P* element repression is dependent on the presence of (a second) *P* element insertion into the subtelomeric heterochromatin of the X chromosome and occurs in the absence of functional HP1. Mutations in *aubergine* were found to disrupt this specific type of *P* element repression (Reiss et al. 2004). *Aubergine* has also been shown to function in the silencing of additional long terminal repeat (LTR) transposons (*mdg1, 1731*), and non-LTR elements (*F* element), as well as the non-coding tandem repeat *mst40* in the germline (Aravin et al. 2001). Lack of a functional copy of *spn-E* alleviates silencing of the heterochromatic *GATE* transposon and increases its expression (Gvozdev et al. 2003). Similar results were obtained for *copia* elements in testes, where mutations in *spn-E* increase expression (Stapleton et al. 2001). In addition, a microarray study comparing gene expression of AGO1-depleted cells with expression levels of AGO2-depleted cells uncovered a common set of mobile elements that is misregulated in both cell lines (Rehwinkel et al. 2006). Thus, at least five RNAi-associated proteins, AGO1, AGO2, SPN-E, AUB, and PIWI, are required for effective retrotransposon silencing, indicating a role for RNAi in maintaining silencing of these repetitive elements. It remains unclear, however, if the reactivation of transposable elements is a direct effect of the defects in the RNAi pathway that impact posttranscriptional silencing, or is a consequence of unraveling the repressive structure of heterochromatin, with associated loss of transcriptional silencing, or both.

Additional insights into the role of RNAi in maintaining transposable elements in a silent state have been gained from recent work on viral invaders and RNAi. While it has been known for some time from work in plants that the RNAi pathway is involved in the degradation of viral RNA and thus the defense against viral infection, evidence for a similar pathway in *Drosophila* is still in its infancy. In a recent study, where *Drosophila* cultures were infected with a birnavirus (*Drosophila* X virus), it was shown that RNAi plays a role in viral defense in *Drosophila* as well. In particular, PIWI, VIG, AUB, ARMI, RM62, R2D2, and AGO2 were all required for the successful initiation of this viral defense pathway (Zambon et al. 2006). Two other classes of viruses, nodaviruses and picorna-like viruses, were used in a second study to challenge wildtype flies and flies mutant in RNAi components to assess their immune response. In this study, *dcr-2*, *r2d2*, and *ago2* mutant flies were shown to have a suppressed immune response, demonstrating the importance of the RNAi pathway (Wang et al. 2006). Finally, the dependence of a successful immune response to viral infection on RNAi was demonstrated for Sindbis virus, a member of the α-virus family, by challenging *dcr-2* mutant flies, which showed much higher mortality than wildtype controls (Galiana-Arnoux et al. 2006).

The role of RNAi in the immune response to viral invaders appears to be conserved from plants to insects and mammals and might offer an explanation for the role of RNAi in maintaining transposable elements in a silent state. Transposable elements are likely derived from ancient viral invaders of the genome, and still carry many characteristics that demonstrate their kinship with viral genomes. The LTR-derived transposons have a dsRNA intermediate, which can serve as a substrate for the RNAi machinery. Thus, the common aspects of viral replication and transposition might explain the multiple roles the RNAi machinery assumes in immune response and the regulation of transposable elements.

Some of these components of the RNAi system also are involved in the regulation of other repeated sequences, for example the *Stellate* locus. *Stellate* is an endogenous locus encompassing multiple tandem arrays of a transcript required for male fertility in *D. melanogaster*. Expression of *Stellate* is regulated by the RNAi pathway through the tandem repeats found at the *Su(Ste)* locus. These repeats represent copies of the *hoppel* transposon, also known as *1360* element, interspersed with a repeated fragment of the *Stellate* gene. The *Su(Ste)* repeats reside in the Y chromosome heterochromatin, while *Stellate* itself is located on the X chromosome. The *Su(Ste)* tandem repeats are expressed in both sense and antisense direction, including regions of identity with the *Stellate* gene (Aravin et al. 2001). Expression in the antisense direction utilizes a promoter from within a copy of the *1360* element. *Spn-E* mutants mimic deficiencies in the *Su(Ste)* locus, allowing for the accumulation of excess *Stellate* transcript (Stapleton et al. 2001). Similarly, *aub* mutations result in the derepression of *Stellate* (Aravin et al. 2001). Lastly, *armi*, encoding a putative ATP-dependent helicase, also disrupts proper *Stellate* regulation through the RNAi pathway, providing yet another link to the various silencing pathways (Tomari et al. 2004). Overall, available evidence at this point is consistent with posttranscriptional regulation of *Stellate* expression through the RNAi pathway. However, the data are not sufficient to exclude the involvement of a transcriptional component to the regulation of *Stellate,* mediated through the RNAi pathway's documented effect on chromatin structure.

While the evidence from *Drosophila* clearly shows that gene silencing is linked to alterations in chromatin structure, and that many instances of gene silencing are impacted by the RNAi pathway, experimental support for a direct connection between RNAi and heterochromatin formation is strongest in other organisms. In *S. pombe,* the relationship between heterochromatin formation and the RNAi machinery has been probed through the use of heterochromatic reporter constructs. These studies examined the effect of mutations in the Argonaute gene *ago1*, the RNase III gene *dcr1*, and the RNA-dependent RNA polymerase gene *rdp1*. When any of these genes is nonfunctional, reporter genes in the pericentric heterochromatin (which are usually silenced) are expressed. In addition, large transcripts from the centromeric regions are recovered in the mutant strains. These large transcripts are absent in wildtype strains. In contrast, large numbers of siRNAs derived from the centromere are present in wildtype but absent in the mutants. The changes in centromeric expression states in the three mutants reflect a biochemical change in chromatin structure. Compared to wildtype, *ago1⁻*, *dcr1⁻*, and *rdp1⁻* lines show higher levels of H3K4 methylation, a mark of transcriptionally active chromatin, as shown by chromatin immunoprecipitation experiments. These regions also show decreased levels of H3K9 methylation, a mark of silenced chromatin, in the mutant lines.

Chromatin immunoprecipitation experiments indicate that the RNA-dependent RNA polymerase RDP1 physically associates with centromeric sequences, suggesting that dsRNA is generated from any transcripts originating at the site (Volpe et al. 2002). Additional data from a study of the *mat* locus confirm the involvement of *ago1*, *dcr1*, and *rdp1* in heterochromatin formation in this domain. Mutations in all three loci lead to loss of silencing and loss of heterochromatic histone marks (Hall et al. 2002). Thus, the data available from *S. pombe* clearly link the RNAi pathway to heterochromatin formation, as mutations in the genes required for RNAi lead to biochemically altered chromatin in normally heterochromatic domains. Further details can be found in other chapters of this book.

In *Arabidopsis*, studies of RNA-directed DNA methylation also have provided a connection between the RNAi pathway and chromatin structure. Similar to *Drosophila* and other organisms, siRNAs homologous to the heterochromatic regions of the *Arabidopsis* genome have been isolated, corresponding, for example, to the 180-bp centromeric repeat and various transposable elements (Llave et al. 2002). Mutations in the RNAi pathway lead to increased transcription of hetero-chromatic sequences such as transposable elements, e.g., *AtSN1*, and a loss of the associated siRNAs (Xie et al. 2004). However, the strongest connection between the RNAi system and chromatin structure is provided by tracking cytosine methyla-tion. Various studies have shown that transgenes processed via the RNAi pathway are targeted for cytosine methylation, and concomitant gene silencing, in a manner dependent on the siRNAs (Aufsatz et al. 2002). Localized H3K9me is also observed in association with cytosine methylation, a further mark of heterochromatin forma-tion in plants (Jackson et al. 2002; Soppe et al. 2002; Tran et al. 2005). Thus, it appears that the RNAi system in *Arabidopsis* is directly involved in targeting hete-rochromatin formation by affecting 5-methylcytosine levels.

While few results have been reported from vertebrates, recent data from chicken-human hybrid cell lines have indicated that Dicer is required for proper sister chro-matid cohesion. Loss of Dicer activity results in increased transcription from centromeric heterochromatin in this system as well. Furthermore, two heterochro-matin-associated proteins are mislocalized in *dicer* deficient cells, the RAD21 cohesion protein and the BubR1 checkpoint protein (Fukagawa et al. 2004). Together, the evidence from *S. pombe* and plants indicates that there is a direct con-nection between heterochromatin formation and the RNAi pathway that is pre-served among diverse eukaryotes. Previous evidence cited above supports the presence of a similar mechanism in *Drosophila*.

4   Experiments Testing an RNAi Connection in *Drosophila*

4.1   Tests Using PEV

The first set of experiments that indicate a possible connection between heterochro-matin and the RNAi pathway in *Drosophila* investigated the impact of mutations in known RNAi components on reporter genes showing PEV. PEV, shown in Fig. 1, can be used as an indicator of heterochromatic packaging as illustrated previously. Thus, the response of a variegating reporter gene to second site mutations has been used to identify genes whose products contribute to chromatin formation. Lines carrying insertions of tandem-repeat reporter constructs are capable of inducing local heterochromatin formation at the insertion site (Dorer and Henikoff 1994; Fanti et al. 1998). These lines as well as lines with single *white* reporter genes inserted within heterochromatin were used to test the involvement of RNAi in PEV. Mutations in the RNAi pathway components *piwi*, *spn-E*, and *aub* relieve silencing of the reporter gene, with *spn-E* showing the strongest effect (Pal-Bhadra et al. 2004). The impact of mutations in RNAi pathway components on PEV has been confirmed with an independent reporter construct (Haynes et al. 2006). In addition, the perturbation of heterochromatin structure was observed by immunohistochemical staining of polytene chromosomes (Pal-Bhadra et al. 2004). Thus, the RNAi pathway proteins PIWI, AUB, and SPN-E affect characteristics of heterochromatin, indicating that the RNAi machinery plays a role in its formation or maintenance in *Drosophila*.

More recently, it has been shown that AGO2, a component of RISC in *Drosophila*, impacts heterochromatin formation as well. In a study of *ago2*-mutant embryos, chromosome segregation was found to be abnormal, as was the localization of the centric histone H3 variant (CID, centromere identifier). This centromere defect was reflected in abnormal HP1 staining of centric heterochromatin on polytene chromosomes. These chromosomes also exhibited defects in H3K9 methylation (Deshpande et al. 2005). Studies of the eye phenotype in flies carrying a *mini-white* reporter gene construct showing PEV confirmed the role of AGO2 in heterochromatin formation. In *ago2/+* heterozygous flies, suppression of PEV is observed, leading to increased expression from the *mini-white* reporter gene (Deshpande et al. 2005). These PEV studies demonstrate the effects of defects in multiple RNAi-associated proteins on heterochromatin formation, linking the two pathways.

4.2   Spectrum of siRNAs

Studies profiling the type and number of small RNA species present within an organism also connect heterochromatin formation and RNAi. In *Drosophila*, a profiling study that cloned and characterized over 4,000 small RNAs identified three kinds of small RNAs. Besides the degradation products of cellular mRNA, which are heterogeneous in size, 21- to 22-nt RNAs and 24- to 26-nt RNAs were also found. These molecules represent miRNAs (based on their structure and annotation in the *Drosophila* genome database) involved in developmental gene control, small interfering RNAs (siRNAs mainly from viral sequences), and repeat-associated small interfering RNAs (rasiRNAs, based on sequence similarity to known repeats). rasiRNAs were recovered from all genomic regions commonly identified as heterochromatin: centromeric repeats, pericentromeric sequences, including transposable elements (retroelements and DNA transposons), and *Su(Ste)* repeats, as well as a number of uncharacterized repeats. The contribution of rasiRNAs to the total small

RNA pool varies over developmental time and is highest in early embryogenesis. In 0- to 2-h and 2- to 4-h embryos, rasiRNAs are as abundant as miRNAs (Aravin et al. 2003). During this same time period, heterochromatin domains are established. While at ca. 100 min after fertilization (cell cycle 10) heterochromatin is not detected by dense staining during interphase, it is easily seen at ca. 130 min after fertilization (nuclear replication cycle 14; Foe et al. 1993). Thus, rasiRNAs are present in high concentrations during the time period critical for heterochromatin establishment and fall off sharply thereafter. These findings are consistent with the idea that these siRNAs might play a role in directing heterochromatin formation.

During recent months, significant progress has been made in the characterization of the three PIWI family members in *Drosophila*, PIWI, AUB, and AGO3. All three function in the germline (Brennecke et al. 2007; Megosh et al. 2006). They associate with small RNAs, which have been termed PIWI-interacting or piRNAs (first observed in rat; Lau et al. 2006). piRNAs may well correspond to the rasiRNA population described in the previous paragraph (Brennecke et al. 2007; Gunawardane et al. 2007; Saito et al. 2006; Vagin et al. 2006). piRNAs differ from siRNAs and miRNAs as they are larger in size and exhibit distinct 3'/5' modifications. The generation of these germline RNAs in *Drosophila* is independent of *dcr-1* and *dcr-2*, but depends on at least three DNA helicases (*rm62*, *spn-E*, and *armi*; Vagin et al. 2006). piRNAs found in complexes with all three PIWI proteins originate from repeated sequences (Brennecke et al. 2007; Saito et al. 2006; Vagin et al. 2006); however, they differ in their orientation. AUB/PIWI-associated piRNAs derive most often from the antisense strand of transposons, while AGO3-associated RNAs derive from the sense strand. In addition, computational analyses indicate that most piRNAs are derived from a relatively small number of master regulatory loci (Brennecke et al. 2007). Based on these data, a model emerges where long transcripts are produced from master regulator loci and are processed into small RNAs by PIWI proteins. The piRNA then serves as guide to target other transcripts for degradation. The different strand specificity of AGO3 and AUB/PIWI piRNAs allows for the possibility of a self-reinforcing loop (ping-pong mechanisms; for details see Brennecke et al. 2007). One interesting hypothesis based on the suggestion that piRNAs may persist in the early embryo is that they may serve to initiate the establishment of a heterochromatic structure at TE locations that then is propagated independently.

4.3 Fourth Chromosome Mapping

Chromosome four of *D. melanogaster* is exceptional in that it exhibits characteristics of both euchromatin and heterochromatin under the classical definition. It is the smallest chromosome at ca. 4.2 Mb (Locke and McDermid 1993). In addition to its centromeric portion and heterochromatic short arm, it has a 1.2-Mb chromosome arm that is replicated in polytene chromosomes to a similar degree as the euchromatic chromosome arms (Celniker and Rubin 2003). With 82 genes, the gene density of this arm is similar to that of other euchromatic chromosome arms. In contrast to the other autosomes, however, the fourth chromosome is late replicating (Barigozzi et al. 1966) and does not undergo meiotic recombination (Sandler and Szauter 1978). The fourth chromosome is strongly associated with HP1 as well as with H3K9 di/trimethylation based on immunofluorescent staining of polytene chromosomes (Haynes et al. 2004; James et al. 1989). Thus, in these latter characteristics the banded portion of the fourth chromosome resembles classical heterochromatin, despite being more like euchromatin in terms of gene density.

The mosaic nature of chromosome four is reflected in studies probing the chromatin domains of the fourth chromosome with a *white* reporter gene driven by an *hsp70* promoter. *Drosophila* lines exhibiting a red-eye phenotype were recovered from reporter gene insertion in four separate, presumably euchromatic, domains on the banded portion of chromosome four. In contrast, over 20 lines with insertions on chromosome four have been recovered with the reporter in heterochromatic domains, as shown by variegating eye phenotype. The chromatin structure of the reporter in variegating lines was found to be less accessible to nucleases. In addition, eye color variegation was suppressed in a *Su(var)2-5* mutant background, indicating that the silencing observed in the variegating lines is dependent on heterochromatin formation, specifically on HP1. Sequence analysis of the insertion sites associated with variegating reporter genes revealed that these sites are often close to genes, most within 2 kb of an annotated expressed gene. Eleven lines with variegating eye phenotype actually have an insertion within the transcribed portion of a gene, raising the possibility that even transcribed regions on the fourth chromosome can have a heterochromatic or silencing effect on the *white* reporter gene. Alternatively, these genes may be active at a different developmental time or in a different tissue, where heterochromatin formation has been circumvented. Further genetic analysis revealed that most variegating inserts are in close proximity to a *1360/hoppel* transposon, suggesting that this element might be a target for heterochromatin formation (Haynes et al. 2004; Sun et al. 2000, 2004). A direct test of the contribution of *1360* to heterochromatin formation was carried out by including a copy of *1360* in a *P* element reporter construct (Haynes et al. 2006). This study found that *1360* alone is insufficient to induce heterochromatin formation in all sequence contexts, but *1360* contributes to heterochromatin formation as its presence can increase the strength of PEV (Haynes et al. 2006).

A comparative analysis of sequences from the fourth chromosome in *D. melanogaster* and its homolog in *D. virilis* has also contributed to our understanding of heterochromatin formation. In contrast to the fourth chromosome in *D. melanogaster*, the *D. virilis* chromosome can be considered euchromatic based on its lack of association with HP1 and H3K9me. Both chromosomes contain a large number of repetitive sequences and exhibit similar gene density. They differ, however, in the density of DNA transposons, with the fourth chromosome of *D. melanogaster* having a significantly higher density of this class of repetitious elements. Interestingly, *1360*, a candidate element for heterochromatin initiation identified in the PEV studies, is among the most common DNA elements in *D. melanogaster*, but appears only rarely in *D. virilis*; the same is true for a second transposon-derived element, *DINE*

(Slawson et al. 2006). This finding again suggests a role for *1360* in heterochromatin formation. siRNAs matching the *1360* element were found among the rasiRNA molecules identified in the *D. melanogaster* small RNA pool (Aravin et al. 2003) as well as among piRNAs (Saito et al. 2006; Vagin et al. 2006). Together, these studies suggest a link between repeated sequences such as *1360*, heterochromatin formation, and RNAi.

4.4 Involvement of RNA Editing via ADAR

Work in recent years has uncovered a link between the RNA editing machinery, DNA repair, and heterochromatin, suggesting the possibility of an interaction with the RNAi pathway as well. The identification of the *dodeca*-satellite binding protein 1 (DDP1) in *Drosophila* provided the first hints of this link. DDP1 is a protein that binds specifically to single-stranded nucleic acids and preferentially interacts with centromeric sequences (Cortes et al. 1999). DDP1 is in the vigilin class of proteins, which contain large numbers of tandem K-homology (KH) domains, thought to be involved in protein-nucleic acid and protein-protein interactions. In *Drosophila*, DDP1 associates with centromeric and pericentromeric heterochromatin based on chromatin immunoprecipitation experiments (ChIP; Wang et al. 2005). It also colocalizes with HP1 on polytene chromosomes (Huertas et al. 2004). When polytene chromosomes from *DDP1* mutants are assayed, a reduction in HP1 staining at the chromocenter is noted, as well as a decrease in H3K9 methylation. In addition, the chromosome structure is altered, and problems with chromosome condensation and segregation occur at a high frequency. These biochemical studies and the finding that mutations in *DDP1* act as dominant suppressors of PEV, indicate that the vigilin class of proteins is involved in heterochromatin formation.

Recent biochemical studies have provided a possible model for the role of vigilin/DDP1 in heterochromatin formation. Using inosine-containing RNA (I-RNA) as bait, vigilin was identified as an I-RNA binding protein, in addition to p54[nrb], PSF, and Matrin. Other components of this complex are Ku86, Ku70, and the DNA-dependent protein kinase DNA-PKcs, as well as the RNA helicase RHA and the ADAR1 protein (Wang et al. 2005). Interestingly, ADAR1 is a dsRNA-specific adenosine deaminase (ADAR). Its activity causes the deamination of adenosines in dsRNA, leading to the formation of I-RNA. Thus, through its association with HP1 and ADAR1, DDP1 provides a link between heterochromatin formation and RNA editing.

The vigilin complex has kinase activity, and its targets include HP1 as well as the histone variant H2AX. The kinase activity of the vigilin complex can be abolished by RNase treatment, indicating a requirement for an RNA entity for part of its function (Wang et al. 2005). However, the localization of DDP1 to the chromocenter of polytene chromosomes is independent of RNA (Cortes et al. 1999). Overall, these results demonstrate that DDP1 and the vigilin complex play a role both in heterochromatin formation and RNA editing. They interact with components of both pathways and provide a link to the RNAi pathway as well, which is involved in heterochromatin formation. Increasingly, experimental evidence suggests that RNA editing, RNAi, and DNA repair mechanisms all can impact heterochromatin formation. It is unclear at this point how exactly these three pathways intersect, but it has been suggested that they all might be part of a genome defense mechanism that originally arose to manage transposable elements (Fernandez et al. 2005).

5 Outlook

In this review, we have summarized the available evidence for a role of RNAi in heterochromatin formation in *D. melanogaster*. While these results provide ample indirect evidence for a link between RNAi and heterochromatin formation, direct evidence is lacking. The isolation of further RISC or RITS-like complexes is needed to clearly establish how the various proteins in the RNAi pathway interact and to identify binding partners. Biochemical studies will provide insights into how the RNAi machinery carries out such different functions as heterochromatin formation and genome defense.

One of the biggest questions remaining concerning heterochromatin formation is how the decision is made to package a given region of the genome as heterochromatin. While our understanding of heterochromatin structure and its maintenance has increased immensely, particularly with the recent focus on histone modifications, very little is known about the initiation or targeting of heterochromatin formation. This initial step leading to heterochromatic packaging is potentially a key step where the RNAi machinery could play a role. RNAi could provide sequence-specificity to target heterochromatin formation by using siRNAs from repetitive regions of the genome as guides. This mechanism is suggested by the data from *S. pombe*, but further experimental work is needed to resolve this issue in *D. melanogaster*.

There is also a question regarding the origin of the various RNAi pathways. It seems likely that RNAi originally arose as a genome defense mechanism to control viral invaders that could be recognized by the dsRNA that they produce. While posttranscriptional gene silencing is sufficient for control of newly invading viruses, transcriptional silencing provides a more permanent means of control for viral particles that are already integrated in the genome. It is unclear how exactly transposable elements are silenced by the RNAi machinery in *D. melanogaster*, whether this is posttranscriptional, transcriptional, or both. It is also possible that new transposable elements are initially posttranscriptionally silenced and then transition to a transcriptionally silenced state. The association of the RNAi pathway with the DNA repair machinery also allows for the possibility that these repetitious elements are actively degraded, leading to a loss of the ability to transpose.

The last question to consider is the role of heterochromatin in genome organization. One of the main consequences of the heterochromatic structure is transcriptional repression, but there are likely additional reasons for the existence of heterochromatin. We know that transcriptional repression can be caused by a number of mechanisms independent of the formation of a heterochromatic structure.

Thus it seems unlikely that transcriptional repression is the ultimate reason for the existence of heterochromatin. The heterochromatic packaging also provides stability for the genome by preventing recombination. Thus, heterochromatin might have a more "structural" role in maintaining a genome. A further role is the contribution of heterochromatin structure to centromere function. It has been demonstrated in yeast that HP1 and the specific chromatin structure it is associated with are required to recruit cohesin to centromeres (Pidoux and Allshire 2005). Although the main significance of heterochromatin is unknown, it is clearly necessary for an organism's ability to successfully manage its genome throughout the life cycle, especially during cell division. Thus, what perhaps started as a viral defense mechanism may have led to a type of chromatin structure that has been co-opted for many roles in the large genomes characteristic of eukaryotes. Indeed, these large genomes are primarily the consequence of large amounts of repetitious DNA; thus, the ability to silence viral invaders may have condemned the organism to carry this DNA along in the genome in an uneasy (and easily perturbed) silent state. Comprehending the role of RNAi in heterochromatin formation will help us to develop an understanding of the significance of heterochromatin in maintaining genome stability and shed light on the origin of this form of chromatin packaging.

Acknowledgements We would like to thank Dr. J.A. Birchler and the members of the Elgin lab for critical review of the manuscript. We would also like to thank K. Huisinga for help with Fig. 3. The authors were supported by National Institutes of Health grants GM68388 and GM073190 to S.C.R.E.

References

Allshire RC, Javerzat JP, Redhead NJ, Cranston G (1994) Position effect variegation at fission yeast centromeres. Cell 76:157-169

Aravin AA, Naumova NM, Tulin AV, Vagin VV, Rozovsky YM, Gvozdev VA (2001) Double-stranded RNA-mediated silencing of genomic tandem repeats and transposable elements in the *D. melanogaster* germline. Curr Biol 11:1017-1027

Aravin AA, Lagos-Quintana M, Yalcin A, Zavolan M, Marks D, Snyder B, Gaasterland T, Meyer J, Tuschl T (2003) The small RNA profile during *Drosophila melanogaster* development. Dev Cell 5:337-350

Ashburner M, Golic KG, Hawley RS (2005) *Drosophila*: a laboratory handbook. Cold Spring Harbor Laboratory Press, Cold Spring Harbor

Aufsatz W, Mette MF, van der Winden J, Matzke AJ, Matzke M (2002) RNA-directed DNA methylation in *Arabidopsis*. Proc Natl Acad Sci U S A 99 [Suppl 4]:16499-16506

Aulner N, Monod C, Mandicourt G, Jullien D, Cuvier O, Sall A, Janssen S, Laemmli UK, Kas E (2002) The AT-hook protein D1 is essential for *Drosophila melanogaster* development and is implicated in position-effect variegation. Mol Cell Biol 22:1218-1232

Bannister AJ, Zegerman P, Partridge JF, Miska EA, Thomas JO, Allshire RC, Kouzarides T (2001) Selective recognition of methylated lysine 9 on histone H3 by the HP1 chromo domain. Nature 410:120-124

Barigozzi C, Dolfini S, Fraccaro M, Raimondi GR, Tiepolo L (1966) *In vitro* study of the DNA replication patterns of somatic chromosomes of *Drosophila melanogaster*. Exp Cell Res 43:231-234

Bernstein E, Caudy AA, Hammond SM, Hannon GJ (2001) Role for a bidentate ribonuclease in the initiation step of RNA interference. Nature 409:363-366

Blumenstiel JP, Hartl DL (2005) Evidence for maternally transmitted small interfering RNA in the repression of transposition in *Drosophila virilis*. Proc Natl Acad Sci U S A 102: 15965-15970

Brennecke J, Aravin AA, Stark A, Dus M, Kellis M, Sachidanandam R, Hannon GJ (2007) Discrete small RNA-generating loci as master regulators of transposon activity in *Drosophila*. Cell 128:1089-1103

Carrozza MJ, Li B, Florens L, Suganuma T, Swanson SK, Lee KK, Shia WJ, Anderson S, Yates J, Washburn MP, Workman JL (2005) Histone H3 methylation by Set2 directs deacetylation of coding regions by Rpd3S to suppress spurious intragenic transcription. Cell 123:581-592

Caudy AA, Myers M, Hannon GJ, Hammond SM (2002) Fragile X-related protein and VIG associate with the RNA interference machinery. Genes Dev 16:2491-2496

Celniker SE, Rubin GM (2003) The *Drosophila melanogaster* genome. Annu Rev Genomics Hum Genet 4:89-117

Celotto AM, Graveley BR (2002) Exon-specific RNAi: a tool for dissecting the functional relevance of alternative splicing. Rna 8:718-724

Cortes A, Huertas D, Fanti L, Pimpinelli S, Marsellach FX, Pina B, Azorin F (1999) DDP1, a single-stranded nucleic acid-binding protein of *Drosophila*, associates with pericentric heterochromatin and is functionally homologous to the yeast Scp160p, which is involved in the control of cell ploidy. EMBO J 18:3820-3833

Cryderman DE, Tang H, Bell C, Gilmour DS, Wallrath LL (1999) Heterochromatic silencing of *Drosophila* heat shock genes acts at the level of promoter potentiation. Nucleic Acids Res 27:3364-3370

Csink AK, Linsk R, Birchler JA (1994) The *Lighten up* (*Lip*) gene of *Drosophila melanogaster*, a modifier of retroelement expression, position effect variegation and white locus insertion alleles. Genetics 138:153-163

Deshpande G, Calhoun G, Schedl P (2005) *Drosophila argonaute-2* is required early in embryogenesis for the assembly of centric/centromeric heterochromatin, nuclear division, nuclear migration, and germ-cell formation. Genes Dev 19:1680-1685

Dimitri P, Corradini N, Rossi F, Mei E, Zhimulev IF, Verni F (2005) Transposable elements as artisans of the heterochromatic genome in *Drosophila melanogaster*. Cytogenet Genome Res 110:165-172

Dorer DR, Henikoff S (1994) Expansions of transgene repeats cause heterochromatin formation and gene silencing in *Drosophila*. Cell 77:993-1002

Eissenberg JC, James TC, Foster-Hartnett DM, Hartnett T, Ngan V, Elgin SC (1990) Mutation in a heterochromatin-specific chromosomal protein is associated with suppression of position-effect variegation in *Drosophila melanogaster*. Proc Natl Acad Sci U S A 87:9923-9927

Eissenberg JC, Morris GD, Reuter G, Hartnett T (1992) The heterochromatin-associated protein HP-1 is an essential protein in *Drosophila* with dosage-dependent effects on position-effect variegation. Genetics 131:345-352

Fanti L, Dorer DR, Berloco M, Henikoff S, Pimpinelli S (1998) Heterochromatin protein 1 binds transgene arrays. Chromosoma 107:286-292

Fernandez HR, Kavi HH, Xie W, Birchler JA (2005) Heterochromatin: on the ADAR radar? Curr Biol 15:R132-R134

Festenstein R, Sharghi-Namini S, Fox M, Roderick K, Tolaini M, Norton T, Saveliev A, Kioussis D, Singh P (1999) Heterochromatin protein 1 modifies mammalian PEV in a dose- and chromosomal-context-dependent manner. Nat Genet 23:457-461

Fire A, Xu S, Montgomery MK, Kostas SA, Driver SE, Mello CC (1998) Potent and specific genetic interference by double-stranded RNA in *Caenorhabditis elegans*. Nature 391: 806-811

Foe VE, Odell GM, Edgar BA (1993) Mitosis and morphogenesis in the *Drosophila* embryo: point and counterpoint. In: Bate M, Arias AM (eds)The development of *Drosophila melanogaster*. Cold Spring Harbor Laboratory Press, Cold Spring Harbor, pp 149-300

Forstemann K, Tomari Y, Du T, Vagin VV, Denli AM, Bratu DP, Klattenhoff C, Theurkauf WE, Zamore PD (2005) Normal microRNA maturation and germ-line stem cell maintenance requires Loquacious, a double-stranded RNA-binding domain protein. PLoS Biol 3:e236

Fukagawa T, Nogami M, Yoshikawa M, Ikeno M, Okazaki T, Takami Y, Nakayama T, Oshimura M (2004) *Dicer* is essential for formation of the heterochromatin structure in vertebrate cells. Nat Cell Biol 6:784-791

Galiana-Arnoux D, Dostert C, Schneemann A, Hoffmann JA, Imler JL (2006) Essential function *in vivo* for Dicer-2 in host defense against RNA viruses in *Drosophila*. Nat Immunol 7:590-597

Gottschling DE, Aparicio OM, Billington BL, Zakian VA (1990) Position effect at *S. cerevisiae* telomeres: reversible repression of Pol II transcription. Cell 63:751-762

Gregory RI, Chendrimada TP, Cooch N, Shiekhattar R (2005) Human RISC couples microRNA biogenesis and posttranscriptional gene silencing. Cell 123:631-640

Grewal SI, Elgin SC (2002) Heterochromatin: new possibilities for the inheritance of structure. Curr Opin Genet Dev 12:178-187

Grimaud C, Bantignies F, Pal-Bhadra M, Ghana P, Bhadra U, Cavalli G (2006) RNAi components are required for nuclear clustering of Polycomb group response elements. Cell 124:957-971

Gunawardane LS, Saito K, Nishida KM, Miyoshi K, Kawamura Y, Nagami T, Siomi H, Siomi MC (2007) A slicer-mediated mechanism for repeat-associated siRNA 5′ end formation in *Drosophila*. Science 315:1587-1590

Gvozdev VA, Aravin AA, Abramov YA, Klenov MS, Kogan GL, Lavrov SA, Naumova NM, Olenkina OM, Tulin AV, Vagin VV (2003) *Stellate* repeats: targets of silencing and modules causing *cis*-inactivation and *trans*-activation. Genetica 117:239-245

Hall IM, Shankaranarayana GD, Noma K, Ayoub N, Cohen A, Grewal SI (2002) Establishment and maintenance of a heterochromatin domain. Science 297:2232-2237

Hamilton AJ, Baulcombe DC (1999) A species of small antisense RNA in posttranscriptional gene silencing in plants. Science 286:950-952

Hammond SM, Boettcher S, Caudy AA, Kobayashi R, Hannon GJ (2001) *Argonaute2*, a link between genetic and biochemical analyses of RNAi. Science 293:1146-1150

Haynes KA, Leibovitch BA, Rangwala SH, Craig C, Elgin SC (2004) Analyzing heterochromatin formation using chromosome 4 of *Drosophila melanogaster*. Cold Spring Harb Symp Quant Biol 69:267-272

Haynes KA, Caudy AA, Collins L, Elgin SC (2006) Element *1360* and RNAi components contribute to HP1-dependent silencing of a pericentric reporter. Curr Biol 16:2222-2227

Hearn MG, Hedrick A, Grigliatti TA, Wakimoto BT (1991) The effect of modifiers of position-effect variegation on the variegation of heterochromatic genes of *Drosophila melanogaster*. Genetics 128:785-797

Heitz E (1928) Das Heterochromatin der Moose. Jb Wiss Bot 69:728-818

Huertas D, Cortes A, Casanova J, Azorin F (2004) *Drosophila* DDP1, a multi-KH-domain protein, contributes to centromeric silencing and chromosome segregation. Curr Biol 14:1611-1620

Jackson JP, Lindroth AM, Cao X, Jacobsen SE (2002) Control of CpNpG DNA methylation by the KRYPTONITE histone H3 methyltransferase. Nature 416:556-560

James TC, Elgin SC (1986) Identification of a nonhistone chromosomal protein associated with heterochromatin in *Drosophila melanogaster* and its gene. Mol Cell Biol 6:3862-3872

James TC, Eissenberg JC, Craig C, Dietrich V, Hobson A, Elgin SC (1989) Distribution patterns of HP1, a heterochromatin-associated nonhistone chromosomal protein of *Drosophila*. Eur J Cell Biol 50:170-180

Jiang F, Ye X, Liu X, Fincher L, McKearin D, Liu Q (2005) Dicer-1 and R3D1-L catalyze micro-RNA maturation in *Drosophila*. Genes Dev 19:1674-1679

Jorgensen RA, Cluster PD, English J, Que Q, Napoli CA (1996) Chalcone synthase cosuppression phenotypes in petunia flowers: comparison of sense vs. antisense constructs and single-copy vs. complex T-DNA sequences. Plant Mol Biol 31:957-973

Kalmykova AI, Klenov MS, Gvozdev VA (2005) Argonaute protein PIWI controls mobilization of retrotransposons in the *Drosophila* male germline. Nucleic Acids Res 33:2052-2059

Keogh MC, Kurdistani SK, Morris SA, Ahn SH, Podolny V, Collins SR, Schuldiner M, Chin K, Punna T, Thompson NJ, Boone C, Emili A, Weissman JS, Hughes TR, Strahl BD, Grunstein M, Greenblatt JF, Buratowski S, Krogan NJ (2005) Cotranscriptional set2 methylation of histone H3 lysine 36 recruits a repressive Rpd3 complex. Cell 123:593-605

Lachner M, O'Carroll D, Rea S, Mechtler K, Jenuwein T (2001) Methylation of histone H3 lysine 9 creates a binding site for HP1 proteins. Nature 410:116-120

Lau NC, Seto AG, Kim J, Kuramochi-Miyagawa S, Nakano T, Bartel DP, Kingston RE (2006) Characterization of the piRNA complex from rat testes. Science 313:363-367

Lee Y, Ahn C, Han J, Choi H, Kim J, Yim J, Lee J, Provost P, Radmark O, Kim S, Kim VN (2003) The nuclear RNase III Drosha initiates microRNA processing. Nature 425:415-419

Lee YS, Nakahara K, Pham JW, Kim K, He Z, Sontheimer EJ, Carthew RW (2004) Distinct roles for *Drosophila* Dicer-1 and Dicer-2 in the siRNA/miRNA silencing pathways. Cell 117:69-81

Leuschner PJ, Obernosterer G, Martinez J (2005) MicroRNAs: Loquacious speaks out. Curr Biol 15:R603-R605

Lin H (2007) piRNAs in the germ line. Science 316:397

Liu Q, Rand TA, Kalidas S, Du F, Kim HE, Smith DP, Wang X (2003) R2D2, a bridge between the initiation and effector steps of the *Drosophila* RNAi pathway. Science 301:1921-1925

Llave C, Kasschau KD, Rector MA, Carrington JC (2002) Endogenous and silencing-associated small RNAs in plants. Plant Cell 14:1605-1619

Locke J, McDermid HE (1993) Analysis of *Drosophila* chromosome 4 using pulsed field gel electrophoresis. Chromosoma 102:718-723

Locke J, Kotarski MA, Tartof KD (1988) Dosage-dependent modifiers of position effect variegation in *Drosophila* and a mass action model that explains their effect. Genetics 120:181-198

Lu BY, Emtage PC, Duyf BJ, Hilliker AJ, Eissenberg JC (2000) Heterochromatin protein 1 is required for the normal expression of two heterochromatin genes in *Drosophila*. Genetics 155:699-708

Lyon MF (1999) X-chromosome inactivation. Curr Biol 9:R235-R237

Marin L, Lehmann M, Nouaud D, Izaabel H, Anxolabehere D, Ronsseray S (2000) *P*-Element repression in *Drosophila melanogaster* by a naturally occurring defective telomeric *P* copy. Genetics 155:1841-1854

Matzke MA, Primig M, Trnovsky J, Matzke AJ (1989) Reversible methylation and inactivation of marker genes in sequentially transformed tobacco plants. EMBO J 8:643-649

Megosh HB, Cox DN, Campbell C, Lin H (2006) The role of PIWI and the miRNA machinery in *Drosophila* germline determination. Curr Biol 16:1884-1894

Metzlaff M, O'Dell M, Cluster PD, Flavell RB (1997) RNA-mediated RNA degradation and chalcone synthase A silencing in petunia. Cell 88:845-854

Miyoshi K, Tsukumo H, Nagami T, Siomi H, Siomi MC (2005) Slicer function of *Drosophila* Argonautes and its involvement in RISC formation. Genes Dev 19:2837-2848

Motamedi MR, Verdel A, Colmenares SU, Gerber SA, Gygi SP, Moazed D (2004) Two RNAi complexes, RITS and RDRC, physically interact and localize to noncoding centromeric RNAs. Cell 119:789-802

Murchison EP, Hannon GJ (2004) miRNAs on the move: miRNA biogenesis and the RNAi machinery. Curr Opin Cell Biol 16:223-229

Napoli C, Lemieux C, Jorgensen R (1990) Introduction of a chimeric chalcone synthase gene into petunia results in reversible co-suppression of homologous genes in *trans*. Plant Cell 2:279-289

Noma K, Sugiyama T, Cam H, Verdel A, Zofall M, Jia S, Moazed D, Grewal SI (2004) RITS acts in *cis* to promote RNA interference-mediated transcriptional and post-transcriptional silencing. Nat Genet 36:1174-1180

Okamura K, Ishizuka A, Siomi H, Siomi MC (2004) Distinct roles for Argonaute proteins in small RNA-directed RNA cleavage pathways. Genes Dev 18:1655-1666

Pal-Bhadra M, Bhadra U, Birchler JA (1997) Cosuppression in *Drosophila*: gene silencing of A*lcohol dehydrogenase* by *white-Adh* transgenes is Polycomb dependent. Cell 90:479-490

Pal-Bhadra M, Bhadra U, Birchler JA (2002) RNAi related mechanisms affect both transcriptional and posttranscriptional transgene silencing in *Drosophila*. Mol Cell 9:315-327

Pal-Bhadra M, Leibovitch BA, Gandhi SG, Rao M, Bhadra U, Birchler JA, Elgin SC (2004) Heterochromatic silencing and HP1 localization in *Drosophila* are dependent on the RNAi machinery. Science 303:669-672

Pidoux AL, Allshire RC (2005) The role of heterochromatin in centromere function. Philos Trans R Soc Lond B Biol Sci 360:569-579

Rehwinkel J, Natalin P, Stark A, Brennecke J, Cohen SM, Izaurralde E (2006) Genome-wide analysis of mRNAs regulated by Drosha and Argonaute proteins in *Drosophila melanogaster*. Mol Cell Biol 26:2965-2975

Reiss D, Josse T, Anxolabehere D, Ronsseray S (2004) *aubergine* mutations in *Drosophila melanogaster* impair P cytotype determination by telomeric *P* elements inserted in heterochromatin. Mol Genet Genomics 272:336-343

Roignant JY, Carre C, Mugat B, Szymczak D, Lepesant JA, Antoniewski C (2003) Absence of transitive and systemic pathways allows cell-specific and isoform-specific RNAi in *Drosophila*. Rna 9:299-308

Ronsseray S, Lehmann M, Nouaud D, Anxolabehere D (1996) The regulatory properties of autonomous subtelomeric P elements are sensitive to a Suppressor of variegation in *Drosophila melanogaster*. Genetics 143:1663-1674

Saito K, Ishizuka A, Siomi H, Siomi MC (2005) Processing of pre-microRNAs by the Dicer-1-Loquacious complex in *Drosophila* cells. PLoS Biol 3:e235

Saito K, Nishida KM, Mori T, Kawamura Y, Miyoshi K, Nagami T, Siomi H, Siomi MC (2006) Specific association of Piwi with rasiRNAs derived from retrotransposon and heterochromatic regions in the *Drosophila* genome. Genes Dev 20:2214-2222

Sandler L, Szauter P (1978) The effect of recombination-defective meiotic mutants on fourth-chromosome crossing over in *Drosophila melanogaster*. Genetics 90:699-712

Sarot E, Payen-Groschene G, Bucheton A, Pelisson A (2004) Evidence for a piwi-dependent RNA silencing of the *gypsy* endogenous retrovirus by the *Drosophila melanogaster* flamenco gene. Genetics 166:1313-1321

Schotta G, Ebert A, Krauss V, Fischer A, Hoffmann J, Rea S, Jenuwein T, Dorn R, Reuter G (2002) Central role of *Drosophila SU(VAR)3-9* in histone H3-K9 methylation and heterochromatic gene silencing. EMBO J 21:1121-1131

Schotta G, Ebert A, Dorn R, Reuter G (2003) Position-effect variegation and the genetic dissection of chromatin regulation in *Drosophila*. Semin Cell Dev Biol 14:67-75

Shaffer CD, Cenci G, Thompson B, Stephens GE, Slawson EE, Adu-Wusu K, Craig C, Gatti M, Elgin SCR (2006) The large isoform of *Drosophila melanogaster* Heterochromatin Protein 2 plays a critical role in gene silencing and chromosome structure. Genetics 174:1189-1204

Slawson EE, Shaffer CD, Malone CD, Leung W, Kellmann E, Shevchek RB, Craig CA, Bloom SM, Bogenpohl J 2nd, Dee J, Morimoto ET, Myoung J, Nett AS, Ozsolak F, Tittiger ME, Zeug A, Pardue ML, Buhler J, Mardis ER, Elgin SC (2006) Comparison of dot chromosome sequences from D. melanogaster and *D. virilis* reveals an enrichment of DNA transposon sequences in heterochromatic domains. Genome Biol 7:R15

Sontheimer EJ (2005) Assembly and function of RNA silencing complexes. Nat Rev Mol Cell Biol 6:127-138

Soppe WJ, Jasencakova Z, Houben A, Kakutani T, Meister A, Huang MS, Jacobsen SE, Schubert I, Fransz PF (2002) DNA methylation controls histone H3 lysine 9 methylation and heterochromatin assembly in *Arabidopsis*. EMBO J 21:6549-6559

Spierer A, Seum C, Delattre M, Spierer P (2005) Loss of the modifiers of variegation Su(var)3-7 or HP1 impacts male X polytene chromosome morphology and dosage compensation. J Cell Sci 118:5047-5057

Stapleton W, Das S, McKee BD (2001) A role of the *Drosophila homeless* gene in repression of *Stellate* in male meiosis. Chromosoma 110:228-240

Sugiyama T, Cam H, Verdel A, Moazed D, Grewal SI (2005) RNA-dependent RNA polymerase is an essential component of a self-enforcing loop coupling heterochromatin assembly to siRNA production. Proc Natl Acad Sci U S A 102:152-157

Sun FL, Cuaycong MH, Craig CA, Wallrath LL, Locke J, Elgin SC (2000) The fourth chromosome of *Drosophila melanogaster*: interspersed euchromatic and heterochromatic domains. Proc Natl Acad Sci U S A 97:5340-5345

Sun FL, Cuaycong MH, Elgin SC (2001) Long-range nucleosome ordering is associated with gene silencing in *Drosophila melanogaster* pericentric heterochromatin. Mol Cell Biol 21:2867-2879

Sun FL, Haynes K, Simpson CL, Lee SD, Collins L, Wuller J, Eissenberg JC, Elgin SC (2004) *cis*-Acting determinants of heterochromatin formation on *Drosophila melanogaster* chromosome four. Mol Cell Biol 24:8210-8220

Tomari Y, Du T, Haley B, Schwarz DS, Bennett R, Cook HA, Koppetsch BS, Theurkauf WE, Zamore PD (2004) RISC assembly defects in the *Drosophila* RNAi mutant *armitage*. Cell 116:831-841

Tran RK, Zilberman D, de Bustos C, Ditt RF, Henikoff JG, Lindroth AM, Delrow J, Boyle T, Kwong S, Bryson TD, Jacobsen SE, Henikoff S (2005) Chromatin and siRNA pathways cooperate to maintain DNA methylation of small transposable elements in *Arabidopsis*. Genome Biol 6:R90

Vagin VV, Sigova A, Li C, Seitz H, Gvozdev V, Zamore PD (2006) A distinct small RNA pathway silences selfish genetic elements in the germline. Science 313:320-324

van der Krol AR, Mur LA, Beld M, Mol JN, Stuitje AR (1990) Flavonoid genes in petunia: addition of a limited number of gene copies may lead to a suppression of gene expression. Plant Cell 2:291-299

Verdel A, Jia S, Gerber S, Sugiyama T, Gygi S, Grewal SI, Moazed D (2004) RNAi-mediated targeting of heterochromatin by the RITS complex. Science 303:672-676

Volpe TA, Kidner C, Hall IM, Teng G, Grewal SI, Martienssen RA (2002) Regulation of heterochromatic silencing and histone H3 lysine-9 methylation by RNAi. Science 297:1833-1837

Wallrath LL (1998) Unfolding the mysteries of heterochromatin. Curr Opin Genet Dev 8:147-153

Wallrath LL, Elgin SC (1995) Position effect variegation in *Drosophila* is associated with an altered chromatin structure. Genes Dev 9:1263-1277

Wang Q, Zhang Z, Blackwell K, Carmichael GG (2005) Vigilins bind to promiscuously A-to-I-edited RNAs and are involved in the formation of heterochromatin. Curr Biol 15:384-391

Wang XH, Aliyari R, Li WX, Li HW, Kim K, Carthew R, Atkinson P, Ding SW (2006) RNA interference directs innate immunity against viruses in adult *Drosophila*. Science 312:452-454

Weiler KS, Wakimoto BT (1995) Heterochromatin and gene expression in *Drosophila*. Annu Rev Genet 29:577-605

Xie Z, Johansen LK, Gustafson AM, Kasschau KD, Lellis AD, Zilberman D, Jacobsen SE, Carrington JC (2004) Genetic and functional diversification of small RNA pathways in plants. PLoS Biol 2:E104

Zambon RA, Vakharia VN, Wu LP (2006) RNAi is an antiviral immune response against a dsRNA virus in *Drosophila melanogaster*. Cell Microbiol 8:880-889

Zhimulev IF, Belyaeva ES, Fomina OV, Protopopov MO, Bolshakov VN (1986) Cytogenetic and molecular aspects of position effect variegation in *Drosophila melanogaster*. I. Morphology and genetic activity of the 2AB region in chromosome rearrangement T(1;2)dorvar7. Chromosoma 94:492-504

RNA-Mediated Transcriptional Gene Silencing in Human Cells

Kevin V. Morris

Abstract The utilization of small interfering RNAs (siRNAs) represents a new paradigm in gene knockout technology. siRNAs can be used to knockdown the expression of a particular gene by targeting the mRNA in a post-transcriptional manner. While there are a plethora of reports applying siRNA-mediated post-transcriptional silencing (PTGS) therapeutically there are apparent limitations such as the duration of the effect and a saturation of the RNA-induced silencing complex (RISC). Recently, data have emerged that indicate an alternative pathway is operative in human cells where siRNAs have been shown, similar to plants, *Drosophila*, *C. elegans*, and *S. Pombe*, to mediate transcriptional gene silencing (TGS). TGS is operative by the antisense strand of the siRNA targeting chromatin remodeling complexes to the specific promoter region(s). This siRNA targeting results in epigenetic modifications that lead to a rewriting of the local histone code, silent state chromatin marks, and ultimately heterochromatization of the targeted gene. The observation that siRNA-directed TGS is operative via epigenetic modifications suggests that similar to plants, and *S. Pombe*, human genes may also be able to be silenced more permanently or for longer periods following a single treatment and may in fact offer a new therapeutic avenue that could prove robust and of immeasurable therapeutic value in the directed control of target gene expression.

Kevin V. Morris

Department of Molecular and Experimental Medicine, The Scripps Research Institute, 10550N, Torrey Pines Road, La Jolla, CA 92037, USA

kmorris@scripps.edu

P.J. Paddison and P.K. Vogt (eds.), *RNA Interference*.
Current Topics in Microbiology and Immunology 320.
© Springer-Verlag Berlin Heidelberg 2008

1 Introduction

1.1 RNAi-Mediated PTGS

RNA interference (RNAi) is the process in which double-stranded small interfering RNAs (siRNAs) modulate gene expression. Termed co-suppression, RNAi was first described in plants (reviewed in Tijsterman et al. 2002). RNAi can suppress gene expression via two distinct pathways involving siRNAs: transcriptional gene silencing (TGS) and post-transcriptional gene silencing (PTGS) (Pal-Bhadra et al. 2002; Sijen et al. 2001). Small interfering RNAs are generated by the action of the ribonuclease (RNase) III-type enzyme Dicer (Bernstein et al. 2001) on double-stranded RNAs (dsRNAs). Dicer is in a complex that also contains the human immunodeficiency virus type 1 (HIV-1) transactivating-response (TAR) RNA-binding protein (TRBP), Argonaute 2 (Ago-2), and the dsRNA-binding protein PACT (Lee et al. 2006; Fig. 1). The dsRNAs are processed by Dicer into siRNAs that are approx. 21–27 bp in length and which can then pair with the complementary target mRNA where cleavage of the mRNA is instigated by the action of Ago-2 (Liu et al. 2004). The Argonaute proteins, specifically Ago-2, constitute the major component of the RNA-induced silencing complex (RISC) and contains three highly conserved domains: the amino-terminal PAZ domain, core conserved domain, and carboxyl-terminal PIWI domain (Song et al. 2004). Ago-2 interacts specifically with the 3′ end of one of the siRNA strands via the Ago-2 conserved PAZ domain (Song et al. 2004). RNAi-mediated PTGS involves siRNA targeting of mRNA and in human cells is operable in both the cytoplasm and nucleus (Langlois et al. 2005; Robb et al. 2005).

1.2 RNAi-Mediated TGS

Double-stranded RNAs can also produce TGS of homologous genomic regions (regions complementary to the siRNAs) in *Arabidopsis*, *Schizosaccharomyces pombe*, *Drosophila*, and mammalian cells (reviewed in Matzke and Birchler 2005). TGS was first observed when doubly transformed tobacco plants surprisingly exhibited a suppressed phenotype of a transgene. Closer examination indicated that observed suppression of the transgene was the result of directed DNA methylation at the transgene loci (Matzke et al. 1989). As it turned out the observed TGS in plants was mediated by dsRNAs, which was substantiated in viroid-infected plants (Wassenegger et al. 1994) and shown to be the result of RNA-dependent DNA methylation (RdDM). The action of RdDM requires a dsRNA that is subsequently processed to yield short RNAs (Wassenegger et al. 1994; Mette et al. 2000). Interestingly, it was these short dsRNAs in the doubly transformed tobacco plant that happened to include sequences that were identical to genomic promoter regions involved in the transgene expression and ultimately led to TGS via methylation of

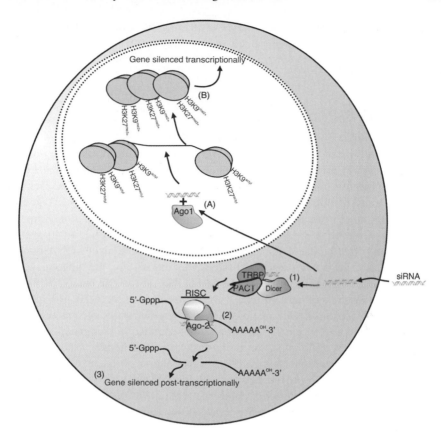

Fig. 1 Post-transcriptional vs transcriptional gene silencing. Synthetic siRNAs transfected directly into the cell can modulate not only post-transcriptional gene silencing (PTGS) via Dicer and RISC but also direct epigenetic modifications to the corresponding genomic loci (the DNA that codes for the targeted mRNA). This nuclear component appears to involve Ago-1. To direct PTGS, the transfected siRNA is processed by Dicer/TRBP/PACT *(1)* and then enters into the Ago-2-containing RISC complex *(2)* where the target mRNA is sliced by the action of Ago-2 *(3)*. Alternatively, synthetic siRNAs can localize to the nucleus in an Ago-1 dependent manner *(A)* and specifically target the homologous genomic sequence to induce chromatin modifications such as $H3K9^{me2+}$ or $H3K27^{me3+}$ *(B)* which are known to result in the conversion of euchromatin to heterochromatin and subsequent transcriptional gene silencing

the homologous promoter and the observed reduction in transgene expression (Matzke et al. 1989). In general, transcriptional gene silencing in plants is carried out by a larger size class of siRNAs, 24–26 nucleotides (nt) in length (Hamilton et al. 2002; Zilberman et al. 2003).

Recently members of the Argonaute protein family in *Arabidopsis* have been shown to play an essential role in RdDM of promoter DNA and transposon silencing (Lippman et al. 2003). Specifically, Ago-4 is known to direct siRNA-mediated silencing, and Ago-4 mutants display reactivation of silent *SUP* alleles, along with a corresponding decrease in both CpNpG DNA and H3K9 methylation (Zilberman et al. 2003). Consequently, in plants, siRNAs that include sequences with homology to genomic promoter regions are capable of directing the methylation of the homologous promoter and subsequent transcriptional gene silencing.

1.3   TGS in S. Pombe

TGS is not solely endogenous in plants. The fission yeast *S. Pombe* also employs TGS via Dicer-generated siRNAs to silence heterochromatic regions that exhibit bi-directional transcription (Fig. 2). Mechanistically, however, *S. Pombe* lacks the epigenetic mechanism of DNA methylation. Instead, *S. Pombe* utilizes Argonaute 1 (Ago-1) to direct histone methylation and heterochromatin formation (Lippman et al. 2003).

In *S. Pombe* and human cells, as well as many other organisms, DNA is packaged into chromatin. Chromatin is basically composed of the genomic DNA wrapped in approx. two full turns, or 146 bp of DNA, around an octameric histone core composed of two of each histone protein (histones: H2A, H2B, H3, and H4) to constitute nucleosomes. Chromatin can exist in various states such as euchromatin or heterochromatin. Typically, euchromatin is depicted as being less condensed and relatively transcriptionally active. Euchromatin is generally associated with acetylated histones and with histone H3 di-methylation on lysine 4 (H3mLys-4), whereas heterochromatin is generally more condensed and relatively transcriptionally inactive. Heterochromatin is generally associated with histone H3 di-methylation on lysine 9 (H3mLys-9) (Lippman et al. 2004). The acetylation of histone tails by histone acetyltransferases (HAT) results in relaxing the chromatin and a disruption of histone-DNA interactions. The relaxing of the histone–DNA interaction is thought to allow for gene activation while the deacetylation of histones by histone deacetylases (HDACs) result in histones that are susceptible to methylation, the condensation of the chromatin, and subsequent transcriptional repression (reviewed in Lusser 2002). Histone H3 Lys-9 di-methylation is generally associated with transcriptional repression and can directly recruit Swi6/HP1 (mammalian heterochromatin protein 1). The recruitment of Swi6/HP1 coincides with spreading in H3 Lys-9 methylation in *cis* (Hall et al. 2002) and subsequent transcriptional suppression and gene silencing.

RNAi-mediated TGS in *S. Pombe* operates specifically through histone 3 lysine-9 methylation (H3K9) (Volpe et al. 2002). In *S. Pombe* mutants in *dcr1* (Dicer homolog) and the only known Argonaute (Ago-1) were shown to be reduced in centromeric repeat H3K9 methylation, which is necessary for centromere function (Volpe et al. 2002). These data suggested a link between RNAi and directed targeting of specific histone modifications to the corresponding genomic sequences, which were homologous to the siRNAs. Thus, *dcr1* and Ago-1 were required to generate the siRNA-directed histone modifications that were required for the secondary recruitment or interaction, with Swi6 resulting in regulation of the heterochromatic state (Volpe et al. 2002).

Additional investigation demonstrated that the *dcr1*-processed dsRNAs, which correspond to centromeric repeats in *S. Pombe*, interact with Ago-1, Chip1 (chromodomain protein), and Tas1 (previously uncharacterized) to form the RNA-induced transcriptional silencing (RITS) complex (Verdel et al. 2004; Fig. 2). The presence of these siRNAs in the RITS complex was shown to require Rdp1, Hrr1 (helicase required for RNA-mediated heterochromatin assembly 1) and Cid12 (a 38-kDa protein involved in mRNA polyadenylation) (Motamedi et al. 2004; Fig. 2). The siRNA-loaded RITS complex then associates with the chromatin-binding factors Swi6 and Clr4 (Suv39H6 human homolog) to silence targeted genomic regions (Verdel et al. 2004) in an RNA polymerase II-dependant fashion (Kato et al. 2005). The siRNA targeting of RITS to the dsRNA-producing genomic region is mechanistically active in silencing by the action of Ago-1-mediated slicing of the centromerically expressed RNAs (Irvine et al. 2006) as well as silencing through the recruitment of histone methylation of the corresponding centromeric region (Fig. 2).

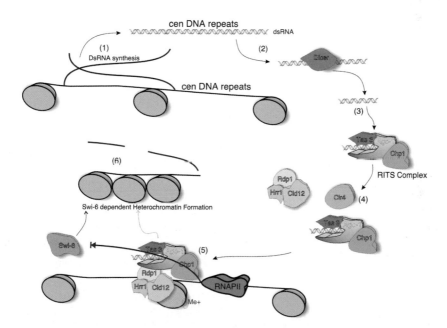

Fig. 2 TGS in *S. Pombe*. DsRNAs are generated from the transcription of centromeric DNA repeats [*cen DNA repeats*, *(1)*] that are then processed by Dicer *(2)* to 21- to 22-bp siRNAs *(3)*. Next, the Dicer-processed siRNAs are loaded into the RITS complex *(4)*. The RITS complex then interacts with the RNA-dependent RNA polymerase complex [RDRC, *(5)*] and the histone methyltransferase Clr4, which can then lead to H3K9 methylation *(5)* and silencing of the siRNA-targeted cen DNA repeat regions and/or swi-6-dependent heterochromatin formation *(6)*. The siRNA-targeted cen DNA repeat RNAs are also targeted by the action of Ago-1 and sliced *(6)*

1.4   *TGS in* C. Elegans, Drosophila, *and* Neurospora

As it turns out, RNAi-mediated TGS is pervasive throughout many biological systems. While the majority of work to date has been performed on *S. Pombe* and plants, other model organisms have demonstrated siRNA-mediated TGS with slight variations in the underlying theme. In the fungi *Neurospora crassa* the silencing of homologous sequences has been termed quelling (Romano 1992). Interestingly, in *Neurospora* the PTGS and TGS pathways both utilize histone 3 Lys-9 di-methylation and moreover appear to be distinct from one another (Chicas et al. 2005), whereas in *Drosophila* the two pathways of RNAi, PTGS and TGS, appear connected via the Piwi protein (Pal-Bhadra et al. 2002). The Piwi family of proteins have several homologs (Piwi/Sign/elF2C/Rde1/Argonaute) and are conserved from plants to animals (Fagard et al. 2000; Tabara et al. 1999; Grishok et al. 2001). Interestingly, in the nematode *Caenorhabditis elegans* the PAZ-Piwi-like protein Rde-1 has been shown to play an essential role in RNA-mediated silencing in the soma of *C. elegans*, whereas other RNA-mediated silencing mechanisms that are operative in the germline do not appear to require Rde-1 (Dernburg et al. 2000; Ketting and Plasterk 2000).

More recently, RNA-mediated transcriptional silencing of somatic transgenes in *C. elegans* has been shown to be the result of ADAR-encoding genes, *adr-1* and *adr-2*, and is dependent on Rde-1 (Grishok et al. 2005). The observed silencing and requirements for both Adr-1 and -2 as well as Rde-1 was the result of siRNA targeting of pre-mRNAs and corresponded with a decrease in both RNA polymerase II and acetylated histones at the targeted genomic region (Grishok et al. 2005). Interestingly, following an RNAi screen in *C. elegans*, genes encoding RNA-binding, Polycomb, and chromodomain proteins as well as histone methyltransferases were detected (Grishok et al. 2005). These data were essentially recapitulated in *C. elegans* in an interesting set of experiments that demonstrated long-term transcriptional gene silencing by RNAi. In essence one dose of siRNAs was capable of inducing gene silencing that was inherited indefinitely in the absence of the original siRNA trigger (Vastenhouw et al. 2006). This long-term inheritance of siRNA-mediated TGS appeared to require had-4 (a class II histone deacetylase), K03D10.3 (a histone acetyltransferase of the MYST family), isw-1 (a homolog of the yeast chromatin-remodeling ATPase ISW1), and mrg-1 (a chromodomain protein) (Vastenhouw et al. 2006). Taken together these data strongly suggest that RNA-mediated TGS in *C. elegans* contains a convergence of pathways that include epigenetic modifying factors as well as RNA. Overall, one cannot help but notice that indeed RNA is more intricately involved in the regulation of gene expression than has previously been envisioned.

1.5   *TGS in Human Cells*

A few commonalities can be discerned from the work performed in Plants, *S. Pombe, C. elegans*, and *Drosophila*. To begin with, siRNAs can (1) direct transcriptional gene silencing in a specific and directed manner, (2) the directed silencing correlates with epigenetic modifications such as histone methylation at the chromatin of the particular siRNA targeted gene, and (3) PIWI-related proteins appear to be involved and required for siRNA-directed TGS. As such, and based on the relative conservation in biology, i.e., the theory of evolution and natural selection, one cannot help but also expect to observe similarities or conserved commonalities between plants, *C. elegans, S. Pombe, Drosophila*, and humans.

Observations of siRNA-mediated TGS in mammalian cells has lagged behind the work done in other model organisms such as *Arabidopsis* (plants) and *S. Pombe* (yeast) (Morris et al. 2004). However, recent studies by our group and others have revealed that siRNA-mediated TGS in mammalian cells does occur and appears to be the result of the siRNA-directed H3K9 and H3K27 methylation, specifically H3K9me2 and H3K27me3, at the corresponding siRNA-targeted promoter (Morris et al. 2004; Castanotto et al. 2005; Bühler et al. 2005; Janowski et al. 2005; Suzuki et al. 2005). While some DNA methylation has also been observed at the siRNA-targeted promoters, the role in which DNA methylation plays in the observed silencing is debatable (Janowski et al. 2005; Park et al. 2004; Svoboda et al. 2004; Ting et al. 2005). Indeed, the ability of siRNAs to direct targeted DNA methylation could result in a much greater duration of suppression, as DNA methylation tends to correlate more robustly with long-term suppressed genes than does histone methylation. However, to date little is known regarding how long siRNA-directed TGS of RNA polymerase II promoters (RNAPII) can persist in human cells. The majority of siRNA-directed TGS experiments in human cells have been carried out so far with synthetic siRNAs targeted to RNAPII promoters (Morris et al. 2004; Castanotto et al. 2005; Janowski et al. 2005; Suzuki et al. 2005; Ting et al. 2005; Janowski et al. 2006; Kim et al. 2006; Weinberg et al. 2005; Zhang et al. 2005) or constitutive-expressing short-hairpin RNA (shRNA) expressing stable lentiviral transduced cell lines (Castanotto et al. 2005). Nonetheless, the observation that siRNA-directed TGS is operative via epigenetic modifications argues favorably for a longer term effect relative to siRNA-directed PTGS, provided the siRNAs are efficiently delivered to the nucleus. However, experimental evidence supporting this claim is still lacking.

While the duration of the siRNA-directed effect remains to be determined, what has become evident recently is that siRNAs directed to RNAPII promoter regions can mediate transcriptional silencing in human cells and that a repressive histone methyl mark is observed at the targeted promoter (Morris et al. 2004; Bühler et al. 2005; Ting et al. 2005; Weinberg et al. 2005). Furthermore, only the antisense strand of the siRNA is required to mediate histone methylation and silencing of the targeted RNAPII promoter (Weinberg et al. 2005). Moreover, RNAPII appears required for siRNA-mediated TGS and DNA methyltransferase 3A (DNMT3a) co-immunoprecipitates (co-IP) with biotin-linked siRNAs at the H3K27^{me3+}-targeted promoter (Weinberg et al. 2005). Recently, Ago-1 (and possibly also Ago-2) has been shown to be involved in siRNA-mediated TGS in human cells (Janowski et al. 2006; Kim et al. 2006). Ago-1 was shown to co-IP with RNAPII, and an enrichment of EZH2 and TRBP has also been observed along with Ago-1 at siRNA-targeted

promoters (Kim et al. 2006). Furthermore, the suppression of Ago-1 functionally
inhibits siRNA-mediated TGS in human cells (Kim et al. 2006). Clearly, in human
cells, similar to observations in other organisms such as *S. Pombe* and *Arabidopsis*,
Argonaute proteins and H3K9 methylation are required for transcriptional silencing, linking the RNAi and chromatin silencing machinery.

1.6   Model of TGS in Human Cells

A model for the mechanism of how siRNA-directed TGS is directed and initiated
in human cells has begun to emerge and appears to exhibit many similarities as well
as some distinct differences with the previously established models for TGS in *S.
Pombe* and plants. Similar to *S. Pombe*, siRNA-mediated TGS in human cells
involves the siRNAs, particularly the antisense strand, RNAPII, and histone methylation (Janowski et al. 2006; Kim et al. 2006; Morris 2005, 2006; Fig. 3A and B).
However, in human cells DNMT3a has been shown to co-immunoprecipitate along
with the antisense strand of the promoter-specific siRNA at the siRNA-targeted
promoter (Weinberg et al. 2005). Interestingly, DNMT3a has also been shown to
bind siRNAs in vitro (Jeffery and Nakielny 2004). Similar to observations in *S.
Pombe* (Kato et al. 2005), TGS in human cells requires RNAPII (Weinberg et al.
2005), possibly suggesting that the promoter region is transcribed and either that an
RNAPII-expressed transcript covers or corresponds with the siRNA-targeted gene/
chromatin (Fig. 3A) or that during transcription RNAPII unwinds the targeted gene
and subsequently allows access of the antisense strand of the siRNA (Fig. 3B) to
the targeted gene. Either mechanism would explain how the antisense strand of the
siRNA can localize to the particular targeted gene promoter region and fundamentally recruit and/or direct chromatin modifications that ultimately result in TGS.

Interestingly, preliminary evidence from siRNA-mediated TGS of the EF1-α
and HIV-1 promoters has demonstrated a paradigm for the underlying mechanism
in which the antisense strand of the siRNA by itself can direct TGS via the induction of a corresponding silent histone methyl-mark at the targeted promoter
(Weinberg et al. 2005). This siRNA- and/or antisense RNA-directed histone methylation is capable of spreading distal in a 5′ to 3′ direction from the original targeted
region corresponding to the homologous siRNA. This observed spreading of histone methylation might be due to an interaction with Ago-1 and RNAPII (Kim et
al. 2006). Furthermore, the observed spreading of histone methylation, specifically
H3K9me2+, and the observed H3K27me3+ methyl mark at the siRNA-targeted promoter, is reminiscent of those phenotypes observed in the X-inactivation-like pathway. One cannot help but wonder if siRNA-mediated RNAi-like responses in the
cell (PTGS and TGS) are simply a remnant of a more ancient pathway utilized by
the cell to deal with competing genes, such as is observed in mammalian
X-inactivation.

The observation that RNAPII is involved in siRNA-mediated TGS in both
S. Pombe and more recently in human cells (Kim et al. 2006; Weinberg et al. 2005)

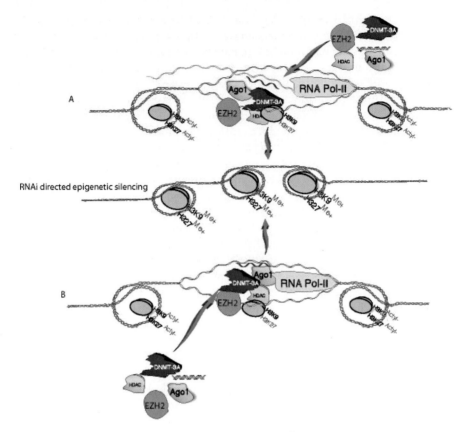

Fig. 3 A, B Proposed mechanisms for TGS in human cells. Two models for siRNA-mediated TGS have been proposed; either an RNA/RNA- or an RNA/DNA-mediated mode of silencing. **A** The RNA/RNA model might operate via the siRNAs interacting with a low-copy, possibly non-coding, RNA transcript that spans the chromatin of the targeted promoter region. One notion is that the siRNAs are unwound, possibly by action of an Ago-1 containing complex (although currently there are no data supporting this function in Ago-1). The unwinding of the siRNA might then allow interactions with a complex also containing DNMT3a. Thus the antisense strand of the siRNA, Ago-1 (Kim et al. 2006) and DNMT3a (Weinberg et al. 2005; Jeffery and Nakielny 2004), as well as factors previously shown to bind DNMT3a such as HDAC-1 and Suv39H1 (Fuks et al. 2001; Fuks et al. 2000) and possibly EZH2 (Viré et al. 2005), might all localize to the targeted promoter region possibly by interacting with a low-copy RNA being produced by RNAPII during transcription of the siRNA-targeted gene. The result of targeting these factors to this region would be the methylation of the local histones, H3K9^{me2+} and H3K27^{mc3+}, ultimately resulting in targeted TGS. **B** Alternatively, siRNA-mediated TGS might function through an RNA/DNA intermediate. The RNA/DNA model would be expected to function by the antisense strand of the siRNA gaining access to the targeted DNA by the effects of RNAPII unwinding the targeted genomic region, which would then allow the Ago-1, DNMT3a (Fuks et al. 2001), HDAC-1, Suv39H1 (Fuks et al. 2003), and possibly EZH2 chromatin remodeling factors to gain access, ultimately leading to gene silencing of the siRNA-targeted promoter

suggests two potential models. The first—the RNA/RNA model—proposes that there is an RNAPII-expressed non-coding transcript that is homologous to the targeted promoter/gene that somehow remains associated with the local chromatin corresponding to the targeted gene (Fig. 3A). This non-coding RNA might somehow remain affiliated with the nucleosome(s)—and as such would permit the RNAi machinery to direct chromatin modifications—or a chromatin-modifying complex to the targeted genomic region, ultimately leading to TGS. This putative non-coding RNA could be envisioned to act as a local "address" to allow chromatin and RNAi modification complexes, guided by siRNAs, access to the targeted gene (Fig. 3A). Supporting the RNA/RNA model is the observation that heterochromatin formation in mouse cells involves HP1 proteins and treatment with RNase causes a dispersion of HP1 proteins from pericentromeric foci (Muchardt et al. 2002) and higher order chromatin structures appear to contain an uncharacterized RNA component that might function as a scaffolding in chromatin remodeling (Maison et al. 2002). Whether such a non-coding RNA exists—if the siRNAs target this non-coding RNA during RNAPII transcription or if the non-coding RNA somehow associates with local chromatin—remains to be determined.

An alternative model, the RNA/DNA model, could also be envisioned to operate in an RNAPII-dependent manner where RNAPII essentially unwinds the targeted DNA and permits the intercalation of the antisense strand of the siRNA as well as RNAi and chromatin remodeling machinery to access to the targeted promoter region (Fig. 3B). Supporting this model is the observation that RNAPII has been shown to associate with complete unfolding of 1.85 out of 3 nucleosomes upstream of the transcription start site for the PH05 promoter (Boeger et al. 2005) and that the siRNA EF52 target site, shown to initiate TGS in human cells, is approx. one nucleosome upstream of the TATAA transcriptional start site (Morris et al. 2004). Moreover, RNA Pol-II is associated with nearly 60 subunits and a mass exceeding 3,000 kDa (Boeger et al. 2005). Overall, these reports suggest, at least in human cells, that a good, albeit speculative, hypothesis for the role of RNAPII in siRNA-mediated TGS might be to essentially unwind the targeted promoter region to allow the promoter-directed siRNAs access to their respective target.

1.7   Endogenous Small RNAs Involved in Gene Regulation

While it is becoming apparent in human cells that there is a mechanism in place by which siRNAs or small, 21-nt-long antisense RNAs can transcriptionally modulate gene expression, it is less clear what the endogenous signal utilizing this pathway might be, i.e., siRNA, small antisense RNAs, microRNAs, etc. In *C. elegans*, deep sequencing has recently revealed a class of 21 U-RNAs that consist of 21-nt-long RNAs containing a uridine 5′-monophosphate and 3′-terminal ribose (Ruby et al. 2006). These 21 U-RNAs were found to correlate with 5,700 genomic loci and were essentially dispersed between regions involved in protein-coding regions (Ruby et al. 2006). Overall, these data suggested that non-coding regions of the genome, while not necessarily coding for a protein, appear to express RNAs that might be involved in gene regulation. As many of these small 21 U-RNAs matched non-coding regions it is possible that they are involved in transcriptional modulation of *C. elegans* gene expression (Ruby et al. 2006). In human cells, however, far less is known, and the majority of inferences have been surmised from computationally based approaches. One recent observation involved the discovery and characterization of a vast array of small (21- to 26-nt), non-coding RNAs that fundamentally suggested that there is an RNA component, possibly involved in gene regulation, i.e., siRNA-mediated TGS, within the basic fabric of human cells (Katayama et al. 2005). Another interesting observation was noted when the intergenic regions of the human genome were assessed. Interestingly, a subset of approx. 127,998 patterns, that were essentially approx. 22 nt in length, was discerned and termed "pykons" (Rigoutsos et al. 2006). Many of these pykons were overlapping genes involved in cell communication, transcription, regulation of transcription, and cell signaling (Rigoutsos et al. 2006). Overall, these data indicate that there may well be another layer of complexity that is operative in the genome of many organisms and supports a paradigm in which RNA is actively involved in the regulation of DNA. One cannot help but contemplate the concept that DNA and genomes are simply repositories of information actively being managed by RNA. Oddly enough, these RNAs are encoded from the DNA/genes that they are actively managing, a sort of chicken and egg scenario.

2 Conclusion

The observation in human cells that siRNAs, particularly the antisense strand alone, can direct TGS and that this event involves DNMT3a, histone methylation, and RNAPII strongly suggests that siRNAs can be used to specifically direct epigenetic modifications in human cells. Indeed, the modification of histone tails, such as via methylation, results in a "histone code." The "histone code" hypothesis argues that the local histone environment (specifically in the nucleosomes) can have an effect on the expression profile of the corresponding local gene (Jenuwein and Allis 2001). These "marked" histone tails are then capable of dictating the recruitment of various specialized chromatin remodeling factors (Strahl et al. 1999; Turner 2000). To date the histone code is best exemplified by the sheer multiplicity of modifications that can occur to histones (reviewed in Fuks et al. 2002). Interestingly, the fundamental underlying mechanism responsible for governing the histone code is not yet well understood. One potential mechanism for regulating the histone code could be mediated by siRNAs and in particular small antisense RNAs. Interestingly, the recent discovery and characterization of a vast array of small (21- to 26-nt) non-coding RNAs suggests that there is an RNA component, possibly involved in gene regulation, i.e., siRNA-mediated TGS, that is weaved into the basic fabric of the cell and has been to date overlooked (Katayama et al. 2005). While it is becoming apparent that RNAi goes beyond the confines of the cytoplasm, the observations with siRNA-mediated TGS are evocative of an antisense-related phenomenon that is deeply seeded in the fabric of the cell. Indeed, one day it may be possible to harness RNA to direct permanent epigenetic modifications resulting in superlative control of the human genome.

Acknowledgements I would like to thank Paula J. Olecki for graphical assistance and John J. Rossi for his comments, criticisms, and valued conversations on siRNA-mediated TGS. This work was supported by NIH HLB R01 HL83473 to K.V.M.

References

Bernstein E, Caudy AA, Hammond SM, Hannon GJ (2001) Role for a bidentate ribonuclease in the initiation step of RNA interference. Nature 409:363–366

Boeger H, Bushnell DA, Davis R, Griesenbeck J, Lorch Y, Strattan JS, Westover KD, Kornberg RD (2005) Structural basis of eukaryotic gene transcription. FEBS Lett 579:899–903

Bühler M, Mohn F, Stalder L, Mühlemann O (2005) Transcriptional silencing of nonsense codon-containing immunoglobulin minigenes. Mol Cell 18:307–317

Castanotto D, Tommasi S, Li M, Li H, Yanow S, Pfeifer GP, Rossi JJ (2005) Short hairpin RNA-directed cytosine (CpG) methylation of the RASSF1A gene promoter in HeLa cells. Mol Ther 12:179–183

Chicas A, Forrest EC, Sepich S, Cogoni C, Macino G (2005) Small interfering RNAs that trigger posttranscriptional gene silencing are not required for the histone H3 Lys9 methylation necessary for transgenic tandem repeat stabilization in Neurospora crassa. Mol Cell Biol 25:3793–3801

Dernburg AF, Zalevsky J, Colaiácovo MP, Villeneuve AM (2000) Transgene-mediated cosuppression in the C. elegans germ line. Genes Dev 14:1578–1583

Fagard M, Boutet S, Morel JB, Bellini C, Vaucheret H (2000) AGO1, QDE-2, and RDE-1 are related proteins required for post-transcriptional gene silencing in plants, quelling in fungi, and RNA interference in animals. Proc Natl Acad Sci U S A 97:11650–11654

Fuks F, Burgers WA, Brehm A, Hughes-Davies L, Kouzarides T (2000) DNA methyltransferase Dnmt1 associates with histone deacetylase activity. Nat Genet 24:88–91

Fuks F, Burgers WA, Godin N, Kasai M, Kouzarides T (2001) Dnmt3a binds deacetylases and is recruited by a sequence-specific repressor to silence transcription. EMBO J 20:2536–2544

Fuks F, Hurd PJ, Deplus R, Kouzarides T (2002) Histone modifications in transcriptional regulation. Curr Opin Genet Dev 12:142–148

Fuks F, Hurd PJ, Deplus R, Kouzarides T (2003) The DNA methyltransferases associate with HP1 and the SUV39H1 histone methyltransferase. Nucleic Acids Res 31:2305–2312

Grishok A, Pasquinelli AE, Conte D, Li N, Parrish S, Ha I, Baillie DL, Fire A, Ruvkun G, Mello CC (2001) Genes and mechanisms related to RNA interference regulate expression of the small temporal RNAs that control C. elegans developmental timing. Cell 106:23–34

Grishok A, Sinskey JL, Sharp PA (2005) Transcriptional silencing of a transgene by RNAi in the soma of C. elegans. Genes Dev 19:683–696

Hall IM, Shankaranarayana GD, Noma K, Ayoub N, Cohen A, Grewal SIS (2002) Establishment and maintenance of a heterochromatin domain. Science 297:2232–2237

Hamilton A, Voinnet O, Chappell L, Baulcombe D (2002) Two classes of short interfering RNA in RNA silencing. EMBO J 21:4671–4679

Irvine DV, Zaratiegui M, Tolia NH, Goto DB, Chitwood DH, Vaughn MW, Joshua-Tor L, Martienssen RA (2006) Argonaute slicing is required for heterochromatic silencing and spreading. Science 313:1134–1137

Janowski BA, Huffman KE, Schwartz JC, Ram R, Hardy D, Shames DS, Minna JD, Corey DR (2005) Inhibiting gene expression at transcription start sites in chromosomal DNA with antigene RNAs. Nat Chem Biol 1:210–215

Janowski BA, Huffman KE, Schwartz JC, Ram R, Nordsell R, Shames DS, Minna JD, Corey DR (2006) Involvement of AGO1 and AGO2 in mammalian transcriptional silencing. Nat Struct Mol Biol 13:787–792

Jeffery L, Nakielny S (2004) Components of the DNA methylation system of chromatin control are RNA-binding proteins. J Biol Chem 279:49479–49487

Jenuwein T, Allis CD (2001) The histone code. Science 293:1074–1080

Katayama S, Tomaru Y, Kasukawa T, Waki K, Nakanishi M, Nakamura M, Nishida H, Yap CC, Suzuki M, Kawai J, Suzuki H, Carninci P, Hayashizaki Y, Wells C, Frith M, Ravasi T, Pang KC, Hallinan J, Mattick J, Hume DA, Lipovich L, Batalov S, Engström PG, Mizuno Y, Faghihi MA, Sandelin A, Chalk AM, Mottagui-Tabar S, Liang Z, Lenhard B, Wahlestedt C, et al (2005) Antisense transcription in the mammalian transcriptome. Science 309:1564–1566

Kato H, Goto DB, Martienssen RA, Urano T, Furukawa K, Murakami Y (2005) RNA polymerase II is required for RNAi-dependent heterochromatin assembly. Science 309:467–469

Ketting RF, Plasterk RH (2000) A genetic link between co-suppression and RNA interference in C. elegans. Nature 404:296–298

Kim DH, Villeneuve LM, Morris KV, Rossi JJ (2006) Argonaute-1 directs siRNA-mediated transcriptional gene silencing in human cells. Nat Struct Mol Biol 13:793–797

Langlois MA, Boniface C, Wang G, Alluin J, Salvaterra PM, Puymirat J, Rossi JJ, Lee NS (2005) Cytoplasmic and nuclear retained DMPK mRNAs are targets for RNA interference in myotonic dystrophy cells. J Biol Chem 280:16949–16954

Lee Y, Hur I, Park SY, Kim YK, Suh MR, Kim VN (2006) The role of PACT in the RNA silencing pathway. EMBO J 25:522–532

Lippman Z, May B, Yordan C, Singer T, Martienssen R (2003) Distinct mechanisms determine transposon inheritance and methylation via small interfering RNA and histone modification. PLoS Biol 1:E67

Lippman Z, Gendrel AV, Black M, Vaughn MW, Dedhia N, McCombie WR, Lavine K, Mittal V, May B, Kasschau KD, Carrington JC, Doerge RW, Colot V, Martienssen R (2004) Role of transposable elements in heterochromatin and epigenetic control. Nature 430:471–476

Liu J, Carmell MA, Rivas FV, Marsden CG, Thomson JM, Song JJ, Hammond SM, Joshua-Tor L, Hannon GJ (2004) Argonaute2 Is the catalytic engine of mammalian RNAi. Science 305:1437–1441

Lusser A (2002) Acetylated, methylated, remodeled: chromatin states for gene regulation. Curr Opin Plant Biol 5:437–443

Maison C, Bailly D, Peters AH, Quivy JP, Roche D, Taddei A, Lachner M, Jenuwein T, Almouzni G (2002) Higher-order structure in pericentric heterochromatin involves a distinct pattern of histone modification and an RNA component. Nat Genet 30:329–334

Matzke MA, Birchler JA (2005) RNAi-mediated pathways in the nucleus. Nat Rev Genet 6:24–35

Matzke MA, Primig M, Trnovsky J, Matzke AJM (1989) Reversible methylation and inactivation of marker genes in sequentially transformed tobacco plants. EMBO J 8:643–649

Mette MF, Aufsatz W, Van der Winden J, Matzke AJM, Matzke MA (2000) Transcriptional silencing and promoter methylation triggered by double-stranded RNA. EMBO J 19:5194–5201

Morris KV (2005) siRNA-mediated transcriptional gene silencing: the potential mechanism and a possible role in the histone code. Cell Mol Life Sci 62:3057–3066

Morris KV (2006) Therapeutic potential of siRNA-mediated transcriptional gene silencing. Biotechniques [Suppl]:7–13

Morris KV, Chan SW, Jacobsen SE, Looney DJ (2004) Small interfering RNA-induced transcriptional gene silencing in human cells. Science 305:1289–1292

Motamedi MR, Verdel A, Colmenares SU, Gerber SA, Gygi SP, Moazed D (2004) Two RNAi complexes, RITS and RDRC, physically interact and localize to noncoding centromeric RNAs. Cell 119:789–802

Muchardt C, Guilleme M, Seeler JS, Trouche D, Dejean A, Yaniv M (2002) Coordinated methyl and RNA binding is required for heterochromatin localization of mammalian HP1alpha. EMBO Rep 3:975–981

Pal-Bhadra M, Bhadra U, Birchler JA (2002) RNAi related mechanisms affect both transcriptional and posttranscriptional transgene silencing in Drosophila. Mol Cell 9:315–327

Park CW, Chen Z, Kren BT, Steer CJ (2004) Double-stranded siRNA targeted to the huntingtin gene does not induce DNA methylation. Biochem Biophys Res Commun 323:275–280

Rigoutsos I, Huynh T, Miranda K, Tsirigos A, McHardy A, Platt D (2006) Short blocks from the noncoding parts of the human genome have instances within nearly all known genes and relate to biological processes. Proc Natl Acad Sci U S A 103:6605–6610

Robb GB, Brown KM, Khurana J, Rana TM (2005) Specific and potent RNAi in the nucleus of human cells. Nat Struct Mol Biol 12:133–137

Romano NG (1992) Macino, Quelling: transient inactivation of gene expression in Neurospora crassa by transformation with homologous sequences. Mol Microbiol 6:3343–3353

Ruby JG, Jan C, Player C, Axtell MJ, Lee W, Nusbaum C, Ge H, Bartel DP (2006) Large-scale sequencing reveals 21U-RNAs and additional microRNAs and endogenous siRNAs in C. Elegans. Cell 127:1193–1207

Sijen T, Vign I, Rebocho A, et al (2001) Transcriptional and posttranscriptional gene silencing are mechanistically related. Curr Biol 11:436–440

Song JJ, Smith SK, Hannon GJ, Joshua-Tor L (2004) Crystal structure of Argonaute and its implications for RISC slicer activity. Science 305:1434–1437

Strahl BD, Ohba R, Cook RG, Allis CD (1999) Methylation of histone H3 at lysine 4 is highly conserved and correlates with transcriptionally active nuclei in tetrahymena. Proc Natl Acad Sci U S A 96:14967–14972

Suzuki K, Shijuuku T, Fukamachi T, Zaunders J, Guillemin G, Cooper D, Kelleher A (2005) Prolonged transcriptional silencing and CpG methylation induced by siRNAs targeted to the HIV-1 promoter region. J RNAi Gene Silencing 1:66–78

Svoboda P, Stein P, Filipowicz W, Schultz RM (2004) Lack of homologous sequence-specific DNA methylation in response to stable dsRNA expression in mouse oocytes. Nucleic Acids Res 32:3601–3606

Tabara H, Sarkissian M, Kelly WG, Fleenor J, Grishok A, Timmons L, Fire A, Mello CC (1999) The rde-1 gene, RNA interference, and transposon silencing in C. elegans. Cell 99:123–132

Tijsterman M, Ketting RF, Plasterk RH (2002) The genetics of RNA silencing. Annu Rev Genet 36:489–519

Ting AH, Schuebel KE, Herman JG, Baylin SB (2005) Short double-stranded RNA induces transcriptional gene silencing in human cancer cells in the absence of DNA methylation. Nat Genet 37:906–910

Turner BM (2000) Histone acetylation and an epigenetic code. BioEssays 22:836–845

Vastenhouw NL, Brunschwig K, Okihara KL, Muller F, Tijsterman M, Plasterk RH (2006) Gene expression: long-term gene silencing by RNAi. Nature 442:882

Verdel A, Jia S, Gerber S, Sugiyama T, Gygi S, Grewal SI, Moazed D (2004) RNAi-mediated targeting of heterochromatin by the RITS complex. Science 303:672–676

Viré E, Brenner C, Deplus R, Blanchon L, Fraga M, Didelot C, Morey L, Van Eynde A, Bernard D, Vanderwinden JM, Bollen M, Esteller M, Di Croce L, de Launoit Y, Fuks F (2005) The Polycomb group protein EZH2 directly controls DNA methylation. Nature 439:871–874

Volpe TA, Kidner C, Hall IM, Teng G, Grewal SIS, Martienssen RA (2002) Regulation of heterochromatic silencing and histone H3 lysine-9 methylation by RNAi. Science 297:1833–1837

Wassenegger M, Graham MW, Wang MD (1994) RNA-directed de novo methylation of genomic sequences in plants. Cell 76:567–576

Weinberg MS, Villeneuve LM, Ehsani A, Amarzguioui M, Aagaard L, Chen Z, Riggs AD, Rossi JJ, Morris KV (2005) The antisense strand of small interfering RNAs directs histone methylation and transcriptional gene silencing in human cells. RNA 12:256–262

Zhang M, Ou H, Shen YH, Wang J, Wang J, Coselli J, Wang XL (2005) Regulation of endothelial nitric oxide synthase by small RNA. Proc Natl Acad Sci U S A 102:16967–16972

Zilberman D, Cao X, Jacobsen SE (2003) Argonaute4 control of locus-specific siRNA accumulation and DNA and histone methylation. Science 299:716–719

RNA Silencing in Mammalian Oocytes and Early Embryos

Petr Svoboda

Abstract RNA silencing is a common term for homology-dependent silencing phenomena found in the majority of eukaryotic species. RNA silencing pathways share several conserved components. The common denominator of these pathways is the presence of specific, short (21-25 nt) RNA molecules generated from different double-stranded RNA substrates by a specific RNase III activity. Short RNA molecules serve as a template for sequence-specific effects including transcriptional silencing, mRNA degradation, and inhibition of translation. This review will discuss possible roles of RNA silencing pathways in mouse oocytes and early embryos as well as the use of RNA silencing for experimental inhibition of gene expression in this model system.

Petr Svoboda
Institute of Molecular Genetics, Czech Academy of Sciences, Videnska 1083,
14220 Prague, Czech Republic
svobodap@img.cas.cz

P.J. Paddison and P.K. Vogt (eds.), *RNA Interference.*
Current Topics in Microbiology and Immunology 320.
© Springer-Verlag Berlin Heidelberg 2008

1 Introduction

Mammalian cells accommodate several pathways that respond to double-stranded RNA (dsRNA). These pathways include the interferon pathway, RNA editing by adenosine deaminases, and RNA silencing (Fig. 1). RNA silencing is a general term for a conserved group of pathways that induce sequence-specific gene silencing by mRNA degradation, translational repression, or transcriptional silencing. The common feature of RNA silencing pathways are *trans*-acting short RNA molecules generated from different dsRNA substrates by Dicer, an RNase III family member.

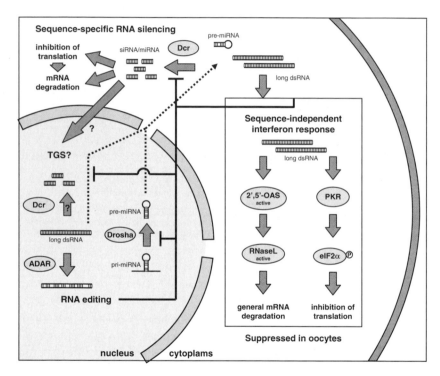

Fig. 1 Pathways responding to dsRNA in mammalian cells. In the sequence-independent interferon response, dsRNA activates protein kinase R (PKR) that catalyzes phosphorylation of translation initiation factor eIF2α, which in turn inhibits translation. PKR is also involved in interferon induction (through NF-κB). Interferon and dsRNA also activate 2′,5′-oligoadenylate synthetase (2′,5′-OAS) that produces 2′,5′ oligoadenylates that subsequently induce activation of RNase L that is responsible for general RNA degradation. Both PKR and 2′, 5′-OAS are essential for the apoptotic response to dsRNA. The sequence-specific RNA silencing is triggered either by long dsRNA or by specific short hairpin microRNA (miRNA) precursors. Processing of primary miRNA transcripts by Drosha occurs in the nucleus, pre-miRNA and long dsRNA substrates are subsequently processed into short RNAs by cytoplasmic Dicer. Short RNAs then guide translational inhibition and/or mRNA degradation. Data on the nuclear role of mammalian Dicer are inconclusive. DsRNA can be also recognized and processed by ADAR (adenosine deaminases that act on RNA), resulting in inhibitory effects on Drosha and Dicer processing as well as prevention of induction of the interferon response

The main goal of this review is to provide a comprehensive picture of RNA silencing in mammalian oocytes and early embryos. The first part provides an introduction to dsRNA-induced pathways in mammals and highlights features of these pathways in oocytes and early embryos. It also covers possible natural roles of RNA silencing. The second part reviews the use of RNA silencing to experimentally inhibit gene expression in order to study gene function in oocytes and early embryos. In addition, interferon response and RNA editing pathways can antagonize, modulate, or mask sequence-specific effects of RNA silencing. Therefore, these two pathways are also briefly discussed.

2 Mechanisms of RNA Silencing

Posttranscriptional RNA silencing pathways, RNA interference (RNAi), and microRNA (miRNA) pathways regulate gene expression by inducing degradation and/or translational repression of target mRNAs. These pathways are initiated by different forms of dsRNA that are processed by Dicer, an RNase III endonuclease, into 21- to 22-nucleotide-long RNA molecules that serve as sequence-specific guides for silencing (reviewed in Sontheimer and Carthew 2005; Zamore and Haley 2005).

2.1 Production of Short RNAs in RNAi and miRNA Pathways

RNAi is induced by a long dsRNA that is cut by Dicer into numerous short interfering RNAs (siRNA), which in turn guide recognition and degradation of base-pairing mRNAs. In invertebrates, such as *Caenorhabditis* and *Drosophila*, RNAi functions as a defense mechanism against viruses and parasitic sequences in the genome (reviewed in Buchon and Vaury 2006; Saumet and Lecellier 2006). RNAi also operates in mammalian cells but its role is not known. In most mammalian cells, long dsRNA triggers the interferon pathway, resulting in a global inhibition of protein synthesis and RNA degradation (reviewed in Wang and Carmichael 2004). However, in mammalian oocytes, early embryos, and a few other cell types, experimental delivery of long dsRNA specifically induces RNAi (Billy et al. 2001; Gan et al. 2002; Svoboda et al. 2000; Wianny and Zernicka-Goetz 2000; Yang et al. 2001).

The vast majority of mammalian Dicer-generated short RNAs found in a cell are miRNAs (Cummins et al. 2006; Mineno et al. 2006). Cloning data provide evidence for hundreds of miRNAs in mammals (Griffiths-Jones et al. 2006). A miRNA originates from a stem-loop structure in a primary endogenous transcripts (pri-miRNA). The stem loop is released as a pre-miRNA after cleavage of pri-miRNA by Drosha, a nuclear RNase III. The pre-miRNA is transported to the cytoplasm where it is processed by the Dicer-containing complex into a short RNA duplex composed of a miRNA and a passenger strand. Mammals have only one Dicer protein producing siRNAs and miRNAs (reviewed in Kim 2005).

The major difference between mammalian RNAi and miRNA pathways is the origin of Dicer products. Both pathways are closely related and, as will be discussed later, the type of posttranscriptional silencing effect depends more on the sequence homology with a cognate mRNA than on the origin of the short RNA. Mammalian RNAi and miRNA pathways can be viewed almost as a single biochemical pathway in which short RNAs of different origins target homologous RNAs through similar, if not identical, effector complexes. However, it should be kept in mind that both pathways have different roles and occasionally (for example in *Drosophila*) have genetically diverged from each other (Lee et al. 2004).

2.2 Effector Complexes in RNAi and miRNA Pathways

Short RNAs produced by Dicer are subsequently incorporated into effector complexes. Dicer interacts with the TRBP (human immunodeficiency virus TAR RNA binding protein), which facilitates loading of short RNAs onto an Argonaute (Ago)-containing effector ribonucleoprotein (RNP) complex, referred to as miRNP or RISC (RNA-induced silencing complex) (Chendrimada et al. 2005; Haase et al. 2005). TRBP has several roles including translational regulation during spermatogenesis (Lee et al. 1996; Zhong et al. 1999) and inhibition of protein kinase R (PKR) (Park et al. 1994), a dsRNA-dependent protein kinase, which is a central player in the interferon response. It has been reported that a robust PKR response correlates with lower levels of TRBP and vice versa (Ong et al. 2005), suggesting that TRBP may also control the balance between RNA silencing and sequence-independent response to dsRNA.

The RISC complex is loaded with a single-stranded short RNA that guides recognition of target mRNAs. The passenger strand is removed and degraded (Matranga et al. 2005). The key components of the RISC are Ago proteins. The mammalian Ago protein family consists of eight members, four of which are ubiquitously expressed (Ago subfamily) while the remaining four (Piwi subfamily) are expressed in germ cells (Hall 2005). All four mammalian Ago proteins, Ago1 through Ago4, associate with miRNAs and are implicated in translational repression (Liu et al. 2004; Meister et al. 2004; Pillai et al. 2004). However, only Ago2 specifically cleaves an mRNA in the middle of the sequence that base-pairs with a short RNA (Liu et al. 2004; Meister et al. 2004; Song et al. 2004).

Whether a short RNA will cause mRNA cleavage via the RNAi mechanism or will act as a miRNA-inducing translational repression depends on the degree of complementarity between the short RNA and mRNA. The Ago2-mediated endonucleolytic cleavage requires formation of a perfect or nearly perfect siRNA-mRNA duplex, while imperfect base-pairing generally results in translational repression (reviewed in Sontheimer 2005). The predicted hybrids between animal miRNAs and their cognate mRNAs typically contain bulges and mismatches and result in translational repression. On the other hand, the extensive pairing of mir-196 with HoxB8 mRNA results in the mRNA cleavage by the RNAi mechanism (Yekta et al. 2004).

Importantly, miRNAs can induce substantial mRNA degradation even in the absence of extensive base-paring to their targets (Bagga et al. 2005; Lim et al. 2005). Repressed mRNAs, miRNAs, and Ago proteins localize to discrete cytoplasmic foci known as P-bodies, likely as a consequence of translational repression (Liu et al. 2005b; Pillai et al. 2005). P-bodies contain mRNA degrading enzymes and it is conceivable that the observed degradation of some miRNA targets is a consequence of their relocation to these structures (reviewed in Anderson and Kedersha 2006; Newbury et al. 2006; Valencia-Sanchez et al. 2006).

2.3 Sequence-Specific Transcriptional Silencing

The RNAi pathway or its components have been linked to transcriptional silencing and heterochromatin formation in fungi, plants, and animals (reviewed in Bayne and Allshire 2005; Matzke and Birchler 2005; Verdel and Moazed 2005). Transcriptional silencing mediated by siRNAs has also been documented in mammalian cells (Morris et al. 2004; Ting et al. 2005). A primary silencing mechanism involves changes in the chromatin structure but not DNA methylation (Ting et al. 2005). The absence of sequence-specific DNA methylation has also been observed in mouse oocytes that show an RNAi effect upon dsRNA expression during oocyte growth (Svoboda et al. 2004b). The natural role of sequence-specific transcriptional silencing is largely unknown. It is likely that regulation of heterochromatin by short RNAs plays a role at specific loci, such as centromeres, as described in embryonic stem (ES) cells lacking Dicer (Kanellopoulou et al. 2005). At the same time, it is unlikely that this mechanism extensively controls expression of protein-coding genes as suggested by the absence of promoter-derived siRNAs in miRNA cloning experiments (Mineno et al. 2006).

3 Other dsRNA-Responding Pathways

3.1 Interferon Pathway

The interferon pathway is the most ubiquitous sequence-independent pathway induced by dsRNA in mammalian cells (reviewed in de Veer et al. 2005). It has been known for over 30 years that an exposure of mammalian cells to dsRNA triggers a global, sequence-independent repression of protein synthesis (Hunter et al. 1975). Exposure of mammalian cells to dsRNA activates PKR that blocks translation by phosphorylating translation initiation factor eIF2α. PKR is also involved in the regulation of nuclear factor (NF)-κB, which plays a key role in interferon induction. Interferon and dsRNA activate 2′,5′-oligoadenylate synthetase (2′,5′-OAS) that produces 2′,5′ oligoadenylates with 5′-terminal triphosphate residues that subsequently induce activation of RNase L; a protein responsible for general RNA degradation (Fig. 1, reviewed in Barber 2001). When RNAi was first discovered in *Caenorhabditis elegans* in 1998 (Fire et al. 1998), the interferon response to dsRNA was a cause of skepticism about the conservation of RNA silencing in mammals. The current view is that some types of RNA-silencing substrates (exogenous dsRNA substrates of different lengths and structures delivered to cells to experimentally silence a gene) can trigger the interferon pathway (reviewed in de Veer et al. 2005). However, there are mammalian cell types, such as oocytes and cells of early embryos, that are refractory to the interferon induction and do not exhibit any sequence-independent dsRNA response (Billy et al. 2001; Stein et al. 2005; Svoboda et al. 2000; Wianny and Zernicka-Goetz 2000; Yang et al. 2001). It should be also noted that experiments documenting that dsRNA induces PKR response are typically based on exposure of cells or lysates to an exogenous dsRNA. The evidence for PKR activation by dsRNA expression is inconclusive. Some reports demonstrate sequence-independent effects such as nonspecific reduction of reporter expression (Yang et al. 2001) or activation of interferon-stimulated genes with certain plasmids expressing short hairpin RNA (shRNA) (Bridge et al. 2003). On the other hand, dsRNA has been detected in somatic cells on several occasions (Kim and Wold 1985; Kramerov et al. 1985; Okano et al. 1991; Schmitt et al. 1986) and dsRNA expressed in NIH 3T3 cells induced a specific knockdown (Wang et al. 2003) while apoptosis mediated by the PKR/interferon response to exogenous dsRNA in NIH 3T3 cells is well documented (McMillan et al. 1995; Srivastava et al. 1998).

PKR and 2′,5′-OAS pathways seem to be suppressed in mouse oocytes as expression levels of PKR proteins and mRNAs of active 2′,5′-OAS isoforms of are low while mRNA levels of inactive 2′,5′-OAS isoforms are enhanced (Stein et al. 2005). These data are in perfect agreement with the Genome Institute of Norvartis Research Foundation (GNF) Symatlas data (Su et al. 2002) for mRNA expression of PKR and 2′,5′-OAS pathway components in oocytes, zygotes, and blastocysts (Fig. 2). Transcript levels of numerous genes inhibiting the PKR and 2′,5′-OAS pathway (Pkrir, Oas1c, Oas1d, Oas1e, and Oas1h) are greatly enhanced in oocytes and zygotes. In fact, inhibitory OAS1 isoforms are among the most abundant transcripts in mouse oocytes. The role (if any) that the suppression of the interferon pathway plays in the oocyte is unclear.

3.2   Adenosine Deamination

The second pathway responding to dsRNA is RNA editing by "adenosine deaminases that act on RNA" (ADAR). ADARs are metazoan RNA editing enzymes that convert adenosine to inosine (which is recognized as guanosine) in double-stranded regions of RNA molecules. RNA editing has been implicated in alternative splicing, RNA stability, codon change, and other processes (reviewed in Bass 2002; Maas et al. 2003). RNA editing by ADARs appears important but nonessential in

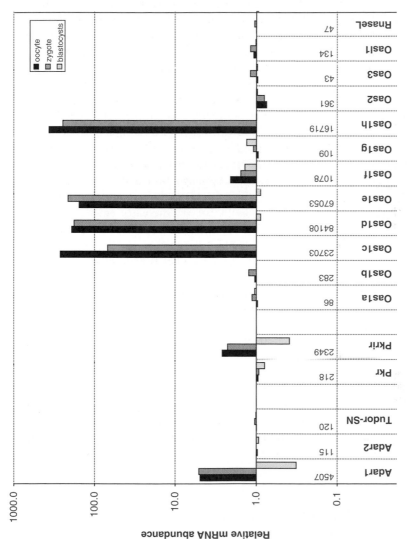

Fig. 2 Relative mRNA expression levels of genes involved in RNA silencing and associated with P-bodies (Anderson and Kedersha 2006). Data were extracted from the gcRMA mouse set in the GNF Symatlas database (Su et al. 2002). Expression levels for oocytes, zygotes, and blastocysts are shown relative to the median expression in 61 mouse tissues, which was set to one. *Numbers below oocyte columns* correspond to raw expression values in oocytes and provide an estimate for mRNA abundance in the oocyte. Intensity values from a chip image are scaled to 200, a number approximately corresponding to average expression in the sample (Su et al. 2002). Values around 50 indicate low abundant transcripts, while values in thousands indicate highly abundant ones. Data for murine Ago1 are not available in the GNF database

Drosophila or *Caenorhabditis*, where strains lacking ADAR activity exhibit behavioral defects (Palladino et al. 2000; Tonkin et al. 2002). Mice lacking ADAR die embryonically (*adar1*$^{-/-}$) or shortly after birth (*adar2*$^{-/-}$) (Higuchi et al. 2000; Wang et al. 2000).

RNA silencing and RNA editing can operate on the same or similar substrates. Several ADAR substrates in *Caenorhabditis* form long hairpin structures in their 3′-untranslated regions (UTRs) (Morse and Bass 1999; Morse et al. 2002). A mammalian ADAR substrate harboring a longer inverted repeat has been also described (Prasanth et al. 2005). The mouse cationic amino acid transporter 2 (mCat2)-transcribed nuclear RNA (CTN-RNA), an alternative product of mCat2, contains an approximately 100-bp stem-loop structure, which is edited but does not induce RNAi (Prasanth et al. 2005). Furthermore, a systematic study of ADAR substrates in mammals (which indirectly provides insight into dsRNA expression in mammals) revealed that the vast majority of editing sites occurs in Alu (92%) sequences (Levanon et al. 2005), where editing typically targets intramolecular duplexes (Athanasiadis et al. 2004). Interestingly, transgenic RNAi in the oocyte is based on a transcript carrying a long dsRNA hairpin (>500 bp) in the 3′-UTR (Stein et al. 2003b). It is not known whether this transcript is targeted by ADARs in the oocyte. In any case, it efficiently enters the RNAi pathway as documented by successful transgenic RNAi experiments in the mouse oocyte (Table 1).

Hyperediting by ADARs can antagonize RNAi. Chemotaxis defects in ADAR-deficient *Caenorhabditis* can be rescued by mutations in the RNAi pathway (Tonkin and Bass 2003). However, ADARs do not always prevent RNAi as shown by RNAi effects in worms expressing long RNA hairpins from a transgene (Tavernarakis et al. 2000). RNA silencing and editing pathways also intersect in mammals. While RNAi and ADAR pathways have antagonistic relationship, they share Tudor staphylococcal nuclease (Tudor-SN). Tudor-SN has been described as a component of unknown function in the RISC complex in *Drosophila*, *Caenorhabditis*, and mammals (Caudy et al. 2003) while it also specifically interacts with and promotes the cleavage of hyperedited dsRNAs (Scadden 2005). Hyperediting of short hairpins of specific miRNA precursors leads to inhibition of the Drosha-mediated cleavage and subsequent degradation of hyperedited pri-miRNA (presumably by Tudor-SN) (Yang et al. 2006). Mature edited miRNAs were also detected (Blow et al. 2006), which could result in a broader range of targets for individual miRNAs. Mammalian ADAR1 RNA also limits siRNA efficacy (Yang et al. 2005). Therefore, it is somewhat counterintuitive that murine ADAR1 mRNA is five times more abundant in the oocyte than in other tissues (Fig. 2). This raises a question of whether ADAR1 antagonizes the endogenous RNAi or miRNA pathways. One hypothesis could be that if miRNAs play a role in removal of maternal mRNAs, miRNA editing could facilitate maternal mRNA clearance by increasing the number of targeted mRNAs. An alternative hypothesis would be that maternal miRNAs themselves need to be degraded and RNA editing is employed in this process.

Table 1 RNAi experiments in mammalian oocytes and early embryos

Gene	Stage	RNAi inducer	Delivery method	RNAi effect	Reference(s)
Mos	Mouse oocyte	dsRNA lhRNA	Microinj. transgene	Null phenotype, parthenogenetic activation of MII eggs	Stein et al. 2003b; Svoboda et al. 2000; Wianny and Zernicka-Goetz 2000
Msy2	Mouse oocyte	dsRNA lhRNA	Micro-inj. transgene	Pleiotropic effect, defects in protein synthesis, abnormal oocytes	Yu et al. 2004
Bnc (basonuclin)	Mouse oocyte	dsRNA lhRNA	Microinj. transgene	Pleiotropic maternal effect phenotype, morphological abnormalities in the oocyte, perturbation of polI and polII transcription, no development beyond two-cell stage	Ma et al. 2006
Wee1b	Mouse oocyte	lhRNA	Microinj. transgene	Relief of meiotic arrest (GVBD induction) in 25% of oocytes	Han et al. 2005
Ctcf	Mouse oocyte	lhRNA	Transgene	Aberrant methylation of H19 imprinting locus	Fedoriw et al. 2004
Fgfr2	Mouse early embryo	shRNA	Transgene	LoxP activated shRNA expression in the germline, embryonic lethal, knockdown was Fgfr2 specific.	Coumoul et al. 2005
Bmp4	Mouse blastocyst	dsRNA	E-poration	70% mRNA reduction at E5.25, range of phenotypes characteristic of Bmp4 null	Soares et al. 2005
Dvl1, Dvl2, Dvl3	Mouse 8-cell, blastocyst	dsRNA	E-poration	Retarded development, morphological abnormalities in simultaneous knockdown of all three genes, 40% did not gastrulate	Soares et al. 2005
Cyclin B1	Rat oocyte	dsRNA	Transfection	No MAPK activation, absence of Mos mRNA polyadenylation	Lazar et al. 2004
Plat (tPA)	Mouse oocyte	dsRNA	Microinj.	95% reduction of PLAT activity	Svoboda et al. 2000
Egfp	Mouse oocyte, zygote	dsRNA	Microinj.	Loss of fluorescence	Svoboda et al. 2004a; Wianny and Zernicka-Goetz 2000
Cdh1 (E-cadherin)	Mouse zygote	dsRNA	Microinj.	70% null phenotype, defect in cavitation	Wianny and Zernicka-Goetz 2000
Itpr1 (IP3R-1)	Mouse oocyte	dsRNA	Microinj.	>90% mRNA reduction, Ca^{2+} oscillations affected	Xu et al. 2003

(continued)

Table 1 (continued)

Gene	Stage	RNAi inducer	Delivery method	RNAi effect	Reference(s)
Doc1r	Mouse oocyte	dsRNA	Microinj.	Aberrant MII spindle	Terret et al. 2003
Miss	Mouse oocyte	dsRNA	Microinj.	Aberrant MII spindle	Lefebvre et al. 2002
Dicer1	Mouse zygote	dsRNA siRNA	Microinj.	>90% mRNA reduction, 60%–90% of RNAi inhibited, increased retrotransposon mRNA	Svoboda et al. 2004a
Atrx	Mouse oocyte	dsRNA siRNA pool	Microinj.	Aberrant alignment of chromosomes on the metaphase II spindle	De La Fuente et al. 2004
Cdc6	Mouse oocyte	dsRNA	Microinj.	Aberrant spindle formation	Anger et al. 2005
Gdf9	Mouse oocyte	dsRNA	Microinj.	Negative effect on cumulus expansion	Gui and Joyce 2005
Bmp15	Mouse oocyte	dsRNA	Microinj.	mRNA knockdown was efficient, used as a control for Gdf9, no phenotype reported	Gui and Joyce 2005
MT-like (Mti7)	Mouse oocyte, zygote	dsRNA	Microinj.	Oocyte microinjection: 43%–53% GV arrest, early PN microinjection: 93% 1-cell arrest, late PN microinjection: 77% 2-cell arrest	Park et al. 2004
Emi1	Mouse oocyte	dsRNA	Microinj.	Morphological defects, large polar bodies, abnormal spindles	Paronetto et al. 2004
hMad2	Human oocyte	dsRNA	Microinj.	85%–92% protein reduction, relief of meiotic arrest (GVBD induction)	Homer et al. 2005
Oct4	Bovine zygote	dsRNA	Microinj.	72% mRNA reduction, reduced number of cells in the ICM	Nganvongpanit et al. 2006
Par3	Mouse 4-cell	dsRNA	Microinj.	Knockdown directed the microinjected blastomere to the inside of the embryo	Plusa et al. 2005
Cdx2	Mouse 2-cell	siRNA	Microinj.	Knock-down in the lagging blastomere caused a failure of trophectoderm formation	Deb et al. 2006
Cox5a, Cox5b, Cox6b1	Mouse zygote	siRNA	Microinj.	Disrupted mitochondrial distribution, increased apoptosis, and lower cell count in blastocysts	Cui et al. 2006
Gpr3	Mouse oocyte	siRNA	Microinj.	Relief of meiotic arrest (GVBD induction) in 73% of oocytes	Mehlmann 2005

dsRNA, long dsRNA; e-poration, electroporation; GV, germinal vesicle; GVBD, GV breakdown; lhRNA, long hairpin RNA, microinj., microinjection; siRNa, shot interfering RNA; PN, pronucleus; ICM, inner cell mass; MII, metaphase II

4 RNA Silencing in Mouse Oocytes and Early Embryos

Mouse oocytes and early embryos were the first mammalian tissues where RNAi was documented (Svoboda et al. 2000; Wianny and Zernicka-Goetz 2000). Features of mammalian RNAi discovered in mouse oocytes include the ability to target untranslated mRNAs (Svoboda et al. 2000; Wianny and Zernicka-Goetz 2000) and the lack of RNA-dependent RNA polymerase (Stein et al. 2003a), which is thought to serve as an amplifier of RNAi in several other species (Sijen et al. 2001). A specific feature of mouse oocytes and early embryos is the apparent absence of interferon response to long dsRNA. Consequently, oocytes and early embryos are the only mammalian cells where long dsRNA is routinely used to trigger RNAi.

Interestingly, GNF Symatlas microarray data (Su et al. 2002) show that mouse oocytes express enhanced levels of Dicer, TRBP2, and several P-body components, but specific miRNA pathway components are not overrepresented (Fig. 3). Dicer mRNA is highly abundant in the oocyte and the relative amount of Dicer mRNA in the oocyte is the highest among all tissues in the GNF dataset (Su et al. 2002). Immunofluorescence and RT-PCR also showed high expression of Dicer in mouse oocytes (M. Drozdz, P. Svoboda, and T. Zoller, unpublished data). Interestingly, Dicer mRNA is also strongly expressed in zebrafish oocytes (Wienholds et al. 2003). Why Dicer expression in mouse oocytes is so high remains a puzzle.

Ago expression seems to be either low (Ago3 and -4) or underrepresented in the mouse oocyte (Ago2). Similarly, mRNA level of GW182, a component of P-bodies required for miRNA-mediated silencing (Jakymiw et al. 2005; Liu et al. 2005a; Rehwinkel et al. 2005), is not different from other tissues. However, mRNAs of several other P-body components are strongly overrepresented. Enhanced mRNA levels of P-body components in the oocyte, thus, seem likely related to an extensive mRNA turnover during maturation and fertilization (Bachvarova et al. 1985) rather than to a higher activity of the miRNA pathway.

The following two sections will discuss the roles of RNA silencing pathways during early mammalian development and the possible biological implications of the domination of an RNAi response to long dsRNA over the interferon pathway.

4.1 *miRNAs Regulating Early Development?*

Direct cloning of miRNAs from mouse oocytes identified a small set of miRNAs (let-7a, -b, -c, -i, miR-20b, miR-320, miR-503) (Watanabe et al. 2006). However, direct cloning of miRNAs is difficult because of the limited amount of obtainable material. Therefore, two other groups opted for analyzing expression of already known miRNAs by RT-PCR-based methods (Murchison et al. 2007; Tang et al. 2007). These data indicate that oocytes (and early embryos) express tens of different miRNAs (Table 2). Cloning experiments from the zebrafish and the *Xenopus* suggest that there are no conserved, abundant, oocyte-specific miRNAs in vertebrates, and miRNAs found in the oocytes are typically found in embryos and tissues

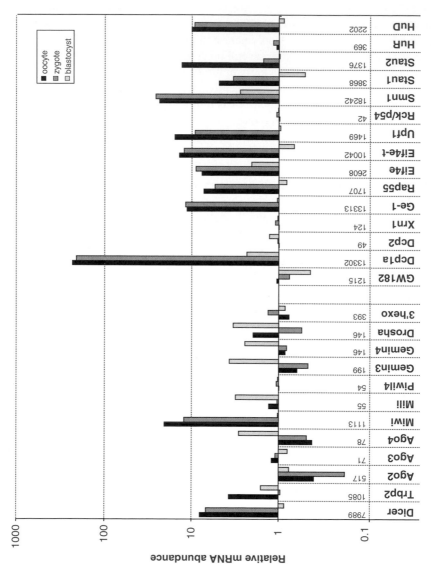

Fig. 3 Relative mRNA expression levels of genes involved in adenosine deamination, PKR, and 2′,5′-OAS pathways. Data were extracted from the gcRMA mouse set in the GNF Symatlas database (Su et al. 2002). Expression levels for oocytes, zygotes, and blastocysts are shown relative to the median expression in 61 mouse tissues, which was set to one. *Numbers below oocyte columns* correspond to raw expression values in oocytes

Table 2 The most abundant miRNAs found in mouse oocytes. Forty microRNAs showing the highest expression in the oocyte (Tang et al. 2007) are listed. Due to different methods used to estimate miRNA expression level, expression for each report was arbitrarily ranked with asterisks[a,b]

miRNA	Accession	Sequence	Expression Murchison et al. 2007[a]	Tang et al. 2007[b]
mmu-let-7a	MIMAT0000521	UGAGGUAGUAGGUUGUAUAGU	**	***
mmu-let-7b	MIMAT0000522	UGAGGUAGUAGGUUGUGUGGUU		**
mmu-let-7c	MIMAT0000523	UGAGGUAGUAGGUUGUAUGGUU		**
mmu-let-7d	MIMAT0000383	AGAGGUAGUAGGUUGCAUAGU	**	***
mmu-let-7d*	MIMAT0000384	CUAUACGACCUGCUGCCUUUCU		*
mmu-let-7e	MIMAT0000524	UGAGGUAGGAGGUUGUAUAGU		***
mmu-let-7f	MIMAT0000525	UGAGGUAGUAGAUUGUAUAGU		***
mmu-let-7g	MIMAT0000121	UGAGGUAGUAGUUUGUACAGU	*	**
mmu-let-7i	MIMAT0000122	UGAGGUAGUAGUUUGUGCUGU		*
mmu-miR-15b	MIMAT0000124	UAGCAGCACAUCAUGGUUUACA	**	*
mmu-miR-16	MIMAT0000527	UAGCAGCACGUAAAAUAUUGGCG	***	*
mmu-miR-17–5p	MIMAT0000649	CAAAGUGCUUACAGUGCAGGUAGU	*	**
mmu-miR-18	MIMAT0000528	UAAGGUGCAUCUAGUGCAGAUA		**
mmu-miR-19a	MIMAT0000651	UGUGCAAAUCUAUGCAAAACUGA	**	***
mmu-miR-19b	MIMAT0000513	UGUGCAAAUCCAUGCAAAACUGA		***
mmu-miR-20a	MIMAT0000529	UAAAGUGCUUAUAGUGCAGGUAG		***
mmu-miR-24	MIMAT0000219	UGGCUCAGUUCAGCAGGAACAG		***
mmu-miR-25	MIMAT0000652	CAUUGCACUUGUCUCGGUCUGA		***
mmu-miR-26a	MIMAT0000533	UUCAAGUAAUCCAGGAUAGGC	**	*
mmu-miR-30a–5p	MIMAT0000128	UGUAAACAUCCUCGACUGGAAG		**
mmu-miR-30b	MIMAT0000130	UGUAAACAUCCUACACUCAGCU	***	**
mmu-miR-30c	MIMAT0000514	UGUAAACAUCCUACACUCUCAGC	***	***
mmu-miR-30d	MIMAT0000515	UGUAAACAUCCCGACUGGAAG	*	*
mmu-miR-92	MIMAT0000539	UAUUGCACUUGUCCCGGCCUG		***
mmu-miR-93	MIMAT0000540	CAAAGUGCUGUUCGUGCAGGUAG		**
mmu-miR-98	MIMAT0000545	UGAGGUAGUAAGUUGUAUUGUU		**
mmu-miR-103	MIMAT0000546	AGCAGCAUUGUACAGGGCUAUGA	**	**

(continued)

P. Svoboda

Table 2 (continued)

miRNA	Accession	Sequence	Expression Murchison et al. 2007[a]	Tang et al. 2007[b]
mmu-miR–106a	MIMAT0000385	CAAAGUGCUAACAGUGCAGGUA		***
mmu-miR–106b	MIMAT0000386	UAAAGUGCUGACAGUGCAGAU		*
mmu-miR–107	MIMAT0000647	AGCAGCAUUGUACAGGGCUAUCA		*
mmu-miR–141	MIMAT0000153	UAACACUGUCUGGUAAAGAUGG	*	*
mmu-miR–182	MIMAT0000211	UUUGGCAAUGGUAGAACUCACA	*	*
mmu-miR–191	MIMAT0000221	CAACGGAAUCCAAAAGCAGCU		*
mmu-miR–200c	MIMAT0000657	UAAUACUGCCGGGUAAUGAUGG	*	**
mmu-miR–222	MIMAT0000670	AGCUACAUCUGGCUACUGGGUCUC	*	*
mmu-miR–292–3p	MIMAT0000370	AAGUGCCGCCAGGUUUUGAGUGU		**
mmu-miR–294	MIMAT0000372	AAAGUGCUUCCCUUUUGUGUGU		*
mmu-miR–296	MIMAT0000374	AGGGCCCCCCUCAAUCCUGU	*	**
mmu-miR–320	MIMAT0000666	AAAAGCUGGGUUGAGAGGGCGAA	*	*
mmu-miR–342	MIMAT0000590	UCUCACACAGAAAUCGCACCCGUC	*	**

[a]miRNAs detected by Murchison et al. (2007) with the Z-score below 1.0 were ranked: *, between 1.0 and 2.0 were ranked **, and above 2.0 were ranked ***. Again, miRNAs ranked *** represent approximately 10% of 30 maternal miRNAs detected (Murchison et al. 2007)

[b]miRNAs detected by Tang et al. (2007) with raw expression values below 100,000 were ranked: *, between 100,000 and 500,000 were ranked **, and above 500,000 were ranked ***. miRNAs ranked *** represent approximately 10% of all 101 maternal miRNAs detected

(Watanabe et al. 2005; Wienholds et al. 2005). Thus, it is likely that miRNAs found in the mouse oocyte-so far-represent a relatively comprehensive set of maternal miRNAs.

Is there a specific role for the miRNA pathway in the oocyte? Although maternal miRNAs are found in other tissues, the loss of Dicer in the oocyte leads to a unique phenotype as Dicer$^{-/-}$ oocytes show defects in spindle formation during meiotic maturation (Murchison et al. 2007; Tang et al. 2007). Numerous transcripts associated with spindle regulation are upregulated in Dicer$^{-/-}$ oocytes and are potential targets for miRNAs detected in the oocyte (Murchison et al. 2007). This result demonstrates that specific roles of the miRNA pathway are given by the combination of miRNAs and their targets and cannot be elucidated just from the set of miRNAs found in a specific cell type.

Is the miRNA pathway also involved in deadenylation and clearance of maternal mRNAs, as has been demonstrated for the miR-430 family in the zebrafish embryo (Giraldez et al. 2006)? Not exactly. There are differences suggesting that the miR-430 family in the zebrafish has adopted a more specialized role compared to its counterparts in mammals.

The miR-430 family is related to several mammalian miRNA families: miR-302, miR-290/372, and miR-17/20/106 (Giraldez et al. 2005). Some of these miRNAs were cloned from murine and human ES cells, which originate from the inner part of the blastocysts (Houbaviy et al. 2003; Suh et al. 2004). In addition, the murine miR-290 family was also found to be highly expressed during preimplantation development (Tang et al. 2007). However, mammalian early development is different from that of the zebrafish and it is unclear if it would require a similar mechanism for removing maternal mRNAs.

The zebrafish development occurs at much faster rate: the zygotic transcription in the zebrafish starts soon after fertilization, the blastocyst stage is reached within several hours, and the embryo is already undergoing segmentation 12 h after fertilization (Kimmel et al. 1995). Zygotic expression of miR-430 is detected 2.5 h after fertilization, at the 256-cell stage, and the subsequent miR-430-driven clearance of maternal transcripts occurs within a few hours (Giraldez et al. 2006). In contrast, a 12 h-old mouse embryo is completing the one-cell stage while the zygotic genome is still silent (reviewed in Schultz 2002). The blastocyst stage is reached within approximately 3.5 days after fertilization (4 h in the zebrafish).

The miR-430 cluster expression is zygotic, not maternal. The zygotic transcription in the zebrafish starts shortly after fertilization while the zygote still contains a high amount of maternal mRNA. In contrast, by the time zygotic transcription is activated in the two-cell mouse embryo, maternal transcripts are already extensively degraded (Bachvarova et al. 1985; Paynton et al. 1988; Schultz 2002). Degradation of maternal mRNAs in the mouse occurs in a step-wise manner, involving induction of degradation by meiotic maturation, fertilization, or both (Alizadeh et al. 2005; Oh et al. 2000; Sakurai et al. 2005), prior to the zygotic genome activation. Since the transition between the maternal and zygotic phases of gene expression is slow in mammals, the pressure to precisely synchronize gene expression in a short time window is not that strong. Therefore, the mouse embryo may not need the miRNA pathway for a rapid, extensive clearance of maternal miRNAs. Zygotic miRNAs, such as the miR-290-295 cluster, may be needed to lower expression of some genes highly expressed in the oocyte, but such function would be different from removing maternal transcripts.

Transition between the oocyte and the two-cell embryo with activated zygotic genome (oocyte-to-zygote transition) occurs without transcription. Thus, any process affecting mRNA stability, such as the miRNA pathway, will contribute to maternal mRNA degradation. However, while maternal miRNAs potentially target hundreds of genes (Murchison et al. 2007; Tang et al. 2007), they likely have only a limited role in direct mRNA degradation during the oocyte-to-zygote transition. Motif analysis of 3′-UTRs from Dicer$^{-/-}$ oocytes (Murchison et al. 2007) indicates that the most enriched motifs associated with destabilization of maternal mRNAs do not represent complements of miRNA seeding regions. The most enriched motifs found in degraded maternal mRNAs are AU-rich, while putative miRNA binding sites show several orders of magnitude lower scores (Murchison et al. 2007). In addition, microarray data related to mRNA stability during oocyte-to-zygote transition indicate that transcripts whose downregulation is a function of time (many of which are presumably candidates for miRNA targets in the oocyte) do not overlap with transcripts downregulated upon resumption of meiosis and fertilization (Puschendorf et al. 2006; Zeng et al. 2004; Zeng and Schultz 2005). Thus, maternal miRNAs contribute to maternal mRNA degradation to some extent, but the bulk of maternal mRNAs is degraded by another mechanism(s).

4.2   Silencing of Mobile Elements and Viruses by RNAi in Mammals?

It has been mentioned previously that, unlike most mammalian cells, oocytes and early embryos apparently suppress interferon response to dsRNA, which efficiently and specifically triggers RNAi in these cells (Billy et al. 2001; Stein et al. 2005; Svoboda et al. 2000; Wianny and Zernicka-Goetz 2000; Yang et al. 2001). Does RNAi recognize endogenous long dsRNA and downregulate homologous transcripts?

RNAi is unlikely involved in antisense regulation of overlapping transcripts. The mammalian genome produces a significant number of overlapping transcripts that, in numerous cases, appear to be functionally related (Shendure and Church 2002; Yelin et al. 2003). However, evidence does not support the processing of naturally occurring sense antisense transcripts by RNAi (Faghihi and Wahlestedt 2006; Houbaviy and Sharp 2002). In addition, a large-scale analysis of small RNAs in postimplantation mouse embryos identified only two repeat sequences, which would fit criteria of an endogenous siRNA (Mineno et al. 2006). It is interesting that strong RNAi mutants in *Caenorhabditis* appear otherwise healthy (Tabara et al. 1999), and a germline RNAi-resistant population of *Caenorhabditis* has been found in the nature (Tijsterman et al. 2002). This further argues against a role of RNAi in regulating expression of bona fide endogenous genes. Nevertheless, the RNAi pathway is found in almost all eukaryotes, suggesting that it provides benefits leading to its conservation through evolution. RNAi in invertebrate species acts as a protecting mechanism against parasitic sequences such as viruses and mobile elements (Kalmykova et al. 2005; Lu et al. 2005; Tabara et al. 1999; Wang et al. 2006; Wilkins et al. 2005). Could this apply to some extent to mammals?

Viruses interact with mammalian RNA silencing machinery, as is evidenced by miRNAs and RNAi suppressors encoded by mammalian viruses (reviewed in Li and Ding 2005). However, it is not clear how important RNAi is in combating viral infection in mammals. Since oocytes (and presumably early developmental stages) exhibit suppressed PKR/interferon response to dsRNA (Stein et al. 2005), it is tempting to speculate that RNAi in these cells substitutes the antiviral interferon response. Ovulated eggs and preimplantation embryos are directly exposed to the external environment in the reproductive tract and could be infected by viruses introduced to the reproductive tract, for example, by the seminal fluid. Evidence exists that viral infection can possibly occur in mammalian oocytes or early embryos, but it is rare and often indirect (Bertrand et al. 2004; Bielanski et al. 2004; Botquin et al. 1994; Devaux et al. 2003; Fray et al. 1998; Papaxanthos-Roche et al. 2004; Richoux et al. 1989). It is interesting to note that some experiments in oocytes or early embryos indicate certain resistance to viruses (Baccetti et al. 1999; Cortez Romero et al. 2006; Tebourbi et al. 2002; Tsuboi and Bielanski 2005). What advantage RNAi would offer over the interferon response is not clear. It is speculated that the interferon response could be more harmful because its activation would have an invariable negative effect on the viability of an embryo while RNAi would provide a chance for blocking the virus while maintaining normal development. If this were the case, RNAi substituting the interferon response would provide a selective advantage.

Mobile elements in the genome represent another candidate target for RNAi in mammalian cells. Approximately 40% of mammalian genomes are sequences of transposable elements (TEs) (Jurka et al. 2005; Lander et al. 2001; Waterston et al. 2002). Most TEs are retroelements that retrotranspose through a "copy and paste" mechanism that utilizes an RNA intermediate. TEs have the capacity to cause deleterious mutations and they are often viewed as harmful parasites (Bestor 1999). Numerous mechanisms operate to silence TEs in animals including transcriptional silencing mediated by DNA methylation (Bourc'his and Bestor 2004; Hata and Sakaki 1997; Walsh et al. 1998), chromatin changes (Huang et al. 2004; Martens et al. 2005), and possibly RNAi.

Interestingly, mRNA level of Miwi, another Ago family member, is enhanced in the oocyte and the zygote (Fig. 3). Miwi and its human ortholog, Hiwi, are related to Ago proteins involved in miRNA silencing, but their expression is restricted to the germline. Unlike Ago proteins, Hiwi does not induce translational repression (Pillai et al. 2004). Piwi, a homolog of Miwi in *Drosophila*, is involved in the repression of retrotransposons (Kalmykova et al. 2005). Miwi is highly expressed in spermatocytes and spermatids and it is essential for spermatogenesis (Deng and Lin 2002). The function of Miwi in the oocyte is unknown. Miwi (−/−) females are viable and fertile but activity of retrotransposons in oocytes lacking Miwi has not been addressed.

Mammalian TEs apparently can generate dsRNA (Kramerov et al. 1985; Peaston et al. 2004; Svoboda et al. 2004a; Svoboda and Cara 2006), and expression of several retrotransposons occurs in mammalian oocytes and early embryos (Park et al. 2004; Peaston et al. 2004; Piko et al. 1984). It has been proposed that function of RNAi in oocytes and early embryos could constrain expression of TEs, thereby limiting their activity in mammalian germ-line cells (Svoboda et al. 2004a). Indeed, inhibiting Dicer in preimplantation mouse embryos or deleting it in ES cells results in an increased abundance of mRNAs of retrotransposons L1, IAP, and MuERV-L (Kanellopoulou et al. 2005; Svoboda et al. 2004a). In addition, putative L1 and IAP siRNAs were cloned from mouse oocytes (Watanabe et al. 2006), while L1 and IAP transcripts showed instability in the oocyte (Puschendorf et al. 2006). However, other data do not provide evidence that RNAi functions in oocytes and early embryos to constrain mobile elements. Increased abundance of TE transcripts was not observed in two independent conditional knockouts of Dicer in the oocyte (Murchison et al. 2007; Tang et al. 2007). Furthermore, increased abundance of TE transcripts was not observed in an independently generated Dicer knockout ES cell line (Murchison et al. 2005; P. Svoboda, unpublished). Therefore, there is currently no conclusive evidence supporting involvement of RNAi in repression of TEs in the oocyte.

5   Experimental Use of RNA Silencing in Mouse Oocytes and Early Embryos

RNAi is the method of choice to inhibit gene expression in many cell types, and numerous sources provide general guidelines for the use of the RNAi approach. This section focuses on the RNAi approach in mammalian oocytes and early embryos, particularly on the use of transgenic RNAi.

5.1   Microinjection of dsRNA

Microinjection of dsRNA (or siRNA) is the most common utilization of RNAi in oocytes or early embryos (reviewed, for example, in Grabarek and Zernicka-Goetz 2003; Svoboda 2004). RNAi induced by dsRNA microinjection is an excellent tool for studying the role of maternal transcripts recruited either during oocyte maturation or embryo development. Recruited transcripts accumulate in the oocyte but are not translated; therefore, the stability of the coded protein does not affect the efficiency of RNAi. Inhibition of oocyte maturation with compounds such as 3-isobutyl-l-methyl-xanthine (IBMX) extends the exposure time to dsRNA, so transcripts that would be recruited during oocyte maturation can be more efficiently degraded (Svoboda et al. 2000). Most experiments published to date (Table 1) used long dsRNA, which is easy and inexpensive to prepare. Briefly, a few hundred nucleotide long fragment of a gene is in vitro transcribed to generate sense and antisense strands which are annealed. Purified dsRNA is diluted to concentrations between 0.2 and 1.0 µg/µl and injected cytoplasmically. A detailed protocol for preparation and microinjection of dsRNA has been described elsewhere (Stein and Svoboda 2003).

5.2   Electroporation of dsRNA

Electroporation is an attractive alternative to dsRNA microinjection. It allows one to simultaneously induce RNAi in a high number of oocytes or early embryos and it also allows for the simultaneous delivery of dsRNA into individual blastomeres of preimplantation embryos (Grabarek et al. 2002). Importantly, Grabarek et al. developed a protocol allowing for electroporation of zona-enclosed embryos. This feature is important for experiments requiring transfer of treated embryos. Electroporation of dsRNA into later stages of early development is suitable for studies of gene function during implantation or shortly after it (Soares et al. 2005). In addition, electroporation of pre-processed siRNA has also been successfully used in early postimplantation embryos (Mellitzer et al. 2002).

5.3   Transfection of dsRNA

Successful transfection of long dsRNA into mammalian oocytes has been described in one report (Lazar et al. 2004). This experiment utilized rat oocytes without zona pellucida, which were transfected with purified dsRNA (33 ng/µl), using cationic liposomes (35 µg/ml) in L-15 medium containing IBMX. After 7 h, the oocytes were transferred to inhibitor-free medium for additional culture. It is possible that rat oocytes are more susceptible to cationic liposome transfection than mouse oocytes. However, our experiments with several commercially available transfection reagents (Fugene, Lipofectamine, Lipofectin) revealed a high toxicity of these reagents in mouse oocytes even after dilution or a short incubation time (Svoboda 2004).

5.4   Expression of dsRNA from a Transgene

The delivery methods described above have limitations in terms of timing of delivery of dsRNA and duration of the RNAi effect. This led to the development of transgenic RNAi, which permits the induction of RNAi already during oocyte development (Stein et al. 2003b). In principle, the choice of a promoter for dsRNA expression allows one to induce RNAi in premeiotic and postmeiotic oocytes, or during preimplantation development. The following will summarize the existing tools for transgenic RNAi and their future development.

5.4.1 Transgenes Expressing Long Hairpin RNA

Because hairpin RNA assures efficient formation of dsRNA, it has been chosen numerous times for induction of RNA silencing via expression from plasmids or transgenes. Different model systems and types of experiments have dictated different vector designs, so today there is an extremely large number of hairpin-expressing RNA systems available for RNA silencing. In general, pol II-driven long RNA hairpins are typically used in small-scale experiments in plants and invertebrates. In mammals, transgenes expressing long RNA hairpins are occasionally used but they have not acquired wider attention than in mouse oocytes (reviewed in Svoboda 2004). The advantage of long hairpin RNA is that it can be combined with a tissue-specific pol II promoter assuring tissue-specific expression of dsRNA. It also delivers a population of different siRNAs that ensure a robust RNAi. However, working with inverted repeats to generate transgenes expressing long hairpin RNA may be difficult. The following will briefly summarize the most common problems and solutions (reviewed in detail in Svoboda 2004) that we (and others) have learned about while producing constructs expressing long hairpin RNAs (>500 bp).

Transgene Design   All reported transgenes for expression of long dsRNA in the oocyte (Table 1) follow a previously developed design (Svoboda et al. 2001), where an inverted repeat is inserted downstream of a ZP3-driven enhanced green fluorescent protein (EGFP) coding sequence (Fig. 4a). Inverted repeats can be produced in two configurations with respect to the cognate mRNA sequence: anti-sense-loop-sense (A-S) or sense-loop-antisense (S-A). Both configurations have been successfully used (Stein et al. 2003b; Yu et al. 2004). Hypothetically, the S-A configuration is likely to function better if activation of a cryptic polyadenylation site in the antisense sequence occurs. At least a partial hairpin can be formed from the S-A configuration, while A-S produces none. In any case, testing of a transiently expressed transgene is recommended prior to producing mice.

Cloning Problems   Problems with cloning can be relieved by growing bacterial clones at room temperature and in special bacterial strains such as Stbl4 (Invitrogen) or Sure (Stratagene). Employing even a short spacer (20-50 bp) in the middle of an inverted repeat increases cloning efficiency. The longer the spacer the easier it is to clone the inverted repeat. Efficient RNAi transgenes in mammals contained inverted repeats with spacers up to 250 bp (Yu et al. 2004). A combination of genomic DNA with introns in the sense arm fused to the antisense arm made of a complementary DNA (cDNA) fragment also facilitates the efficiency of cloning (Kalidas and Smith 2002). Similarly, using an intron as a spacer enhances cloning efficiency and produces intron-less hairpins, which were shown to have outstanding efficiency of silencing in plants (Wesley et al. 2001).

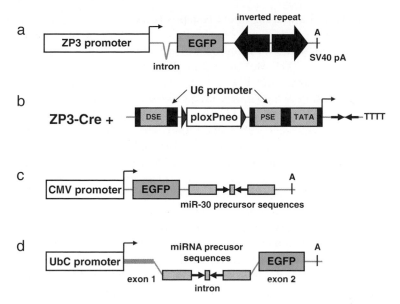

Fig. 4a-d Design of transgenes, which can be used directly (**a, b**) or after a minor modification (**c, d**) for transgenic RNAi in mammalian oocytes and early embryos. **a** Transgenes expressing long dsRNA from the oocyte-specific ZP3 promoter. This design was successfully used on several occasions (Table 1). **b** Pol III-driven short hairpin expressing transgene activated upon Cre-mediated recombination (Coumoul et al. 2005). This design can be directly used in combination with the ZP3-Cre transgene (Lewandoski et al. 1997) to induce mRNA knockdown in oocytes. **c, d** Pol II-driven short hairpin transgenes expressing a GFP reporter and a short hairpin modeled after a miRNA precursor. **c** pPRIME lentiviral vectors utilize siRNA sequences embedded in mir-30 sequences located in an exon (Stegmeier et al. 2005). With an oocyte-specific specific promoter, this vector could be used to knock down genes in oocytes in transgenic mice produced either via classical microinjection or by infection of one-cell embryos by lentiviruses (Lois et al. 2002). **d** Precursors for short hairpins modeled after miR-155 or miR-30 were also placed into an intron. (Chung et al. 2006; Xia et al. 2006)

Despite all possible pitfalls listed above, transgenic RNAi in mouse oocytes has produced functional knockdown on numerous occasions (Fedoriw et al. 2004; Han et al. 2005; Ma et al. 2006; Stein et al. 2003b; Yu et al. 2004; see also Table 1). Phenotypes in knockdown mice (Table 1) were fairly robust, except for the Wee1B knockdown, where approximately 25% of oocytes showed a phenotype and Wee1B mRNA was not knocked down as much as transcripts in other knockdown experiments (Han et al. 2005). The cause of a weaker knockdown is not clear. It is possible that the double-stranded hairpin did not form properly. This would be consistent with well-detectable EGFP fluorescence (Han et al. 2005), while EGFP in other transgenic experiments was barely detectable, suggesting efficient dsRNA formation and processing (Stein et al. 2003b; Yu et al. 2004).

5.4.2 Transgenes Expressing Short Hairpin RNA

Gene silencing with shRNA was introduced by several different groups in 2002 (Brummelkamp et al. 2002; McManus et al. 2002; Paddison et al. 2002; Yu et al. 2002; Zeng et al. 2002) and it was subsequently used in transgenic animals (reviewed in Prawitt et al. 2004). According to the hairpin structure, short hairpin systems fall into two classes: class I hairpins, which are based on linking strands of functional siRNA sequences with a small loop. The minimal class I hairpin contains a 19-bp dsRNA stem and a 4- to 9-nt loop, and it is probably not processed like a classical miRNA (Brummelkamp et al. 2002; McManus et al. 2002; Paddison et al. 2002; van de Wetering et al. 2003). Class II hairpins are directly modeled after miRNA precursors (Zeng et al. 2002).

Both RNA polymerases, RNA pol II and III, can be used to produce a functional silencing hairpin. The majority of the shRNA vectors use pol III promoters, typically U6 or H1. Both promoters appear comparably efficient in transgenic mice, although differences have also been reported (Seibler et al. 2005; Wooddell et al. 2005). The key feature of pol III systems is termination of transcription at a stretch of thymidines, leaving 1-4 uridines at the 3′ terminus, which makes one end of the self-annealed transcript similar to an siRNA. Pol III systems are used efficiently for transient or constitutive expression in cell culture. A tetracycline-inducible pol III system was also developed (van de Wetering et al. 2003).

The major disadvantage for using pol III-driven shRNA expression is the absence of tissue specificity of pol III transcription. This problem is partially solved by using a loxP recombination activating pol III (Coumoul et al. 2005; Fritsch et al. 2004; Fig. 4b). It is functional and versatile because one targeting transgene can be combined with existing animals expressing Cre recombinase in different tissues. However, the loxP strategy may sometimes be too complicated, as it requires crossing of two transgenes and a screening for recombination. It may be faster and easier to generate transgenic animals with pol II-driven tissue-specific shRNA expression than to produce animals with a loxP transgene, which has to be crossed to Cre animals to reveal which founder lines provide the best knockdown. If one wants to study one gene in different tissues, then adopting the Cre system has clear advantages. However, if one is interested in analyzing numerous genes only in the oocyte, then designing a pol II-driven transgene would be more suitable.

The pioneering work of Zeng et al. has showed that pol II can also be used to produce a functional silencing hairpin (Zeng et al. 2002). The pol II strategy is based on placing an siRNA sequence into a pri-miRNA-like transcript, which is then processed by miRNA pathway (Fig. 4c, d). This allows for generating constructs harboring shRNA within a reporter (such as EGFP), allowing for tissue-specific delivery and simple screening for the presence of the active transgene (Chung et al. 2006; Stegmeier et al. 2005; Xu et al. 2003). Pol II-driven shRNA transgenes provide the same tissue specificity as the pol II-driven long hairpins described in the previous section, thus eliminating the major advantage the long hairpin system has had so far. In addition, short hairpins are much easier to generate and manipulate and most likely will become the preferred design for transgenic RNAi in oocytes or early embryos.

6 Conclusions

Mouse oocytes and early embryos represent an interesting model system that can be approached with various RNAi-based tools. Experimental RNAi provides an unprecedented tool. Compared to other methods, it is fast, specific, simple, and is becoming the preferred tool to inhibit gene function in the oocyte or early embryos. At the same time, it is a unique model for studies of RNA silencing itself. Mouse oocytes provide an interesting example of the integration of RNA silencing and other dsRNA-responding pathways.

Acknowledgements I thank Jody Filkowski for help during preparation of the manuscript and Richard Schultz and Paula Stein for helpful discussions. This work was supported by the EMBO SDIG program, project 1483.

References

Alizadeh Z, Kageyama S, Aoki F (2005) Degradation of maternal mRNA in mouse embryos: selective degradation of specific mRNAs after fertilization. Mol Reprod Dev 72:281-290

Anderson P, Kedersha N (2006) RNA granules. J Cell Biol 172:803-808

Anger M, Stein P, Schultz RM (2005) CDC6 requirement for spindle formation during maturation of mouse oocytes. Biol Reprod 72:188-194

Athanasiadis A, Rich A, Maas S (2004) Widespread A-to-I RNA editing of Alu-containing mRNAs in the human transcriptome. PLoS Biol 2:e391

Baccetti B, Benedetto A, Collodel G, Crisá N, di Caro A, Garbuglia AR, Piomboni P (1999) Failure of HIV-1 to infect human oocytes directly. J Acquir Immune Defic Syndr 21:355-361

Bachvarova R, De Leon V, Johnson A, Kaplan G, Paynton BV (1985) Changes in total RNA, polyadenylated RNA, and actin mRNA during meiotic maturation of mouse oocytes. Dev Biol 108:325-331

Bagga S, Bracht J, Hunter S, Massirer K, Holtz J, Eachus R, Pasquinelli AE (2005) Regulation by let-7 and lin-4 miRNAs results in target mRNA degradation. Cell 122:553-563

Barber GN (2001) Host defense, viruses and apoptosis. Cell Death Differ 8:113-126

Bass BL (2002) RNA editing by adenosine deaminases that act on RNA. Annu Rev Biochem 71:817-846

Bayne EH, Allshire RC (2005) RNA-directed transcriptional gene silencing in mammals. Trends Genet 21:370-373

Bertrand E, Zissis G, Marissens D, Gérard M, Rozenberg S, Barlow P, Delvigne A (2004) Presence of HIV-1 in follicular fluids, flushes and cumulus oophorus cells of HIV-1-seropositive women during assisted-reproduction technology. AIDS 18:823-825

Bestor TH (1999) Sex brings transposons and genomes into conflict. Genetica 107:289-295

Bielanski A, Larochelle R, Algire J, Magar R (2004) Distribution of PCV-2 DNA in the reproductive tract, oocytes and embryos of PCV-2 antibody-positive pigs. Vet Rec 155:597-598

Billy E, Brondani V, Zhang H, Müller U, Filipowicz W (2001) Specific interference with gene expression induced by long, double-stranded RNA in mouse embryonal teratocarcinoma cell lines. Proc Natl Acad Sci U S A 98:14428-14433

Blow MJ, Grocock RJ, van Dongen S, Enright AJ, Dicks E, Futreal PA, Wooster R, Stratton MR (2006) RNA editing of human microRNAs. Genome Biol 7:R27

Botquin V, Cid-Arregui A, Schlehofer JR (1994) Adeno-associated virus type 2 interferes with early development of mouse embryos. J Gen Virol 75:2655-2662

Bourc'his D, Bestor TH (2004) Meiotic catastrophe and retrotransposon reactivation in male germ cells lacking Dnmt3L. Nature 431:96-99

Bridge AJ, Pebernard S, Ducraux A, Nicoulaz AL, Iggo R (2003) Induction of an interferon response by RNAi vectors in mammalian cells. Nat Genet 34:263-264

Brummelkamp TR, Bernards R, Agami R (2002) A system for stable expression of short interfering RNAs in mammalian cells. Science 296:550-553

Buchon N, Vaury C (2006) RNAi: a defensive RNA-silencing against viruses and transposable elements. Heredity 96:195-202

Caudy AA, Ketting RF, Hammond SM, Denli AM, Bathoorn AM, Tops BB, Silva JM, Myers MM, Hannon GJ, Plasterk RH (2003) A micrococcal nuclease homologue in RNAi effector complexes. Nature 425:411-414

Chendrimada TP, Gregory RI, Kumaraswamy E, Norman J, Cooch N, Nishikura K, Shiekhattar R (2005) TRBP recruits the Dicer complex to Ago2 for microRNA processing and gene silencing. Nature 436:740-744

Chung KH, Hart CC, Al-Bassam S, Avery A, Taylor J, Patel PD, Vojtek AB, Turner DL (2006) Polycistronic RNA polymerase II expression vectors for RNA interference based on BIC/miR-155. Nucleic Acids Res 34:e53

Cortez Romero C, Fieni F, Roux C, Russo P, Guibert JM, Guiguen F, Chebloune Y, Pépin M, Pellerin JL (2006) Detection of ovine lentivirus in the cumulus cells, but not in the oocytes or follicular fluid, of naturally infected sheep. Theriogenology 66:1131-1139

Coumoul X, Shukla V, Li C, Wang RH, Deng CX (2005) Conditional knockdown of Fgfr2 in mice using Cre-LoxP induced RNA interference. Nucleic Acids Res 33:e102

Cui XS, Li XY, Jeong YJ, Jun JH, Kim NH (2006) Gene expression of cox5a, 5b, or 6b1 and their roles in preimplantation mouse embryos. Biol Reprod 74:601-610

Cummins JM, He Y, Leary RJ, Pagliarini R, Diaz LA Jr, Sjoblom T, Barad O, Bentwich Z, Szafranska AE, Labourier E, Raymond CK, Roberts BS, Juhl H, Kinzler KW, Vogelstein B, Velculescu VE (2006) The colorectal microRNAome. Proc Natl Acad Sci U S A 103:3687-3692

De La Fuente R, Viveiros MM, Wigglesworth K, Eppig JJ (2004) ATRX, a member of the SNF2 family of helicase/ATPases, is required for chromosome alignment and meiotic spindle organization in metaphase II stage mouse oocytes. Dev Biol 272:1-14

de Veer MJ, Sledz CA, Williams BR (2005) Detection of foreign RNA: implications for RNAi. Immunol Cell Biol 83:224-228

Deb K, Sivaguru M, Yong HY, Roberts RM (2006) Cdx2 gene expression and trophectoderm lineage specification in mouse embryos. Science 311:992-996

Deng W, Lin H (2002) miwi, a murine homolog of piwi, encodes a cytoplasmic protein essential for spermatogenesis. Dev Cell 2:819-830

Devaux A, Soula V, Sifer C, Branger M, Naouri M, Porcher R, Poncelet C, Neuraz A, Alvarez S, Benifla JL, Madelenat P, Brun-Vezinet F, Feldmann G (2003) Hepatitis C virus detection in follicular fluid, culture media from HCV+ women, and viral risk during IVF procedures. Hum Reprod 18:2342-2349

Faghihi MA, Wahlestedt C (2006) RNA interference is not involved in natural antisense mediated regulation of gene expression in mammals. Genome Biol 7:R38

Fedoriw AM, Stein P, Svoboda P, Schultz RM, Bartolomei MS (2004) Transgenic RNAi reveals essential function for CTCF in H19 gene imprinting. Science 303:238-240

Fire A, Xu S, Montgomery MK, Kostas SA, Driver SE, Mello CC (1998) Potent and specific genetic interference by double-stranded RNA in Caenorhabditis elegans. Nature 391:806-811

Fray MD, Prentice H, Clarke MC, Charleston B (1998) Immunohistochemical evidence for the localization of bovine viral diarrhea virus, a single-stranded RNA virus, in ovarian oocytes in the cow. Vet Pathol 35:253-259

Fritsch L, Martinez LA, Sekhri R, Naguibneva I, Gérard M, Vandromme M, Schaeffer L, Harel-Bellan A (2004) Conditional gene knock-down by CRE-dependent short interfering RNAs. EMBO Rep 5:178-182

Gan L, Anton KE, Masterson BA, Vincent VA, Ye S, Gonzalez-Zulueta M (2002) Specific interference with gene expression and gene function mediated by long dsRNA in neural cells. J Neurosci Methods 121:151-157

Giraldez AJ, Cinalli RM, Glasner ME, Enright AJ, Thomson JM, Baskerville S, Hammond SM, Bartel DP, Schier AF (2005) MicroRNAs regulate brain morphogenesis in zebrafish. Science 308:833-838

Giraldez AJ, Mishima Y, Rihel J, Grocock RJ, Van Dongen S, Inoue K, Enright AJ, Schier AF (2006) Zebrafish MiR-430 promotes deadenylation and clearance of maternal mRNAs. Science 312:75-79

Grabarek JB, Zernicka-Goetz M (2003) RNA interference in mammalian systems-a practical approach. Adv Exp Med Biol 544:205-216

Grabarek JB, Plusa B, Glover DM, Zernicka-Goetz M (2002) Efficient delivery of dsRNA into zona-enclosed mouse oocytes and preimplantation embryos by electroporation. Genesis 32:269-276

Griffiths-Jones S, Grocock RJ, van Dongen S, Bateman A, Enright AJ (2006) miRBase: microRNA sequences, targets and gene nomenclature. Nucleic Acids Res 34:D140-D144

Gui LM, Joyce IM (2005) RNA interference evidence that growth differentiation factor-9 mediates oocyte regulation of cumulus expansion in mice. Biol Reprod 72:195-199

Haase AD, Jaskiewicz L, Zhang H, Lainé S, Sack R, Gatignol A, Filipowicz W (2005) TRBP, a regulator of cellular PKR, HIV-1 virus expression, interacts with Dicer and functions in RNA silencing. EMBO Rep 6:961-967

Hall TM (2005) Structure and function of argonaute proteins. Structure 13:1403-1408

Han SJ, Chen R, Paronetto MP, Conti M (2005) Wee1B is an oocyte-specific kinase involved in the control of meiotic arrest in the mouse. Curr Biol 15:1670-1676

Hata K, Sakaki Y (1997) Identification of critical CpG sites for repression of L1 transcription by DNA methylation. Gene 189:227-234

Higuchi M, Maas S, Single FN, Hartner J, Rozov A, Burnashev N, Feldmeyer D, Sprengel R, Seeburg PH (2000) Point mutation in an AMPA receptor gene rescues lethality in mice deficient in the RNA-editing enzyme ADAR2. Nature 406:78-81

Homer HA, McDougall A, Levasseur M, Murdoch AP, Herbert M (2005) RNA interference in meiosis I human oocytes: towards an understanding of human aneuploidy. Mol Hum Reprod 11:397-404

Houbaviy HB, Sharp PA (2002) Small RNA Northerns suggest that RNA interference is not involved in the downregulation of Xist by Tsix. Keystone Symposia 2002, RNA Interference, Cosuppression and Related Phenomena. Taos, New Mexico

Houbaviy HB, Murray MF, Sharp PA (2003) Embryonic stem cell-specific MicroRNAs. Dev Cell 5:351-358

Huang J, Fan T, Yan Q, Zhu H, Fox S, Issaq HJ, Best L, Gangi L, Munroe D, Muegge K (2004) Lsh, an epigenetic guardian of repetitive elements. Nucleic Acids Res 32:5019-5028

Hunter T, Hunt T, Jackson RJ, Robertson HD (1975) The characteristics of inhibition of protein synthesis by double-stranded ribonucleic acid in reticulocyte lysates. J Biol Chem 250:409-417

Jakymiw A, Lian S, Eystathioy T, Li S, Satoh M, Hamel JC, Fritzler MJ, Chan EK (2005) Disruption of GW bodies impairs mammalian RNA interference. Nat Cell Biol 7: 1267-1274

Jurka J, Kapitonov VV, Pavlicek A, Klonowski P, Kohany O, Walichiewicz J (2005) Repbase Update, a database of eukaryotic repetitive elements. Cytogenet Genome Res 110:462-467

Kalidas S, Smith DP (2002) Novel genomic cDNA hybrids produce effective RNA interference in adult Drosophila. Neuron 33:177-184

Kalmykova AI, Klenov MS, Gvozdev VA (2005) Argonaute protein PIWI controls mobilization of retrotransposons in the Drosophila male germline. Nucleic Acids Res 33:2052-2059

Kanellopoulou C, Muljo SA, Kung AL, Ganesan S, Drapkin R, Jenuwein T, Livingston DM, Rajewsky K (2005) Dicer-deficient mouse embryonic stem cells are defective in differentiation and centromeric silencing. Genes Dev 19:489-501

Kim SK, Wold BJ (1985) Stable reduction of thymidine kinase activity in cells expressing high levels of anti-sense RNA. Cell 42:129-138

Kim VN (2005) MicroRNA biogenesis: coordinated cropping and dicing. Nat Rev Mol Cell Biol 6:376-385

Kimmel CB, Ballard WW, Kimmel SR, Ullmann B, Schilling TF (1995) Stages of embryonic development of the zebrafish. Dev Dyn 203:253-310

Kramerov DA, Bukrinsky MI, Ryskov AP (1985) DNA sequences homologous to long double-stranded RNA, Transcription of intracisternal A-particle genes and major long repeat of the mouse genome. Biochim Biophys Acta 826:20-29

Lander ES, Linton LM, Birren B, Nusbaum C, Zody MC, Baldwin J, Devon K, Dewar K, Doyle M, FitzHugh W, Funke R, Gage D, Harris K, Heaford A, Howland J, Kann L, Lehoczky J, LeVine R, McEwan P, McKernan K, Meldrim J, Mesirov JP, Miranda C, Morris W, Naylor J, Raymond C, Rosetti M, Santos R, Sheridan A, Sougnez C, Stange-Thomann N, Stojanovic N, Subramanian A, Wyman D, Rogers J, Sulston J, Ainscough R, Beck S, Bentley D, Burton J, Clee C, Carter N, Coulson A, Deadman R, Deloukas P, Dunham A, Dunham I, Durbin R, French L, Grafham D, Gregory S, Hubbard T, Humphray S, Hunt A, Jones M, Lloyd C, McMurray A, Matthews L, Mercer S, Milne S, Mullikin JC, Mungall A, Plumb R, Ross M, Shownkeen R, Sims S, Waterston RH, Wilson RK, Hillier LW, McPherson JD, Marra MA, Mardis ER, Fulton LA, Chinwalla AT, Pepin KH, Gish WR, Chissoe SL, Wendl MC, Delehaunty KD, Miner TL, Delehaunty A, Kramer JB, Cook LL, Fulton RS, Johnson DL, Minx PJ, Clifton SW, Hawkins T, Branscomb E, Predki P, Richardson P, Wenning S, Slezak T, Doggett N, Cheng JF, Olsen A, Lucas S, Elkin C, Uberbacher E, Frazier M, Gibbs RA, Muzny DM, Scherer SE, Bouck JB, Sodergren EJ, Worley KC, Rives CM, Gorrell JH, Metzker ML, Naylor SL, Kucherlapati RS, Nelson DL, Weinstock GM, Sakaki Y, Fujiyama A, Hattori M, Yada T, Toyoda A, Itoh T, Kawagoe C, Watanabe H, Totoki Y, Taylor T, Weissenbach J, Heilig R, Saurin W, Artiguenave F, Brottier P, Bruls T, Pelletier E, Robert C, Wincker P, Smith DR, Doucette-Stamm L, Rubenfield M, Weinstock K, Lee HM, Dubois J, Rosenthal A, Platzer M, Nyakatura G, Taudien S, Rump A, Yang H, Yu J, Wang J, Huang G, Gu J, Hood L, Rowen L, Madan A, Qin S, Davis RW, Federspiel NA, Abola AP, Proctor MJ, Myers RM, Schmutz J, Dickson M, Grimwood J, Cox DR, Olson MV, Kaul R, Raymond C, Shimizu N, Kawasaki K, Minoshima S, Evans GA, Athanasiou M, Schultz R, Roe BA, Chen F, Pan H, Ramser J, Lehrach H, Reinhardt R, McCombie WR, de la Bastide M, Dedhia N, Blöcker H, Hornischer K, Nordsiek G, Agarwala R, Aravind L, Bailey JA, Bateman A, Batzoglou S, Birney E, Bork P, Brown DG, Burge CB, Cerutti L, Chen HC, Church D, Clamp M, Copley RR, Doerks T, Eddy SR, Eichler EE, Furey TS, Galagan J, Gilbert JG, Harmon C, Hayashizaki Y, Haussler D, Hermjakob H, Hokamp K, Jang W, Johnson LS, Jones TA, Kasif S, Kaspryzk A, Kennedy S, Kent WJ, Kitts P, Koonin EV, Korf I, Kulp D, Lancet D, Lowe TM, McLysaght A, Mikkelsen T, Moran JV, Mulder N, Pollara VJ, Ponting CP, Schuler G, Schultz J, Slater G, Smit AF, Stupka E, Szustakowski J, Thierry-Mieg D, Thierry-Mieg J, Wagner L, Wallis J, Wheeler R, Williams A, Wolf YI, Wolfe KH, Yang SP, Yeh RF, Collins F, Guyer MS, Peterson J, Felsenfeld A, Wetterstrand KA, Patrinos A, Morgan MJ, de Jong P, Catanese JJ, Osoegawa K, Shizuya H, Choi S, Chen YJ; International Human Genome Sequencing Consortium (2001) Initial sequencing and analysis of the human genome. Nature 409:860-921

Lazar S, Gershon E, Dekel N (2004) Selective degradation of cyclin B1 mRNA in rat oocytes by RNA interference (RNAi). J Mol Endocrinol 33:73-85

Lee K, Fajardo MA, Braun RE (1996) A testis cytoplasmic RNA-binding protein that has the properties of a translational repressor. Mol Cell Biol 16:3023-3034

Lee YS, Nakahara K, Pham JW, Kim K, He Z, Sontheimer EJ, Carthew RW (2004) Distinct roles for Drosophila Dicer-1 and Dicer-2 in the siRNA/miRNA silencing pathways. Cell 117:69-81

Lefebvre C, Terret ME, Djiane A, Rassinier P, Maro B, Verlhac MH (2002) Meiotic spindle stability depends on MAPK-interacting, spindle-stabilizing protein (MISS), a new MAPK substrate. J Cell Biol 157:603-613

Levanon EY, Hallegger M, Kinar Y, Shemesh R, Djinovic-Carugo K, Rechavi G, Jantsch MF, Eisenberg E (2005) Evolutionarily conserved human targets of adenosine to inosine RNA editing. Nucleic Acids Res 33:1162-1168

Lewandoski M, Wassarman KM, Martin GR (1997) Zp3-cre, transgenic mouse line for the activation or inactivation of loxP-flanked target genes specifically in the female germ line. Curr Biol 7:148-151

Li HW, Ding SW (2005) Antiviral silencing in animals. FEBS Lett 579:5965-5973

Lim LP, Lau NC, Garrett-Engele P, Grimson A, Schelter JM, Castle J, Bartel DP, Linsley PS, Johnson JM (2005) Microarray analysis shows that some microRNAs downregulate large numbers of target mRNAs. Nature 433:769-773

Liu J, Carmell MA, Rivas FV, Marsden CG, Thomson JM, Song JJ, Hammond SM, Joshua-Tor L, Hannon GJ (2004) Argonaute2 is the catalytic engine of mammalian RNAi. Science 305:1437-1441

Liu J, Rivas FV, Wohlschlegel J, Yates JR 3rd, Parker R, Hannon GJ (2005a) A role for the P-body component GW182 in microRNA function. Nat Cell Biol 7:1261-1266

Liu J, Valencia-Sanchez MA, Hannon GJ, Parker R (2005b) MicroRNA-dependent localization of targeted mRNAs to mammalian P-bodies. Nat Cell Biol 7:719-723

Lois C, Hong EJ, Pease S, Brown EJ, Baltimore D (2002) Germline transmission and tissue-specific expression of transgenes delivered by lentiviral vectors. Science 295:868-872

Lu R, Maduro M, Li F, Li HW, Broitman-Maduro G, Li WX, Ding SW (2005) Animal virus replication and RNAi-mediated antiviral silencing in Caenorhabditis elegans. Nature 436:1040-1043

Ma J, Zeng F, Schultz RM, Tseng H (2006) Basonuclin: a novel mammalian maternal-effect gene. Development 133:2053-2062

Maas S, Rich A, Nishikura K (2003) A-to-I RNA editing: recent news and residual mysteries. J Biol Chem 278:1391-1394

Martens JH, O'Sullivan RJ, Braunschweig U, Opravil S, Radolf M, Steinlein P, Jenuwein T (2005) The profile of repeat-associated histone lysine methylation states in the mouse epigenome. EMBO J 24:800-812

Matranga C, Tomari Y, Shin C, Bartel DP, Zamore PD (2005) Passenger-strand cleavage facilitates assembly of siRNA into Ago2-containing RNAi enzyme complexes. Cell 123:607-620

Matzke MA, Birchler JA (2005) RNAi-mediated pathways in the nucleus. Nat Rev Genet 6:24-35

McManus MT, Petersen CP, Haines BB, Chen J, Sharp PA (2002) Gene silencing using microRNA designed hairpins. Rna 8:842-850

McMillan NA, Carpick BW, Hollis B, Toone WM, Zamanian-Daryoush M, Williams BR (1995) Mutational analysis of the double-stranded RNA (dsRNA) binding domain of the dsRNA-activated protein kinase, PKR. J Biol Chem 270:2601-2606

Mehlmann LM (2005) Oocyte-specific expression of Gpr3 is required for the maintenance of meiotic arrest in mouse oocytes. Dev Biol 288:397-404

Meister G, Landthaler M, Patkaniowska A, Dorsett Y, Teng G, Tuschl T (2004) Human Argonaute2 mediates RNA cleavage targeted by miRNAs and siRNAs. Mol Cell 15:185-197

Mellitzer G, Hallonet M, Chen L, Ang SL (2002) Spatial and temporal 'knock down' of gene expression by electroporation of double-stranded RNA and morpholinos into early postimplantation mouse embryos. Mech Dev 118:57-63

Mineno J, Okamoto S, Ando T, Sato M, Chono H, Izu H, Takayama M, Asada K, Mirochnitchenko O, Inouye M, Kato I (2006) The expression profile of microRNAs in mouse embryos. Nucleic Acids Res 34:1765-1771

Morris KV, Chan SW, Jacobsen SE, Looney DJ (2004) Small interfering RNA-induced transcriptional gene silencing in human cells. Science 305:1289-1292

Morse DP, Bass BL (1999) Long RNA hairpins that contain inosine are present in Caenorhabditis elegans poly(A)+ RNA. Proc Natl Acad Sci U S A 96:6048-6053

Morse DP, Aruscavage PJ, Bass BL (2002) RNA hairpins in noncoding regions of human brain and Caenorhabditis elegans mRNA are edited by adenosine deaminases that act on RNA. Proc Natl Acad Sci U S A 99:7906-7911

Murchison EP, Partridge JF, Tam OH, Cheloufi S, Hannon GJ (2005) Characterization of Dicer-deficient murine embryonic stem cells. Proc Natl Acad Sci U S A 102:12135-12140

Murchison EP, Stein P, Xuan Z, Pan H, Zhang MQ, Schultz RM, Hannon GJ (2007) Critical roles for Dicer in the female germline. Genes Dev 21:682-693

Newbury SF, Muhlemann O, Stoecklin G (2006) Turnover in the Alps: an mRNA perspective: Workshops on mechanisms and regulation of mRNA turnover. EMBO Rep 7:143-148

Nganvongpanit K, Müller H, Rings F, Hoelker M, Jennen D, Tholen E, Havlicek V, Besenfelder U, Schellander K, Tesfaye D (2006) Selective degradation of maternal and embryonic transcripts in in vitro produced bovine oocytes and embryos using sequence specific double-stranded RNA. Reproduction 131:861-874

Oh B, Hwang S, McLaughlin J, Solter D, Knowles BB (2000) Timely translation during the mouse oocyte-to-embryo transition. Development 127:3795-3803

Okano H, Aruga J, Nakagawa T, Shiota C, Mikoshiba K (1991) Myelin basic protein gene and the function of antisense RNA in its repression in myelin-deficient mutant mouse. J Neurochem 56:560-567

Ong CL, Thorpe JC, Gorry PR, Bannwarth S, Jaworowski A, Howard JL, Chung S, Campbell S, Christensen HS, Clerzius G, Mouland AJ, Gatignol A, Purcell DF (2005) Low TRBP levels support an innate human immunodeficiency virus type 1 resistance in astrocytes by enhancing the PKR antiviral response. J Virol 79:12763-12772

Paddison PJ, Caudy AA, Bernstein E, Hannon GJ, Conklin DS (2002) Short hairpin RNAs (shRNAs) induce sequence-specific silencing in mammalian cells. Genes Dev 16:948-958

Palladino MJ, Keegan LP, O'Connell MA, Reenan RA (2000) A-to-I pre-mRNA editing in Drosophila is primarily involved in adult nervous system function and integrity. Cell 102:437-449

Papaxanthos-Roche A, Trimoulet P, Commenges-Ducos M, Hocké C, Fleury HJ, Mayer G (2004) PCR-detected hepatitis C virus RNA associated with human zona-intact oocytes collected from infected women for ART. Hum Reprod 19:1170-1175

Park CE, Shin MR, Jeon EH, Lee SH, Cha KY, Kim K, Kim NH, Lee KA (2004) Oocyte-selective expression of MT transposon-like element, clone MTi7 and its role in oocyte maturation and embryo development. Mol Reprod Dev 69:365-374

Park H, Davies MV, Langland JO, Chang HW, Nam YS, Tartaglia J, Paoletti E, Jacobs BL, Kaufman RJ, Venkatesan S (1994) TAR RNA-binding protein is an inhibitor of the interferon-induced protein kinase PKR. Proc Natl Acad Sci U S A 91:4713-4717

Paronetto MP, Giorda E, Carsetti R, Rossi P, Geremia R, Sette C (2004) Functional interaction between p90Rsk2 and Emi1 contributes to the metaphase arrest of mouse oocytes. EMBO J 23:4649-4659

Paynton BV, Rempel R, Bachvarova R (1988) Changes in state of adenylation and time course of degradation of maternal mRNAs during oocyte maturation and early embryonic development in the mouse. Dev Biol 129:304-314

Peaston AE, Evsikov AV, Graber JH, de Vries WN, Holbrook AE, Solter D, Knowles BB (2004) Retrotransposons regulate host genes in mouse oocytes and preimplantation embryos. Dev Cell 7:597-606

Piko L, Hammons MD, Taylor KD (1984) Amounts, synthesis, and some properties of intracisternal A particle-related RNA in early mouse embryos. Proc Natl Acad Sci U S A 81:488-492

Pillai RS, Artus CG, Filipowicz W (2004) Tethering of human Ago proteins to mRNA mimics the miRNA-mediated repression of protein synthesis. Rna 10:1518-1525

Pillai RS, Bhattacharyya SN, Artus CG, Zoller T, Cougot N, Basyuk E, Bertrand E, Filipowicz W (2005) Inhibition of translational initiation by Let-7 MicroRNA in human cells. Science 309:1573-1576

Plusa B, Frankenberg S, Chalmers A, Hadjantonakis AK, Moore CA, Papalopulu N, Papaioannou VE, Glover DM, Zernicka-Goetz M (2005) Downregulation of Par3 and aPKC function directs cells towards the ICM in the preimplantation mouse embryo. J Cell Sci 118:505-515

Prasanth KV, Prasanth SG, Xuan Z, Hearn S, Freier SM, Bennett CF, Zhang MQ, Spector DL (2005) Regulating gene expression through RNA nuclear retention. Cell 123:249-263

Prawitt D, Brixel L, Spangenberg C, Eshkind L, Heck R, Oesch F, Zabel B, Bockamp E (2004) RNAi knock-down mice: an emerging technology for post-genomic functional genetics. Cytogenet Genome Res 105:412-421

Puschendorf M, Stein P, Oakeley EJ, Schultz RM, Peters AH, Svoboda P (2006) Abundant transcripts from retrotransposons are unstable in fully grown mouse oocytes. Biochem Biophys Res Commun 347:36-43

Rehwinkel J, Behm-Ansmant I, Gatfield D, Izaurralde E (2005) A crucial role for GW182 and the DCP1:DCP2 decapping complex in miRNA-mediated gene silencing. Rna 11:1640-1647

Richoux V, Panthier JJ, Salmon AM, Condamine H (1989) Acquisition of endogenous ecotropic MuLV can occur before the late one-cell stage in the genital tract of SWR/J-RF/J hybrid females. J Exp Zool 252:96-100

Sakurai T, Sato M, Kimura M (2005) Diverse patterns of poly(A) tail elongation and shortening of murine maternal mRNAs from fully grown oocyte to 2-cell embryo stages. Biochem Biophys Res Commun 336:1181-1189

Saumet A, Lecellier CH (2006) Anti-viral RNA silencing: do we look like plants? Retrovirology 3:3

Scadden AD (2005) The RISC subunit Tudor-SN binds to hyper-edited double-stranded RNA and promotes its cleavage. Nat Struct Mol Biol 12:489-496

Schmitt HP, Kuhn B, Alonso A (1986) Characterization of cloned sequences complementary to F9 cell double-stranded RNA and their expression during differentiation. Differentiation 30:205-210

Schultz RM (2002) The molecular foundations of the maternal to zygotic transition in the preimplantation embryo. Hum Reprod Update 8:323-331

Seibler J, Küter-Luks B, Kern H, Streu S, Plum L, Mauer J, Kühn R, Brüning JC, Schwenk F (2005) Single copy shRNA configuration for ubiquitous gene knockdown in mice. Nucleic Acids Res 33:e67

Shendure J, Church GM (2002) Computational discovery of sense-antisense transcription in the human and mouse genomes. Genome Biol 3:RESEARCH0044

Sijen T, Fleenor J, Simmer F, Thijssen KL, Parrish S, Timmons L, Plasterk RH, Fire A (2001) On the role of RNA amplification in dsRNA-triggered gene silencing. Cell 107:465-476

Soares ML, Haraguchi S, Torres-Padilla ME, Kalmar T, Carpenter L, Bell G, Morrison A, Ring CJ, Clarke NJ, Glover DM, Zernicka-Goetz M (2005) Functional studies of signaling pathways in peri-implantation development of the mouse embryo by RNAi. BMC Dev Biol 5:28

Song JJ, Smith SK, Hannon GJ, Joshua-Tor L (2004) Crystal structure of Argonaute and its implications for RISC slicer activity. Science 305:1434-1437

Sontheimer EJ (2005) Assembly and function of RNA silencing complexes. Nat Rev Mol Cell Biol 6:127-138

Sontheimer EJ, Carthew RW (2005) Silence from within: endogenous siRNAs and miRNAs. Cell 122:9-12

Srivastava SP, Kumar KU, Kaufman RJ (1998) Phosphorylation of eukaryotic translation initiation factor 2 mediates apoptosis in response to activation of the double-stranded RNA-dependent protein kinase. J Biol Chem 273:2416-2423

Stegmeier F, Hu G, Rickles RJ, Hannon GJ, Elledge SJ (2005) A lentiviral microRNA-based system for single-copy polymerase II-regulated RNA interference in mammalian cells. Proc Natl Acad Sci U S A 102:13212-13217

Stein P, Svoboda P (2003) Guide to RNAi in mouse oocytes and preimplantation embryos. In: Hannon J (ed) RNAi: A guide to gene silencing. Cold Spring Harbor Press, Cold Spring Harbor, pp 313-343

Stein P, Svoboda P, Anger M, Schultz RM (2003a) RNAi: mammalian oocytes do it without RNA-dependent RNA polymerase. Rna 9:187-192

Stein P, Svoboda P, Schultz RM (2003b) Transgenic RNAi in mouse oocytes: a simple and fast approach to study gene function. Dev Biol 256:187-193

Stein P, Zeng F, Pan H, Schultz RM (2005) Absence of non-specific effects of RNA interference triggered by long double-stranded RNA in mouse oocytes. Dev Biol 286:464-471

Su AI, Cooke MP, Ching KA, Hakak Y, Walker JR, Wiltshire T, Orth AP, Vega RG, Sapinoso LM, Moqrich A, Patapoutian A, Hampton GM, Schultz PG, Hogenesch JB (2002) Large-scale analysis of the human and mouse transcriptomes. Proc Natl Acad Sci U S A 99:4465-4470

Suh MR, Lee Y, Kim JY, Kim SK, Moon SH, Lee JY, Cha KY, Chung HM, Yoon HS, Moon SY, Kim VN, Kim KS (2004) Human embryonic stem cells express a unique set of microRNAs. Dev Biol 270:488-498

Svoboda P (2004) Long dsRNA and silent genes strike back: RNAi in mouse oocytes and early embryos. Cytogenet Genome Res 105:422-434

Svoboda P, Cara AD (2006) Hairpin RNA: a secondary structure of primary importance. Cell Mol Life Sci 63:901-908

Svoboda P, Stein P, Hayashi H, Schultz RM (2000) Selective reduction of dormant maternal mRNAs in mouse oocytes by RNA interference. Development 127:4147-4156

Svoboda P, Stein P, Schultz RM (2001) RNAi in mouse oocytes and preimplantation embryos: effectiveness of Hairpin dsRNA. Biochem Biophys Res Commun 287:1099-1104

Svoboda P, Stein P, Anger M, Bernstein E, Hannon GJ, Schultz RM (2004a) RNAi and expression of retrotransposons MuERV-L and IAP in preimplantation mouse embryos. Dev Biol 269:276-285

Svoboda P, Stein P, Filipowicz W, Schultz RM (2004b) Lack of homologous sequence-specific DNA methylation in response to stable dsRNA expression in mouse oocytes. Nucleic Acids Res 32:3601-3606

Tabara H, Sarkissian M, Kelly WG, Fleenor J, Grishok A, Timmons L, Fire A, Mello CC (1999) The rde-1 gene, RNA interference, transposon silencing in C. elegans. Cell 99:123-132

Tang F, Kaneda M, O'Carroll D, Hajkova P, Barton SC, Sun YA, Lee C, Tarakhovsky A, Lao K, Surani MA (2007) Maternal microRNAs are essential for mouse zygotic development. Genes Dev 21:644-648

Tavernarakis N, Wang SL, Dorovkov M, Ryazanov A, Driscoll M (2000) Heritable and inducible genetic interference by double-stranded RNA encoded by transgenes. Nat Genet 24:180-183

Tebourbi L, Testart J, Cerutti I, Moussu JP, Loeuillet A, Courtot AM (2002) Failure to infect embryos after virus injection in mouse zygotes. Hum Reprod 17:760-764

Terret ME, Lefebvre C, Djiane A, Rassinier P, Moreau J, Maro B, Verlhac MH (2003) DOC1R: a MAP kinase substrate that control microtubule organization of metaphase II mouse oocytes. Development 130:5169-5177

Tijsterman M, Okihara KL, Thijssen K, Plasterk RH (2002) PPW-1, a PAZ/PIWI protein required for efficient germline RNAi is defective in a natural isolate of C. elegans. Curr Biol 12:1535

Ting AH, Schuebel KE, Herman JG, Baylin SB (2005) Short double-stranded RNA induces transcriptional gene silencing in human cancer cells in the absence of DNA methylation. Nat Genet 37:906-910

Tonkin LA, Bass BL (2003) Mutations in RNAi rescue aberrant chemotaxis of ADAR mutants. Science 302:1725

Tonkin LA, Saccomanno L, Morse DP, Brodigan T, Krause M, Bass BL (2002) RNA editing by ADARs is important for normal behavior in Caenorhabditis elegans. EMBO J 21:6025-6035

Tsuboi T, Bielanski A (2005) Resistance of immature bovine oocytes to non-cytopathogenic bovine viral diarrhoea virus in vitro. Vet Rec 156:546-548

Valencia-Sanchez MA, Liu J, Hannon GJ, Parker R (2006) Control of translation and mRNA degradation by miRNAs and siRNAs. Genes Dev 20:515-524

van de Wetering M, Oving I, Muncan V, Pon Fong MT, Brantjes H, van Leenen D, Holstege FC, Brummelkamp TR, Agami R, Clevers H (2003) Specific inhibition of gene expression using a stably integrated, inducible small-interfering-RNA vector. EMBO Rep 4:609-615

Verdel A, Moazed D (2005) RNAi-directed assembly of heterochromatin in fission yeast. FEBS Lett 579:5872-5878

Walsh CP, Chaillet JR, Bestor TH (1998) Transcription of IAP endogenous retroviruses is constrained by cytosine methylation. Nat Genet 20:116-117

Wang J, Tekle E, Oubrahim H, Mieyal JJ, Stadtman ER, Chock PB (2003) Stable and controllable RNA interference: investigating the physiological function of glutathionylated actin. Proc Natl Acad Sci U S A 100:5103-5106

Wang Q, Carmichael GG (2004) Effects of length and location on the cellular response to double-stranded RNA. Microbiol Mol Biol Rev 68:432-452

Wang Q, Khillan J, Gadue P, Nishikura K (2000) Requirement of the RNA editing deaminase ADAR1 gene for embryonic erythropoiesis. Science 290:1765-1768

Wang XH, Aliyari R, Li WX, Li HW, Kim K, Carthew R, Atkinson P, Ding SW (2006) RNA interference directs innate immunity against viruses in adult Drosophila. Science 312:452-454

Watanabe T, Takeda A, Mise K, Okuno T, Suzuki T, Minami N, Imai H (2005) Stage-specific expression of microRNAs during Xenopus development. FEBS Lett 579:318-324

Watanabe T, Takeda A, Tsukiyama T, Mise K, Okuno T, Sasaki H, Minami N, Imai H (2006) Identification and characterization of two novel classes of small RNAs in the mouse germline: retrotransposon-derived siRNAs in oocytes and germline small RNAs in testes. Genes Dev 20:1732-1743

Waterston RH, Lindblad-Toh K, Birney E, Rogers J, Abril JF, Agarwal P, Agarwala R, Ainscough R, Alexandersson M, An P, Antonarakis SE, Attwood J, Baertsch R, Bailey J, Barlow K, Beck S, Berry E, Birren B, Bloom T, Bork P, Botcherby M, Bray N, Brent MR, Brown DG, Brown SD, Bult C, Burton J, Butler J, Campbell RD, Carninci P, Cawley S, Chiaromonte F, Chinwalla AT, Church DM, Clamp M, Clee C, Collins FS, Cook LL, Copley RR, Coulson A, Couronne O, Cuff J, Curwen V, Cutts T, Daly M, David R, Davies J, Delehaunty KD, Deri J, Dermitzakis ET, Dewey C, Dickens NJ, Diekhans M, Dodge S, Dubchak I, Dunn DM, Eddy SR, Elnitski L, Emes RD, Eswara P, Eyras E, Felsenfeld A, Fewell GA, Flicek P, Foley K, Frankel WN, Fulton LA, Fulton RS, Furey TS, Gage D, Gibbs RA, Glusman G, Gnerre S, Goldman N, Goodstadt L, Grafham D, Graves TA, Green ED, Gregory S, Guigó R, Guyer M, Hardison RC, Haussler D, Hayashizaki Y, Hillier LW, Hinrichs A, Hlavina W, Holzer T, Hsu F, Hua A, Hubbard T, Hunt A, Jackson I, Jaffe DB, Johnson LS, Jones M, Jones TA, Joy A, Kamal M, Karlsson EK, Karolchik D, Kasprzyk A, Kawai J, Keibler E, Kells C, Kent WJ, Kirby A, Kolbe DL, Korf I, Kucherlapati RS, Kulbokas EJ, Kulp D, Landers T, Leger JP, Leonard S, Letunic I, Levine R, Li J, Li M, Lloyd C, Lucas S, Ma B, Maglott DR, Mardis ER, Matthews L, Mauceli E, Mayer JH, McCarthy M, McCombie WR, McLaren S, McLay K, McPherson JD, Meldrim J, Meredith B, Mesirov JP, Miller W, Miner TL, Mongin E, Montgomery KT, Morgan M, Mott R, Mullikin JC, Muzny DM, Nash WE, Nelson JO, Nhan MN, Nicol R, Ning Z, Nusbaum C, O'Connor MJ, Okazaki Y, Oliver K, Overton-Larty E, Pachter L, Parra G, Pepin KH, Peterson J, Pevzner P, Plumb R, Pohl CS, Poliakov A, Ponce TC, Ponting CP, Potter S, Quail M, Reymond A, Roe BA, Roskin KM, Rubin EM, Rust AG, Santos R, Sapojnikov V, Schultz B, Schultz J, Schwartz MS, Schwartz S, Scott C, Seaman S, Searle S, Sharpe T, Sheridan A, Shownkeen R, Sims S, Singer JB, Slater G, Smit A, Smith DR, Spencer B, Stabenau A, Stange-Thomann N, Sugnet C, Suyama M, Tesler G, Thompson J, Torrents D, Trevaskis E, Tromp J, Ucla C, Ureta-Vidal A, Vinson JP, Von Niederhausern AC, Wade CM, Wall M, Weber RJ, Weiss RB, Wendl MC, West AP, Wetterstrand K, Wheeler R, Whelan S, Wierzbowski J, Willey D, Williams S, Wilson RK, Winter E, Worley KC, Wyman D, Yang S, Yang SP, Zdobnov EM, Zody MC, Lander ES (2002) Initial sequencing and comparative analysis of the mouse genome. Nature 420:520-562

Wesley SV, Helliwell CA, Smith NA, Wang MB, Rouse DT, Liu Q, Gooding PS, Singh SP, Abbott D, Stoutjesdijk PA, Robinson SP, Gleave AP, Green AG, Waterhouse PM (2001) Construct design for efficient, effective and high-throughput gene silencing in plants. Plant J 27:581-590

Wianny F, Zernicka-Goetz M (2000) Specific interference with gene function by double-stranded RNA in early mouse development. Nat Cell Biol 2:70-75

Wienholds E, Koudijs MJ, van Eeden FJ, Cuppen E, Plasterk RH (2003) The microRNA-producing enzyme Dicer1 is essential for zebrafish development. Nat Genet 35:217-218

Wienholds E, Kloosterman WP, Miska E, Alvarez-Saavedra E, Berezikov E, de Bruijn E, Horvitz HR, Kauppinen S, Plasterk RH (2005) MicroRNA expression in zebrafish embryonic development. Science 309:310-311

Wilkins C, Dishongh R, Moore SC, Whitt MA, Chow M, Machaca K (2005) RNA interference is an antiviral defence mechanism in Caenorhabditis elegans. Nature 436:1044-1047

Wooddell CI, Van Hout CV, Reppen T, Lewis DL, Herweijer H (2005) Long-term RNA interference from optimized siRNA expression constructs in adult mice. Biochem Biophys Res Commun 334:117-127

Xia XG, Zhou H, Samper E, Melov S, Xu Z (2006) Pol II-expressed shRNA knocks down Sod2
    gene expression and causes phenotypes of the gene knockout in mice. PLoS Genet 2:e10
Xu Z, Williams CJ, Kopf GS, Schultz RM (2003) Maturation-associated increase in IP3 receptor
    type 1: role in conferring increased IP3 sensitivity and Ca^{2+} oscillatory behavior in mouse eggs.
    Dev Biol 254:163-171
Yang S, Tutton S, Pierce E, Yoon K (2001) Specific double-stranded RNA interference in undif-
    ferentiated mouse embryonic stem cells. Mol Cell Biol 21:7807-7816
Yang W, Wang Q, Howell KL, Lee JT, Cho DS, Murray JM, Nishikura K (2005) ADAR1 RNA
    deaminase limits short interfering RNA efficacy in mammalian cells. J Biol Chem
    280:3946-3953
Yang W, Chendrimada TP, Wang Q, Higuchi M, Seeburg PH, Shiekhattar R, Nishikura K (2006)
    Modulation of microRNA processing and expression through RNA editing by ADAR deami-
    nases. Nat Struct Mol Biol 13:13-21
Yekta S, Shih IH, Bartel DP (2004) MicroRNA-directed cleavage of HOXB8 mRNA. Science
    304:594-596
Yelin R, Dahary D, Sorek R, Levanon EY, Goldstein O, Shoshan A, Diber A, Biton S, Tamir Y,
    Khosravi R, Nemzer S, Pinner E, Walach S, Bernstein J, Savitsky K, Rotman G (2003)
    Widespread occurrence of antisense transcription in the human genome. Nat Biotechnol
    21:379-386
Yu J, Deng M, Medvedev S, Yang J, Hecht NB, Schultz RM (2004) Transgenic RNAi-mediated
    reduction of MSY2 in mouse oocytes results in reduced fertility. Dev Biol 268:195-206
Yu JY, DeRuiter SL, Turner DL (2002) RNA interference by expression of short-interfering RNAs
    and hairpin RNAs in mammalian cells. Proc Natl Acad Sci U S A 99:6047-6052
Zamore PD, Haley B (2005) Ribo-gnome: the big world of small RNAs. Science 309:1519-1524
Zeng F, Schultz RM (2005) RNA transcript profiling during zygotic gene activation in the preim-
    plantation mouse embryo. Dev Biol 283:40-57
Zeng F, Baldwin DA, Schultz RM (2004) Transcript profiling during preimplantation mouse
    development. Dev Biol 272:483-496
Zeng Y, Wagner EJ, Cullen BR (2002) Both natural and designed micro RNAs can inhibit the
    expression of cognate mRNAs when expressed in human cells. Mol Cell 9:1327-1333
Zhong J, Peters AH, Lee K, Braun RE (1999) A double-stranded RNA binding protein required
    for activation of repressed messages in mammalian germ cells. Nat Genet 22:171-174

Identifying Human MicroRNAs

Isaac Bentwich, MD

Abstract   MicroRNAs are a recently discovered group of short, non-coding RNA regulatory genes found in many species including humans. Originally viewed as a rare curiosity, over a thousand peer-reviewed publications have now established their major role in health and disease. MicroRNA discovery approaches, both biological and computational, have played an important role in this enfolding drama, and have led to the discovery of many hundreds of novel microRNAs. These different discovery and validation approaches are briefly reviewed here, as are the challenges and questions that lie ahead.

1   Introduction

MicroRNAs are a recently discovered, extensive class of short (~22 nucleotides), non-coding RNA regulatory genes, found in many species including humans, and shown to play a major role in health and disease (Bartel 2004; Johnston and Hobert 2003; Lim et al. 2003a; Poy et al. 2004). Their main documented mode of action is repressing translation of target proteins, by binding complementarily to mRNAs of these targets (Lee et al. 1993; Kloosterman et al. 2004; Brennecke et al. 2005; Kiriakidou et al. 2004). MicroRNAs are processed from a 'hairpin' shaped precursor, a feature which has become an important criterion to identification of microRNAs (Ambros et al. 2003).

Isaac Bentwich, MD
Rosetta Genomics Ltd., 10 Plaut Street, 76706 Rehovot, Israel
bentwich@rosettagenomics.com

P.J. Paddison and P.K. Vogt (eds.), *RNA Interference.*
Current Topics in Microbiology and Immunology 320.
© Springer-Verlag Berlin Heidelberg 2008

The discovery of microRNAs and their scope is something of an unfolding drama. The first microRNA, *lin-4*, was discovered in the worm *Caenorhabditis elegans* in 1993 (Lee et al. 1993), and for 7 years was considered a lone, peculiar phenomenon specific to worms. Only in 2000 was a second microRNA discovered, *let-7*, which like *lin-4* was also involved in controlling timing of the development of the worm, and hence both genes were then termed stRNA (short temporal RNA) (Reinhart et al. 2000). Several months later, *let-7* was shown to be strikingly evolutionarily conserved in a broad range of species including human, suggesting for the first time a much broader role (Pasquinelli et al. 2000). In 2001, 95 new such genes were discovered, including 58 in *C. elegans*, 16 in *Drosophila melanogaster*, and 21 in humans, and the term microRNA was coined (Lau et al. 2001; Lee and Ambros 2001; Lagos-Quintana et al. 2001).

Initial efforts to discover microRNAs relied on a biological approach of cloning and sequencing (Lau et al. 2001; Lee and Ambros 2001; Lagos-Quintana et al. 2001; Lagos-Quintana et al. 2002). Informatics played a limited role in these efforts, verifying that the cloned sequences are part of a hairpin structure, typical of microRNA precursors (Ambros et al. 2003). Informatics was also used to find putative micro RNAs—microRNAs that were sequenced in other species and were informatically found to be conserved in the human genome, but could not be cloned in man. By early 2003, such efforts have led to identification of 109 human microRNAs (Lim et al. 2003a).

It was apparent, however, that such biological approaches might be limited in their ability to detect rare microRNAs, and are of course limited to the tissues examined. This, together with the fact that microRNA precursors share a common secondary 'hairpin'-shaped structure, has led to the development of increasingly sophisticated computational approaches, which attempted to identify possible microRNAs.

Predictions made by one of these early algorithms in early 2003 led to a conclusion that the number of vertebrate microRNAs cannot exceed 255, and that most of these have already been identified (Lim et al. 2003a). Interestingly, this assessment of the number of human microRNAs continued to be widely accepted throughout 2003 and 2004 (Lagos-Quintana et al. 2003; Grad et al. 2004; Ambros 2004).

In 2005 we described a novel approach for identification of human microRNAs, which integrated a novel computational approach with novel biological validation techniques (Bentwich et al. 2005). Using this approach, we were able to report 89 new human microRNAs, doubling the number of human microRNAs sequenced in man at that time. Our approach allowed us, for the first time, to discover non-conserved microRNAs, and provided strong evidence that the number of human microRNAs is much larger than previously believed, and that hundreds of conserved and non-conserved microRNAs remain to be discovered.

The following sections review the principles of microRNA prediction and validation, and describe the perspective of on-going trends in microRNA identification and discovery.

2   Bioinformatic MicroRNA Prediction: Principles and Challenges

Computerized identification of novel microRNAs is a difficult pattern-recognition challenge. MicroRNAs have certain properties in common, notably the fact that they are 'diced' from a hairpin-shaped precursor, which in principle allows for computerized prediction of novel microRNAs. However, no one property (e.g. free-energy, sequence pattern) is sufficient for accurately detecting microRNAs. Even when assessing multiple such properties, rigid thresholds of such property-values are also insufficiently sensitive. Rather, it is the combination of multiple properties, with a suitably different weighting of these different properties, that provides a more desirable accuracy.

Bioinformatic prediction of microRNAs utilizes machine learning algorithms that are 'trained' on a 'training set' of known microRNAs and their hairpin-shaped precursors, such that the resulting algorithm can correctly identify novel postulated microRNA sequences. Typically, such algorithms use as a 'control group' a large group of hairpin sequences randomly selected from the genome. The vast majority of these hairpins are assumed not to be microRNA precursors. The training and control sets are then studied for properties which effectively distinguish the known microRNAs from the control group of random genomic hairpins. The resulting algorithm uses these distinguishing properties to assess unrecognized hairpin sequences, and grade each such sequence for the probability that it is a valid novel microRNA.

In general, distinctive properties include (1) structural features, such as hairpin length, hairpin-loop length, thermodynamic stability, base-pairing, bulge size and location, and distance of the microRNA from the loop of its hairpin precursor, and (2) sequence features such as nucleotide content and location, sequence complexity, repeat elements and internal and inverted sequence repeats. An iterative process is used to check and improve the accuracy of the algorithm, by repeatedly training the algorithm on a subset of the known microRNAs, and then checking its scoring accuracy on a separate subset of the known microRNAs against a control group of random hairpins. The computer does not 'know' this second subset, and hence scores them as it would any unknown sequences. These scores may therefore be assessed for their sensitivity and specificity. This methodology is depicted in Fig. 1.

Most predictor algorithms depend on evolutionary conservation of microRNA sequences between different species. Such algorithms receive as input sequences that are homologous in two species, and use various approaches to detect microRNAs that are conserved in these two species. This approach allows the filtering out of many of the false-positive candidates, but is obviously limited to detecting conserved microRNAs.

Once novel potential microRNAs have been bioinformatically predicted, an attempt is made to validate their expression in various tissues or cell cultures (or both). This too is challenging since failure to biologically validate the expression of a predicted microRNA does not necessarily imply that the bioinformatic prediction

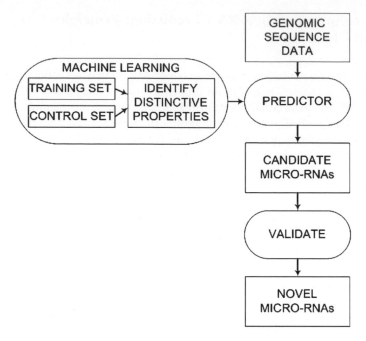

Fig. 1 Machine learning prediction of microRNAs. Machine learning algorithms are used to identify distinctive properties that differentiate between a training set of known microRNAs and a control set of genomic hairpins. Based on these, a predictor is used to identify candidate micro-RNAs from genomic sequence data. Finally, biological validation determines which of these candidates are valid novel microRNAs

was incorrect: It may be that the microRNA is not expressed in the examined tissues, is expressed only in certain cell phases, or is expressed in low abundance which escapes detection by the technique used. This latter cause is especially problematic with microRNAs, which are often very similar in sequence to one another. Expression of an abundant microRNA may therefore mask the expression of a rare one that is very similar in sequence, especially when using PCR amplification.

These difficulties in biologically validating predicted microRNAs lead to an interesting 'circular' challenge. How does one attempt to informatically detect microRNAs that are expressed at such low concentrations that they go undetected by currently available biological detection approaches? Even if an algorithm is developed which seems to be capable of identifying such low-abundance microR-NAs, how do we know if the algorithm is correct? To do so, a novel biological detection assay must be developed, which is more sensitive than the ones currently used. But then how does one test such a biological validation assay, which is capable of identifying a postulated microRNA that is not detected by any existing biological assay? Such methodological difficulties are not insurmountable, but do point to the challenges facing the development of novel microRNA detection methodologies.

3   A Novel, 'Integrated' Approach to MicroRNA Identification

Seven years ago, several years before the heightened interest in microRNAs, we set out to develop a novel bioinformatic approach that would allow us to effectively discover human microRNA genes. Our motivation to do so was the biological theory formulated below, which predicted the existence of many hundreds, possibly thousands, of microRNA-like genes involved in differentiation (Bentwich 2005).

As we started developing and applying microRNA discovery algorithms, we quickly realized that bioinformatics may be augmented by powerful effective biological validation techniques, including high-throughput validation, in order to be effective. High-throughput validation is important, as it allows us to deal effectively with large groups of hairpins that have a relatively high percentage of false-positives. At the time, high-density microarrays for detecting expression of microRNAs were not available, so we had to develop that methodology (Barad et al. 2004).

We further realized that microarrays alone would not provide sufficient biological validation, because of their limited specificity of hybridization. This is especially problematic when dealing with microRNAs, which are very short in length (~22 nucleotides) and are often very similar in sequence (some microRNAs differ by only a single nucleotide). Simple PCR-amplified sequencing techniques used at the time to validate microRNAs turned out to be insufficiently specific. Using such sequencing techniques, an abundant microRNA can 'mask' the expression of a rare microRNA that is very similar (but not identical) in sequence. This was a major problem, since we typically were interested in those microRNAs expressed at low levels, and not in the abundant ones that have already been discovered. And so we had to develop a novel microRNA sequencing technique that was more specific than existing methodologies.

These efforts eventually led to our success in developing a novel microRNA detection approach that integrated a novel algorithmic approach with the above-mentioned high-throughput validation technique and a novel biological validation technique we developed (Bentwich et al. 2005). This approach and our findings are briefly summarized here.

Our approach may be likened to a discovery 'funnel': a step-wise process that starts out very broad and then applies more specific validation techniques on incrementally smaller groups of candidates to eventually validate a relatively small number of microRNAs (Fig. 2).

We started out by computationally scanning the entire human genome for hairpin structures. This was a daunting computational task that had not been attempted before. We then scored each hairpin for its similarity to known microRNAs, using PalGrade, a novel algorithm we developed. Next, we determined the expression levels of high-scoring postulated microRNAs in six tissues (placenta, testis, thymus, brain and prostate). Finally, we validated microRNAs, the expression of which was detected by the microarray, using a novel sensitive sequencing technique we developed. This sequencing technique uses a specific biotinylated capture oligonucleotide, designed for the predicted microRNA to be cloned, to 'fish out' the

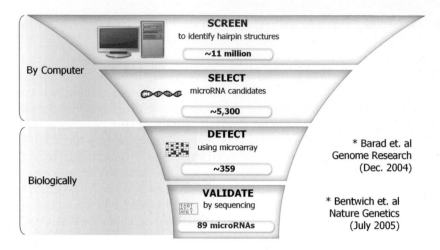

Fig. 2 MicroRNA discovery 'funnel'. Initial folding of the entire human genome resulted in approx. 11 million hairpins. High-throughput microarray experiments were used to test the expression of approx. 5,300 of the high-scoring candidates. Of these, 886 were found to be expressed in one of six tissues tested. Of these, 359 were subjected to validation by sequencing, resulting in 89 novel validated microRNAs (including 33 that are similar or adjacent to the microRNAs sought)

complementary sequence from the microRNA-enriched libraries, which are then amplified, cloned and sequenced.

Computational scanning the entire human genome identified approx. 11 million hairpins. Of these, an initial group of 434,239 candidate microRNAs were identified that passed a minimal hairpin score threshold (PalGrade>0) and were not on repetitive elements. This group contained 86% of the known microRNAs, suggesting that if systematically scanned, 86% of all microRNAs would be revealed. From this initial candidate group we selected approx. 5,300 predicted microRNA sequences for high-throughput expression validation by microarray, together with a control group of 7,500 non-microRNA hairpin controls. Microarray experiments in the above-mentioned six tissues resulted in 886 candidate microRNAs with significant signals of at least one of their two predicted mature microRNAs. Finally, we subjected 359 of these to sequence validation using our new sequence-directed cloning and sequencing method. With this approach we successfully cloned and sequenced 89 novel human microRNAs (56 were part of the original 359 sample, and 33 were either similar or adjacent to the microRNAs originally sought). Reassuringly, only one of the 89 novel microRNAs we found originated from the extremely large control group.

Hairpin structures were found by folding the entire human genome using the Vienna package (Hofacker 2003), in windows of 1,000 nucleotides in length with an overlap of 150 nucleotides, and accepting only hairpins that are at least 55 nucleotides in length and have a loop of no more than 20 nucleotides. Hairpins were assigned a high stability score, if they appeared in many folding configurations, as indicated by the Vienna package partition function graph. The PalGrade algorithm we used was developed by comparing features of known microRNA precursors to those of a background set of 10,000 randomly selected hairpins found in non-protein coding regions. The hairpin *structural* characteristics used were: (1) hairpin length, (2) loop length, (3) stability score (as described above), (4) free energy per nucleotide, (5) matching base pairs, and (6) maximal bulge size. The hairpin sequence characteristics used were: (1) sequence repetitiveness (abundance of any dinucleotide, AA, AT, etc.), (2) regular internal repeat, (3) inverted internal repeat (i.e. internal repeat in opposite orientation within the hairpin), (4) free energy (accounting for nucleotide composition), and (5) GC content. Different weights were assigned to these different features so as to achieve maximum distinguishing between true microRNA precursors and the background set. Figure 3 shows the effectiveness of PalGrade in distinguishing real microRNA precursors from random genomic hairpins (most of which are not microRNA precursors).

MicroRNAs validation was performed using a sequence-directed cloning method we developed (Fig. 4). A population of single-stranded molecules derived from a microRNA-enriched library (Elbashir et al. 2001) is mixed with the biotinylated capture oligonucleotide. After hybridization, streptavidin bound to magnetic beads is added, and the mixture is loaded into a column mounted on a strong

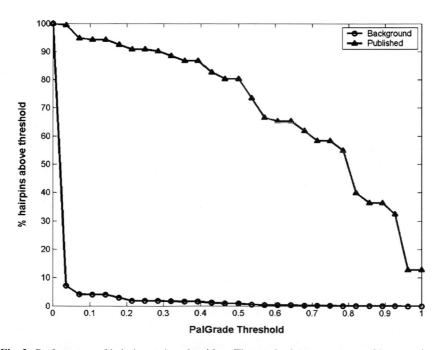

Fig. 3 Performance of hairpin scoring algorithm. The graph plots percentages of known microRNA hairpins (*triangles*) and of random genomic hairpins (*circles*) above or equal to different PalGrade thresholds (*x* axis). The large separation indicates the high sensitivity and specificity of the scoring method

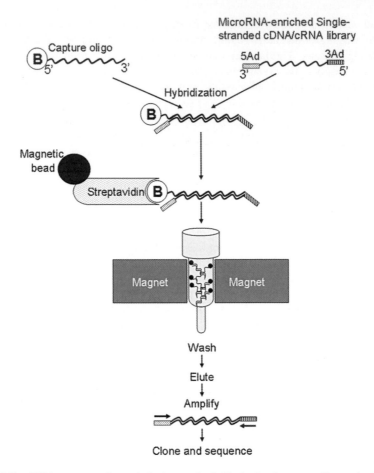

Fig. 4 MicroRNA sequence-directed cloning method. Biotinylated capture oligonucleotides are hybridized with a microRNA-enriched library. Streptavidin bound to magnetic beads is used to separate the microRNAs of interest, which are then amplified, cloned and sequenced

magnet. The column is then washed stringently to remove non-bound or weakly hybridized molecules. The specifically bound molecules are eluted, amplified, cloned and sequenced. This methodology allowed us to validate low-abundance microRNAs, which when using other validation methodologies were 'masked' by abundant microRNAs of a similar sequence.

Our findings helped establish the notion that the number of human microRNAs is significantly larger than previously believed, and that many of these microRNAs are not conserved beyond primates. We assessed the number of both conserved and non-conserved human micro-RNAs by calculating the validation success rate in samples from each PalGrade score group (ignoring similar and adjacent micro-RNAs to avoid positive bias) and then multiplying this validation success rate by the number of hairpins in the genome belonging to that group. Reassuringly, this assessment was further supported by an independent assessment based on probabilistic arguments based informatic data alone. Using this approach we showed that the number of conserved microRNAs is at least roughly 400–500, and that the total number of microRNAs is at least 800.

4 On-going Trends in MicroRNA Discovery

MicroRNA discovery continues to be an exciting, dynamically changing frontier, with different algorithmic approaches, the utilization of an enhanced understanding of the biogenesis of microRNA, new massive sequencing techniques, and the discovery of new classes of 'microRNA-like' genes.

The initial few microRNA detection algorithms are now being joined by a rapidly growing number of different microRNA discovery approaches. Lim et al. developed MirScan, a sophisticated algorithm capable of identifying microRNAs that are conserved in at least two different species (Lim et al. 2003a, b). Using this algorithm, the authors identified 30 conserved microRNAs in *C. elegans* and 38 conserved human microRNAs. Grad et al. used a similar approach to detect and validate 14 microRNAs in *C. elegans* (Grad et al. 2003). Berezikov et al. used a phylogenetic-shadowing approach to identify 16 human microRNAs, and they list several hundred potential candidate microRNAs (Berezikov et al. 2005). This approach identifies microRNAs based on the finding that nucleotides in the stem of the microRNA hairpin precursor are more conserved than those in its loop. Xie et al. used evolutionarily conserved 3′ untranslated region (UTR) motifs as a means of identifying potential microRNA binding sites and their corresponding microRNAs, and they validated six such novel human microRNAs (Xie et al. 2005). Nam et al. developed a microRNA predictor that utilizes a probabilistic co-learning model of sequence and structure (Nam et al. 2006). Ge et al. used serial analysis of gene expression (SAGE) to identify mammalian microRNA (Ge et al. 2006). Sewer at al. sought microRNAs in the proximity of known microRNAs, and which can be identified independently in two or more species (Sewer et al. 2005). Helvik et al. utilized a refined prediction of the 5′ processing site of microRNAs by the Drosha enzyme to achieve enhanced microRNA prediction accuracy (Helvik et al. 2006).

Importantly, advances in the understanding of microRNA's biogenesis leads to improvements in computational microRNA prediction. Initially, processing of microRNA from its precursor has been shown to be largely dependent on its distance from the loop of the microRNA's hairpin precursor, as demonstrated by Zeng et al. (2005) and others. This has served as an important feature in the computational prediction of microRNAs by several different algorithms. More recently, however, Han et al. showed that the single-stranded segments adjacent to the microRNA precursor hairpin are important for its processing, and hence its computational prediction, perhaps more so than the distance from the loop (Han et al. 2006). Observations such as this are bound to improve microRNA prediction.

Following recent technological advances, massive sequencing techniques are poised to play a central role in the discovery of microRNAs and other short RNAs. Cummins et al. (in collaboration with our group) catalogued the colorectal cancer microRNome using a methodology they developed that is based in part on the SAGE methodology (Velculescu et al. 1995), which they optimized for short RNAs (Cummins et al. 2006). This methodology allowed the cloning of over 270,000 clones, 100-fold more than previous human microRNA cloning attempts, leading to identification of 168 microRNA candidates (35 of which we had independently identified). Massively parallel signature sequencing (MPSS) technology (Brenner et al. 2000) is now taking the 'deep sequencing' approach to new heights. Lu et al. used such an approach to extract and analyse over 2 millions sequences in the model plant *Arabidopsis thaliana*, leading to the identification of several new microRNAs (Lu et al. 2005). Mineno et al. obtained approx. 500,000 sequence signatures, leading to the identification of 195 new microRNAs in mouse (Mineno et al. 2006). And recently, Ruby at al. have adapted the use of high-throughput pyrosequencing (Margulies et al. 2005) to clone approx. 400,000 sequences in *C. elegans*, leading to the identification of 18 novel microRNAs (Ruby et al. 2006).

Such massive cloning efforts have also resulted in the surprising discovery of two (thus far) very large new groups of short RNA genes, which appear to be somewhat related to microRNAs, but are clearly not microRNAs. Several months ago Grivna et al. (2006) and Aravin et al. (2006) reported a novel class of short RNA genes, called piRNA (PIWI binding RNAs), expressed in mouse spermatogenesis. Over 1,000 such piRNA have been reported to date. They are 26–31 nucleotides in length, and are related to the microRNA machinery. Recently, Ruby et al. have identified another class of short RNAs, called 21U-RNAs in *C. elegans* and have sequenced over 5,700 such genes (Ruby et al. 2006). This is a group of RNA genes which are all exactly 21 nucleotides in length, start with a uridine, are preceded by two short sequence motifs, and do not have the hairpin structure typical of microRNAs. The discovery of these new groups of short 'microRNA-like' genes might broaden the definition and scope of microRNA discovery tools to encompass other short RNAs.

The discovery of many hundreds of microRNA genes and now of thousands of new 'microRNA-like' genes raises intriguing questions. What could be the role of these genes? Why would the body need thousands of these short sequences? What is the reason for the similarity between these different groups of genes? The continued development of improved tools for the discovery and functional assessment of microRNAs and other short RNA genes will clearly be of help in addressing these and other questions. Several years ago I presented a theoretical model that predicted the existence of thousands of short RNA genes, often to be found in clusters, and argued that they are part of a genomic 'language' or code that effects cellular differentiation (Bentwich 2005). It will be interesting to see if indeed these different RNA gene groups involve such a 'hidden' genomic differentiation-coding 'language'.

References

Ambros V (2004) The functions of animal microRNAs. Nature 431:350–355

Ambros V, Bartel B, Bartel DP, Burge CB, Carrington JC, Chen X, Dreyfuss G, Eddy SR, Griffiths-Jones S, Marshall M, Matzke M, Ruvkun G, Tuschl T (2003) A uniform system for microRNA annotation. Rna 9:277–279

Aravin A, Gaidatzis D, Pfeffer S, Lagos-Quintana M, Landgraf P, Iovino N, Morris P, Brownstein MJ, Kuramochi-Miyagawa S, Nakano T, Chien M, Russo JJ, Ju J, Sheridan R, Sander C, Zavolan M, Tuschl T (2006) A novel class of small RNAs bind to MILI protein in mouse testes. Nature 442:203–207

Barad O, Meiri E, Avniel A, Aharonov R, Barzilai A, Bentwich I, Einav U, Gilad S, Hurban P, Karov Y, Lobenhofer EK, Sharon E, Shiboleth YM, Shtutman M, Bentwich Z, Einat P (2004) MicroRNA expression detected by oligonucleotide microarrays: system establishment and expression profiling in human tissues. Genome Res 14:2486–2494

Bartel DP (2004) MicroRNAs: genomics, biogenesis, mechanism, and function. Cell 116:281–297

Bentwich I (2005) A postulated role for microRNA in cellular differentiation. FASEB J 19:875–879

Bentwich I, Avniel A, Karov Y, Aharonov R, Gilad S, Barad O, Barzilai A, Einat P, Einav U, Meiri E, Sharon E, Spector Y, Bentwich Z (2005) Identification of hundreds of conserved and nonconserved human microRNAs. Nat Genet 37:766–770

Berezikov E, Guryev V, van de Belt J, Wienholds E, Plasterk RH, Cuppen E (2005) Phylogenetic shadowing and computational identification of human microRNA genes. Cell 120:21–24

Brennecke J, Stark A, Russell RB, Cohen SM (2005) Principles of microRNA-target recognition. PLoS Biol 3:e85

Brenner S, Johnson M, Bridgham J, Golda G, Lloyd DH, Johnson D, Luo S, McCurdy S, Foy M, Ewan M, Roth R, George D, Eletr S, Albrecht G, Vermaas E, Williams SR, Moon K, Burcham T, Pallas M, DuBridge RB, Kirchner J, Fearon K, Mao J, Corcoran K (2000) Gene expression analysis by massively parallel signature sequencing (MPSS) on microbead arrays. Nat Biotechnol 18:630–634

Cummins JM, He Y, Leary RJ, Pagliarini R, Diaz LA Jr, Sjoblom T, Barad O, Bentwich Z, Szafranska AE, Labourier E, Raymond CK, Roberts BS, Juhl H, Kinzler KW, Vogelstein B, Velculescu VE (2006) The colorectal microRNAome. Proc Natl Acad Sci U S A 103:3687–3692

Elbashir SM, Lendeckel W, Tuschl T (2001) RNA interference is mediated by 21- and 22-nucleotide RNAs. Genes Dev 15:188–200

Ge X, Wu Q, Wang SM (2006) SAGE detects microRNA precursors. BMC Genomics 7:285

Grad Y, Aach J, Hayes GD, Reinhart BJ, Church GM, Ruvkun G, Kim J (2003) Computational and experimental identification of C. elegans microRNAs. Mol Cell 11:1253–1263

Grad Y, Aach J, Hayes GD, Reinhart BJ, Church GM, Ruvkun G, Kim J (2004) Human microRNA targets. PLoS Biol 2:e363

Grivna ST, Beyret E, Wang Z, Lin H (2006) A novel class of small RNAs in mouse spermatogenic cells. Genes Dev 20:1709–1714

Han J, Lee Y, Yeom KH, Nam JW, Heo I, Rhee JK, Sohn SY, Cho Y, Zhang BT, Kim VN (2006) Molecular basis for the recognition of primary microRNAs by the Drosha-DGCR8 complex. Cell 125:887–901

Helvik SA, Snøve O Jr, Saetrom P (2006) Reliable prediction of Drosha processing sites improves microRNA gene prediction. Bioinformatics 23:142–149

Hofacker IL (2003) Vienna RNA secondary structure server. Nucleic Acids Res 31:3429–3431

Johnston RJ, Hobert O (2003) A microRNA controlling left/right neuronal asymmetry in Caenorhabditis elegans. Nature 426:845–849

Kiriakidou M, Nelson PT, Kouranov A, Fitziev P, Bouyioukos C, Mourelatos Z, Hatzigeorgiou A (2004) A combined computational-experimental approach predicts human microRNA targets. Genes Dev 18:1165–1178

Kloosterman WP, Wienholds E, Ketting RF, Plasterk RH (2004) Substrate requirements for let-7 function in the developing zebrafish embryo. Nucleic Acids Res 32:6284–6291

Lagos-Quintana M, Rauhut R, Lendeckel W, Tuschl T (2001) Identification of novel genes coding for small expressed RNAs. Science 294:853–858

Lagos-Quintana M, Rauhut R, Yalcin A, Meyer J, Lendeckel W, Tuschl T (2002) Identification of tissue-specific microRNAs from mouse. Curr Biol 12:735–739

Lagos-Quintana M, Rauhut R, Meyer J, Borkhardt A, Tuschl T (2003) New microRNAs from mouse and human. Rna 9:175–179

Lau NC, Lim LP, Weinstein EG, Bartel DP (2001) An abundant class of tiny RNAs with probable regulatory roles in Caenorhabditis elegans. Science 294:858–862

Lee RC, Ambros V (2001) An extensive class of small RNAs in Caenorhabditis elegans. Science 294:862–864

Lee RC, Feinbaum RL, Ambros V (1993) The C. elegans heterochronic gene lin-4 encodes small RNAs with antisense complementarity to lin-14. Cell 75:843–854

Lim LP, Glasner ME, Yekta S, Burge CB, Bartel DP (2003) Vertebrate microRNA genes. Science 299:1540

Lim LP, Lau NC, Weinstein EG, Abdelhakim A, Yekta S, Rhoades MW, Burge CB, Bartel DP (2003b) The microRNAs of Caenorhabditis elegans. Genes Dev 17:991–1008

Lu C, Tej SS, Luo S, Haudenschild CD, Meyers BC, Green PJ (2005) Elucidation of the small RNA component of the transcriptome. Science 309:1567–1569

Margulies M, Egholm M, Altman WE, Attiya S, Bader JS, Bemben LA, Berka J, Braverman MS, Chen YJ, Chen Z, Dewell SB, Du L, Fierro JM, Gomes XV, Godwin BC, He W, Helgesen S, Ho CH, Irzyk GP, Jando SC, Alenquer ML, Jarvie TP, Jirage KB, Kim JB, Knight JR, Lanza JR, Leamon JH, Lefkowitz SM, Lei M, Li J, Lohman KL, Lu H, Makhijani VB, McDade KE, McKenna MP, Myers EW, Nickerson E, Nobile JR, Plant R, Puc BP, Ronan MT, Roth GT, Sarkis GJ, Simons JF, Simpson JW, Srinivasan M, Tartaro KR, Tomasz A, Vogt KA, Volkmer GA, Wang SH, Wang Y, Weiner MP, Yu P, Begley RF, Rothberg JM (2005) Genome sequencing in microfabricated high-density picolitre reactors. Nature 437:376–380

Mineno J, Okamoto S, Ando T, Sato M, Chono H, Izu H, Takayama M, Asada K, Mirochnitchenko O, Inouye M, Kato I (2006) The expression profile of microRNAs in mouse embryos. Nucleic Acids Res 34:1765–1771

Nam JW, Kim J, Kim SK, Zhang BT (2006) ProMiR II: a web server for the probabilistic prediction of clustered, nonclustered, conserved and nonconserved microRNAs. Nucleic Acids Res 34:W455–W458

Pasquinelli AE, Reinhart BJ, Slack F, Martindale MQ, Kuroda MI, Maller B, Hayward DC, Ball EE, Degnan B, Müller P, Spring J, Srinivasan A, Fishman M, Finnerty J, Corbo J, Levine M, Leahy P, Davidson E, Ruvkun G (2000) Conservation of the sequence and temporal expression of let-7 heterochronic regulatory RNA. Nature 408:86–89

Poy MN, Eliasson L, Krutzfeldt J, Kuwajima S, Ma X, Macdonald PE, Pfeffer S, Tuschl T, Rajewsky N, Rorsman P, Stoffel M (2004) A pancreatic islet-specific microRNA regulates insulin secretion. Nature 432:226–230

Reinhart BJ, Slack FJ, Basson M, Pasquinelli AE, Bettinger JC, Rougvie AE, Horvitz HR, Ruvkun G (2000) The 21-nucleotide let-7 RNA regulates developmental timing in Caenorhabditis elegans. Nature 403:901–906

Ruby JG, Jan C, Player C, Axtell MJ, Lee W, Nusbaum C, Ge H, Bartel DP (2006) Large-scale sequencing reveals 21U-RNAs and additional microRNAs, endogenous siRNAs in C. elegans. Cell 127:1193–1207

Sewer A, Paul N, Landgraf P, Aravin A, Pfeffer S, Brownstein MJ, Tuschl T, van Nimwegen E, Zavolan M (2005) Identification of clustered microRNAs using an ab initio prediction method. BMC Bioinformatics 6:267

Velculescu VE, Zhang L, Vogelstein B, Kinzler KW (1995) Serial analysis of gene expression. Science 270:484–487

Xie X, Lu J, Kulbokas EJ, Golub TR, Mootha V, Lindblad-Toh K, Lander ES, Kellis M (2005) Systematic discovery of regulatory motifs in human promoters and 3′ UTRs by comparison of several mammals. Nature 434:338–345

Zeng Y, Yi R, Cullen BR (2005) Recognition and cleavage of primary microRNA precursors by the nuclear processing enzyme Drosha. EMBO J 24:138–148

Index

Current Topics in Microbiology and Immunology

Volumes published since 1989

Vol. 295: **Sullivan, David J.; Krishna Sanjeew (Eds.):** Malaria: Drugs, Disease and Post-genomic Biology. 2005. 40 figs., XI, 446 pp. ISBN 3-540-25363-7

Vol. 296: **Oldstone, Michael B. A. (Ed.):** Molecular Mimicry: Infection Induced Autoimmune Disease. 2005. 28 figs., VIII, 167 pp. ISBN 3-540-25597-4

Vol. 297: **Langhorne, Jean (Ed.):** Immunology and Immunopathogenesis of Malaria. 2005. 8 figs., XII, 236 pp. ISBN 3-540-25718-7

Vol. 298: **Vivier, Eric; Colonna, Marco (Eds.):** Immunobiology of Natural Killer Cell Receptors. 2005. 27 figs., VIII, 286 pp. ISBN 3-540-26083-8

Vol. 299: **Domingo, Esteban (Ed.):** Quasispecies: Concept and Implications. 2006. 44 figs., XII, 401 pp. ISBN 3-540-26395-0

Vol. 300: **Wiertz, Emmanuel J.H.J.; Kikkert, Marjolein (Eds.):** Dislocation and Degradation of Proteins from the Endoplasmic Reticulum. 2006. 19 figs., VIII, 168 pp. ISBN 3-540-28006-5

Vol. 301: **Doerfler, Walter; Böhm, Petra (Eds.):** DNA Methylation: Basic Mechanisms. 2006. 24 figs., VIII, 324 pp. ISBN 3-540-29114-8

Vol. 302: **Robert N. Eisenman (Ed.):** The Myc/Max/Mad Transcription Factor Network. 2006. 28 figs., XII, 278 pp. ISBN 3-540-23968-5

Vol. 303: **Thomas E. Lane (Ed.):** Chemokines and Viral Infection. 2006. 14 figs. XII, 154 pp. ISBN 3-540-29207-1

Vol. 304: **Stanley A. Plotkin (Ed.):** Mass Vaccination: Global Aspects – Progress and Obstacles. 2006. 40 figs. X, 270 pp. ISBN 3-540-29382-5

Vol. 305: **Radbruch, Andreas; Lipsky, Peter E. (Eds.):** Current Concepts in Autoimmunity. 2006. 29 figs. IIX, 276 pp. ISBN 3-540-29713-8

Vol. 306: **William M. Shafer (Ed.):** Antimicrobial Peptides and Human Disease. 2006. 12 figs. XII, 262 pp. ISBN 3-540-29915-7

Vol. 307: **John L. Casey (Ed.):** Hepatitis Delta Virus. 2006. 22 figs. XII, 228 pp. ISBN 3-540-29801-0

Vol. 308: **Honjo, Tasuku; Melchers, Fritz (Eds.):** Gut-Associated Lymphoid Tissues. 2006. 24 figs. XII, 204 pp. ISBN 3-540-30656-0

Vol. 309: **Polly Roy (Ed.):** Reoviruses: Entry, Assembly and Morphogenesis. 2006. 43 figs. XX, 261 pp. ISBN 3-540-30772-9

Vol. 310: **Doerfler, Walter; Böhm, Petra (Eds.):** DNA Methylation: Development, Genetic Disease and Cancer. 2006. 25 figs. X, 284 pp. ISBN 3-540-31180-7

Vol. 311: **Pulendran, Bali; Ahmed, Rafi (Eds.):** From Innate Immunity to Immunological Memory. 2006. 13 figs. X, 177 pp. ISBN 3-540-32635-9

Vol. 312: **Boshoff, Chris; Weiss, Robin A. (Eds.):** Kaposi Sarcoma Herpesvirus: New Perspectives. 2006. 29 figs. XVI, 330 pp. ISBN 3-540-34343-1

Vol. 313: **Pandolfi, Pier P.; Vogt, Peter K. (Eds.):** Acute Promyelocytic Leukemia. 2007. 16 figs. VIII, 273 pp. ISBN 3-540-34592-2

Vol. 314: **Moody, Branch D. (Ed.):** T Cell Activation by CD1 and Lipid Antigens, 2007, 25 figs. VIII, 348 pp. ISBN 978-3-540-69510-3

Vol. 315: **Childs, James, E.; Mackenzie, John S.; Richt, Jürgen A. (Eds.):** Wildlife and Emerging Zoonotic Diseases: The Biology, Circumstances and Consequences of Cross-Species Transmission. 2007. 49 figs. VII, 524 pp. ISBN 978-3-540-70961-9

Vol. 316: **Pitha, Paula M. (Ed.):** Interferon: The 50th Anniversary. 2007. VII, 391 pp. ISBN 978-3-540-71328-9

Vol. 317: **Dessain, Scott K. (Ed.):** Human Antibody Therapeutics for Viral Disease. 2007. XI, 202 pp. ISBN 978-3-540-72144-4

Vol. 318: **Rodriguez, Moses (Ed.):** Advances in Multiple Sclerosis and Experimental Demyelinating Diseases. 2008. XIV, 376 pp. ISBN 978-3-540-73679-9

Vol. 319: **Manser, Tim (Ed.):** Specialization and Complementation of Humoral Immune Responses to Infection. 2008. XII, 174 pp. ISBN 978-3-540-73899-2

Vol. 320: **Paddison, Patrick J; Vogt, Peter K. (Eds.):** RNA Interference. 2008. VIII, 274 pp. ISBN 978-3-540-75156-4

Printing: Krips bv, Meppel, The Netherlands
Binding: Stürtz, Würzburg, Germany